FIFTH EDITION

ESSENTIAL MEDICAL GENETICS

Michael Connor

MD, DSc, FRCP
*Professor of Medical Genetics,
University of Glasgow
and Director of the West of Scotland
Regional Genetics Service,
Institute of Medical Genetics,
Yorkhill, Glasgow*

Malcolm Ferguson-Smith

MB ChB, FRCPath, FRCP, FRSE, FRS
*Professor of Pathology,
University of Cambridge
and Honorary Consultant in Medical Genetics,
East Anglian Regional Genetics Service,
Addenbrooke's Hospital,
Cambridge*

Blackwell
Science

© 1984, 1987, 1991, 1993, 1997 by
Blackwell Science Ltd
Editorial Offices:
Osney Mead, Oxford OX2 0EL
25 John Street, London WC1N 2BL
23 Ainslie Place, Edinburgh EH3 6AJ
350 Main Street, Malden
    MA 02148-5018, USA
54 University Street, Carlton
    Victoria 3053, Australia
10, rue Casimlr Delavigne
    75006 Paris, France

Other Editorial Offices:
Blackwell Wissenschafts-Verlag GmbH
    Kurfürstendamm 57
    10707 Berlin, Germany

Blackwell Science KK
MG Kodenmacho Building
7-10 Kodenmacho Nihombashi
Chuo-ku, Tokyo 104, Japan

Iowa State University Press
A Blackwell Science Company
2121 S. State Avenue
Ames, Iowa 50014-8300, USA

The right of the Author to be
identified as the Author of this work
has been asserted in accordance
with the Copyright, Designs and
Patents Act 1988.

Set by Excel Typesetters Co, Hong Kong
Printed and bound in Great Britain
by the Alden Press Ltd.

The Blackwell Science logo is a
trade mark of Blackwell Science Ltd,
registered at the United Kingdom
Trade Marks Registry

First published 1984
Reprinted 1986
Second edition 1987
Third edition 1991
Fourth edition 1993
Four Dragons edition 1993
Fifth edition 1997
International edition 1997
Reprinted 2002.

DISTRIBUTORS

Marston Book Services Ltd
PO Box 269
Abingdon
Oxon OX14 4YN
(*Orders*: Tel: 01235 465500
        Fax: 01235 465555)

The Americas
Blackwell Publishing
c/o AIDC
PO Box 20
50 Winter Sport Lane
Williston, VT 05495-0020
(*Orders*: Tel: 800 216 2522
        Fax: 802 864 7626)

Australia
Blackwell Science Pty Ltd
54 University Street
Carlton, Victoria 3053
(*Orders*: Tel: 03 9347 0300
        Fax: 03 9349 5001)

A catalogue record for this title
is available from the British Library

ISBN 0-86542-666-X (BSL)
ISBN 0-632-04158-7 (International edition)

Library of Congress
Cataloging-in-publication Data

Connor, J. M. (James Michael), 1951–
    Essential medical genetics /
    J. Michael Connor,
    Malcolm A. Ferguson-Smith. – 5th ed.
        p.   cm.
    Includes bibliographical
    references and index.
    ISBN 0-86542-666-X
    1. Medical genetics.
    I. Ferguson-Smith, M. A.
(Malcolm Andrew)
    II. Title.
    [DNLM: 1. Genetics, Medical.
QZ 50 C752e 1997]
RB 155.C66   1997
616'.042–dc21
DNLM/DLC
for Library of Congress   96-45181
                                    CIP

ESSENTIAL
MEDICAL

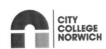

Contents

Preface ix

Acknowledgements x

PART 1 · BASIC PRINCIPLES

1 · Medical Genetics in Perspective, 3

SCIENTIFIC BASIS OF MEDICAL
   GENETICS 3
Mendel's contribution 3
Chromosomal basis of inheritance 4
Chemical basis of inheritance 4
Chromosomal disorders 4
Mitochondrial disorders 5
Single gene disorders 5
Multifactorial (part-genetic) disorders 6
Somatic cell genetic (cumulative genetic) disorders 6
CLINICAL APPLICATIONS OF
   MEDICAL GENETICS 6
Genetic assessment and counselling 7
Prenatal diagnosis 8
Treatment and prevention of genetic disease 8

2 · Nucleic Acid Structure and Function, 9

NUCLEIC ACID STRUCTURE 9
NUCLEIC ACID FUNCTION 12
Gene regulation 14
DNA REPLICATION 14
MUTATION 17
Length mutations 17
Point mutations 20
Molecular pathology of single gene disorders 23

3 · DNA Analysis, 24

INDIRECT MUTANT GENE TRACKING 24
Techniques for demonstration of DNA
   polymorphisms 26
DIRECT MUTANT GENE ANALYSIS 27

4 · Chromosomes, 33

CHROMOSOME ANALYSIS
   (KARYOTYPING) 33
The normal human karyotype 34
Flow karyotyping 37
CHROMOSOME HETEROMORPHISMS 37
CHROMOSOMES IN OTHER SPECIES 42
MITOCHONDRIAL CHROMOSOMES 43
MITOSIS 43

5 · Gametogenesis, 46

MEIOSIS 46
First meiotic division (reduction division) 46
Second meiotic division 47
SPERMATOGENESIS 48
OOGENESIS 48
FERTILIZATION 50
LYONIZATION 50
SEX DETERMINATION AND
   DIFFERENTIATION 53
GENOMIC IMPRINTING
   (PARENTAL IMPRINTING) 54

6 · Chromosome Aberrations, 55

NUMERICAL ABERRATIONS 55
Aneuploidy 55
Polyploidy 56
STRUCTURAL ABERRATIONS 57
IDENTIFICATION OF THE
  CHROMOSOMAL ORIGIN OF
  COMPLEX STRUCTURAL
  REARRANGEMENTS 65
OTHER ABERRATIONS 67
Mosaic 67
Chimaera 67
Uniparental disomy and isodisomy 68

7 · Autosomal Inheritance, 69

AUTOSOMAL SINGLE GENE
  INHERITANCE 69
AUTOSOMAL DOMINANT
  INHERITANCE 69
AUTOSOMAL RECESSIVE
  INHERITANCE 71
AUTOSOMAL CODOMINANT
  INHERITANCE 74
SUMMARY OF AUTOSOMAL
  INHERITANCE 75

8 · Sex-linked Inheritance, 76

Y-LINKED INHERITANCE
  (HOLANDRIC INHERITANCE) 76
X-LINKED RECESSIVE INHERITANCE 77
Other X-linked recessive conditions 79
X-LINKED DOMINANT INHERITANCE 79
X-LINKED CODOMINANT
  INHERITANCE 81

9 · Genomics, 82

FAMILY LINKAGE STUDIES 82
IN SITU HYBRIDIZATION 86
INTERSPECIFIC SOMATIC CELL
  HYBRIDIZATION 87
FLOW SORTED CHROMOSOME DOT-BLOT
  ANALYSES 90
STRUCTURE AND ORGANIZATION OF
  THE GENOME 90

10 · Non-Mendelian Inheritance, 91

MULTIFACTORIAL DISORDERS 91
TWIN CONCORDANCE STUDIES 91
Determination of concordance 92
Results of twin studies 92
FAMILY CORRELATION STUDIES 93
CONTINUOUS MULTIFACTORIAL
  TRAITS 93
DISCONTINUOUS MULTIFACTORIAL
  TRAITS 95
ANALYSIS OF MULTIFACTORIAL
  TRAITS 96
SOMATIC CELL GENETIC DISORDERS 96
MITOCHONDRIAL DISORDERS 97

11 · Medical Genetics in Populations, 98

SELECTION FOR SINGLE GENE
  DISORDERS 98
FOUNDER EFFECT FOR SINGLE
  GENE DISORDERS 100
ALTERED MUTATION RATE FOR
  SINGLE GENE DISORDERS 100

PART 2 · CLINICAL APPLICATIONS

12 · Genetic Assessment and Counselling, 103

COMMUNICATION OF ADVICE 103
History and pedigree construction 103
Clinical examination 103
Confirmation of diagnosis 105
Counselling 106
Follow-up 107
LEGAL ASPECTS 108
SPECIAL POINTS IN COUNSELLING 108

13 · Chromosomal Disorders, 116

TRANSLOCATIONS 116
PERICENTRIC INVERSIONS 117
TRISOMY 21 (MONGOLISM, DOWN
  SYNDROME) 118
47,XYY 120
47,XXY (KLINEFELTER SYNDROME) 120
47,XXX 121
46,XX MALES 121
45,X (TURNER SYNDROME) 121

TRISOMY 18 (EDWARDS SYNDROME). 122
TRISOMY 13 (PATAU SYNDROME) 123
TRIPLOIDY. 123
DELETIONS AND DUPLICATIONS 124
MARKER CHROMOSOMES 125
PRADER–WILLI SYNDROME 126
ANGELMAN SYNDROME
    (HAPPY PUPPET SYNDROME) 126
OTHER MICRODELETION DISORDERS 129

14 · Single Gene Disorders, 130

15 · Immunogenetics, 150

GENETICS OF THE NORMAL
    IMMUNE SYSTEM 150
INHERITED IMMUNODEFICIENCY 151
Genetic susceptibility/resistance to particular infections . . 151
BLOOD GROUPS. 152
ABO blood group 152
Rhesus blood group system 153
HAEMOLYTIC DISEASE OF
    THE NEWBORN. 153
NEONATAL ALLOIMMUNE
    THROMBOCYTOPENIA 154
MAJOR HISTOCOMPATIBILITY
    COMPLEX (MHC). 154
TRANSPLANTATION 155
Blood transfusion 156
Other tissues 156

16 · Genetics of Common Diseases, 157

17 · Cancer Genetics, 162

TUMOUR SUPPRESSOR GENES 162
ONCOGENES 163
GENES INVOLVED IN DNA-REPAIR
    MECHANISMS 165
OTHER GENES 166
CLINICAL RELEVANCE OF GENETIC
    STUDIES IN CANCER 167
GENETIC COUNSELLING ASPECTS OF
    CANCER 169
SINGLE GENE CAUSES OF CANCER 171

18 · Congenital Malformations, 177

Incidence 177
Aetiology 178
MINOR CONGENITAL MALFORMATIONS 178
MAJOR CONGENITAL MALFORMATIONS 178
Central nervous system 179
Heart. 184
Gastrointestinal tract 184
Kidney and urinary tract. 186
Limbs 188
Thyroid 189
MULTIPLE CONGENITAL
    MALFORMATIONS AND
    DYSMORPHIC SYNDROMES 189
Multiple malformations due to known teratogens 194

19 · Prenatal Diagnosis, 197

AMNIOCENTESIS 197
Fetal sexing 197
Fetal karyotyping. 198
Fetal enzyme assay 199
Amniotic fluid biochemistry. 199
Fetal DNA diagnosis 200
Risks of amniocentesis 200
CHORIONIC VILLUS SAMPLING (CVS). 200
CORDOCENTESIS, FETAL SKIN
    BIOPSY, FETAL LIVER BIOPSY. 202
ULTRASONOGRAPHY 202
FETAL CELLS IN THE MATERNAL
    CIRCULATION 203

20 · Population Screening, 204

PRENATAL SCREENING 204
Maternal AFP screening for neural tube defects 204
Screening for fetal chromosomal abnormalities 206
Ultrasound screening 206
NEONATAL SCREENING. 207
Phenylketonuria 208
Congenital hypothyroidism 208
SCREENING FOR CARRIER DETECTION 208
Beta-thalassaemia 208
Sickle cell disease 209
Tay–Sachs disease 209
Cystic fibrosis 209
PRESYMPTOMATIC SCREENING OF
    ADULTS. 209

21 · Prevention and Treatment, 210

OVERALL IMPACT OF GENETIC
   DISEASE 210
TYPES OF GENETIC DISEASE 211
TREATMENT OF GENETIC DISEASE 211
Chromosomal disorders 211
Single gene disorders 211
Multifactorial disorders 212
Mitochondrial disorders 212
Somatic cell genetic disorders 212
SECONDARY PREVENTION OF
   GENETIC DISEASE 212
Chromosomal disorders 212
Single gene disorders 214
Multifactorial disorders 214
PRIMARY PREVENTION OF GENETIC
   DISEASE 214
Chromosomal disorders 214
Single gene disorders 214
Multifactorial disorders 214

Answers to Figure Questions, 215

Further Reading, 216

APPENDICES

1 · Odds and Probabilities, 219

2 · Applications of Bayes' Theorem, 220

3 · Calculation of the Coefficients of Relationship and Inbreeding, 222

4 · Population Genetics of Single Gene Disorders, 223

Glossary, 225

Index, 229

Colour plates appear between pp. 86 and 87

Preface

This book has been written for those to whom an understanding of modern medical genetics is important in their practice as clinicians, scientists, counsellors and teachers. It is based on the authors' personal experience in both clinical and laboratory aspects of busy regional genetics services over a period of 35 years. This period has seen the emergence of modern cytogenetics and molecular genetics alongside the development of medical genetics from a purely academic discipline into a clinical speciality of relevance to every branch of medicine. As in our undergraduate education programmes, we emphasize the central role of the chromosome and the human genome in understanding the molecular mechanisms involved in the pathogenesis of genetic disease. Within the term genetic disease we include not only the classic Mendelian and chromosomal disorders but also the commoner disorders of adulthood with a genetic predisposition and somatic cell genetic disorders, such as cancer.

Since the fourth edition major developments have occurred which include: production of the first physical map of the human genome; cloning of many important genes, including several genes for breast and colon cancer; identification of genetic determinants of some of the common chronic disorders of adulthood, including presenile and senile dementia; and continued development of clinical service applications, most notably in the fields of genetic risk prediction using DNA analysis and in cancer genetics counselling. These changes have been incorporated and the text updated throughout. None the less, we have maintained our principle of passing on what is essential within modern medical genetics and look to the continued generosity of our readers in helping to correct our misconceptions and omissions.

The role of genetic counselling, prenatal diagnosis, carrier detection and other forms of genetic screening in the prevention of genetic disease is now well-established, and this is reflected in the increasing provision of genetic services throughout the world. It is hoped that our book will be useful to those in training for this important task.

J.M.C., M.A.F.-S.

Acknowledgements

We wish to thank many people who have influenced the production of this book. These include particularly:

Victor McKusick, with whom we both spent the formative periods of our early training in medical genetics.

Our colleagues and students at the Institute of Medical Genetics and at the Cambridge University Centre for Medical Genetics.

We are grateful for permission to reproduce the following figures:

Fig. 2.4: Susan Lindsay

Figs 3.3, 3.6, 19.3 and 19.4: Su Loughlin

Fig. 3.5: Anne Hughes

Fig. 3.7: Paul Debenham (Cellmark Diagnostics)

Fig. 3.11: Joan Lavinha

Fig. 3.12: Carolyn Williams, Edward Mayall and Bob Williamson

Fig. 3.14: Sanjay Bidichandani

Figs 4.2–4.5, 6.6, 6.8, 8.6(b), 13.11, 13.12, 13.13(b) and 14.4: Elizabeth Boyd

Figs 4.8 and 9.9: Nigel Carter

Fig. 4.13: The Editor, *Birth Defects Original Article Series*

Fig. 4.14: The Editior, *Annales de Genetique*

Fig. 4.15: Peter Pearson

Figs 5.2, 5.3, 5.9 and 6.9: The Editor, *Excerpta Medica*

Figs 5.8 and 6.4(d): Anne Chandley

Fig. 6.2: James Galt

Figs 6.4(b) and 6.4(c): The Editor, *Journal of Medical Genetics*

Fig. 6.15: Maj Hulten and N. Saadallah

Figs 6.16 and 6.17: The Editor, *Cytogenetics and Cell Genetics*

Fig. 7.6: Brenda Gibson

Figs 7.10 and 7.11: Steve Humphries

Figs 8.3, 8.6(a), 13.2: Douglas Wilcox

Fig. 8.9: Susan Holder

Fig. 9.8: The Editor, *Karger*

Fig. 13.4: Blackwell Scientific Publications

Figs 13.14 and 14.8: John Tolmie

Fig. 13.15: Sue Malcolm

Fig. 14.10: Reed Pyeritz

Figs 17.5, 17.7–17.9: Janet Stewart

Fig. 18.12: Robin Winter

Figs 19.5 and 19.6: Jennifer Lambert

Figs 20.1 and 20.2: Nick Wald

Figs 20.3–20.6, 21.3 and 21.4: David Aitken and Jenny Crossley

Plate 2: Marie Boyd

Plate 3: E. Stefan Mueller

Plate 6: Evelyn Schröck and Thomas Ried

Plates 7, 8 and 9a: Margaret Leversha

Plate 9b: Fentaug Yang

Plate 11: Lionel Willatt

Plate 12: Douglas Higgs and Richard Gibbons

Plate 13: Aspasia Divane

PART 1

BASIC PRINCIPLES

Medical Genetics in Perspective

C O N T E N T S

SCIENTIFIC BASIS OF MEDICAL GENETICS   3
Mendel's contribution   3
Chromosomal basis of inheritance   4
Chemical basis of inheritance   4
Chromosomal disorders   4
Mitochondrial disorders   5
Single gene disorders   5

Multifactorial (part-genetic) disorders   6
Somatic cell genetic (cumulative genetic) disorders   6
CLINICAL APPLICATIONS OF MEDICAL GENETICS. . .   6
Genetic assessment and counselling   7
Prenatal diagnosis   8
Treatment and prevention of genetic disease   8

Medical genetics is the science of human biological variation as it relates to health and disease. Although people have long been aware that individuals differ, that children tend to resemble their parents and that certain diseases tend to run in families, the scientific basis for these observations was only discovered during the past 125 years. The clinical applications of this knowledge are even more recent, with most progress confined to the past 35 years.

SCIENTIFIC BASIS OF MEDICAL GENETICS

Mendel's contribution

Prior to Mendel, parental characteristics were believed to blend in the offspring. Whilst this was acceptable for continuous traits such as height or skin pigmentation, it was clearly difficult to account for the family patterns of discontinuous traits such as haemophilia or albinism. Mendel studied clearly defined pairs of contrasting characters in the offspring of the garden pea (*Pisum sativum*). These peas were, for example, either round or wrinkled and were either yellow or green. Pure bred strains for each of these characteristics were available but when cross bred (the first filial or F_1 progeny) were all round or yellow. If F_1 progeny were bred then each characteristic was re-observed in a ratio of approximately 3 round to 1 wrinkled or 3 yellow to 1 green (in the second filial or F_2 progeny). Mendel concluded that inheritance of these characteristics must be particulate with pairs of hereditary elements (now called genes). In these two examples one characteristic (or trait) was dominant to the other (i.e. all F_1 showed it). The fact that both characteristics were observed in the F_2 progeny entailed *segregation of each pair of genes with one member to one gamete and one to another gamete (Mendel's first law)*.

Figures 1.1 and 1.2 illustrate these experiments with upper case letters used for the dominant characteristic and lower case used for the masked (or recessive) characteristic. If the pair of genes are identical then this is termed homozygous (for the dominant or recessive trait) whereas a heterozygote has one gene of each type.

In his next series of experiments Mendel crossed pure bred strains with two characteristics, e.g. pure bred round/yellow with pure bred wrinkled/green. The F_1 showed only the two dominant characteristics — in this case round/yellow. The F_2 showed four combinations: the original two, namely round/yellow and wrinkled/green, in a ratio of approximately 9 : 1 and two new combinations —wrinkled/yellow and round/green in a ratio of approximately 3 : 3 (Fig. 1.3).

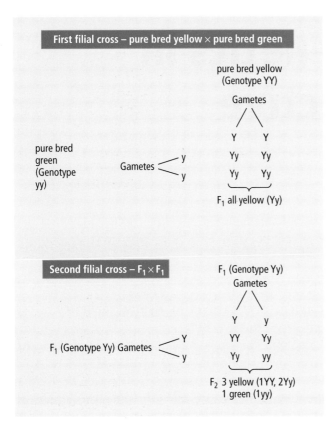

Fig. 1.1 Example of Mendel's breeding experiments for a single trait (yellow or green peas).

In these experiments there was thus no tendency for the genes arising from one parent to stay together in the offspring. In other words *members of different gene pairs assort to gametes independently of one another (Mendel's second law).*

Although Mendel presented and published his work in 1865 the significance of his discoveries was not realized until the early 1900s when three plant breeders, De Vries, Correns and Tschermak, confirmed his findings.

Chromosomal basis of inheritance

In 1839 Schleiden and Schwann established the concept of cells as the fundamental living units. Hereditary transmission through the sperm and egg was known by 1860, and in 1868 Haeckel, noting that the sperm was largely nuclear material, postulated that the nucleus was responsible for heredity. Flemming identified chromosomes within the nucleus in 1882, and in 1903 Sutton and Boveri independently realized that the behaviour of chromosomes during the production of gametes paralleled the behaviour of Mendel's hereditary elements. Thus the chromosomes were discovered to carry the genes. However, at that time, although the chromosomes were known to consist of protein and nucleic acid, it was not clear which component was the hereditary material.

Chemical basis of inheritance

Pneumococci are of two genetically distinct strains: rough or non-encapsulated (non-virulent) and smooth or encapsulated (virulent). Griffith in 1928 added heat-killed smooth bacteria to live rough and found that some of the rough pneumococci were transformed to the smooth, virulent type. Avery, MacLeod and McCarty repeated this experiment in 1944 and showed that nucleic acid was the transforming agent. Thus nucleic acid was shown to carry hereditary information. This stimulated intense interest in the composition of nucleic acids which culminated in Watson and Crick's discovery of the double helical structure for deoxyribonucleic acid (DNA) in 1953.

Chromosomal disorders

By 1890 it was known that one human chromosome (the X

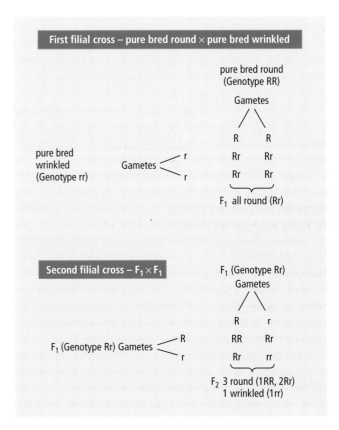

Fig. 1.2 Example of Mendel's breeding experiments for a single trait (round or wrinkled peas).

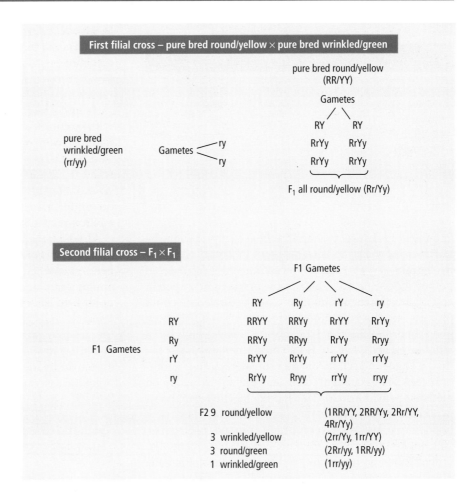

Fig. 1.3 Example of Mendel's breeding experiments for two traits (yellow or green and round or wrinkled peas).

chromosome) did not always have a partner, and in 1905 Wilson and Stevens extended this observation by establishing the pattern of human sex chromosomes. At this time there were believed to be 48 chromosomes in each somatic cell. Tjio and Levan refuted this in 1956 when they showed the normal human chromosome number to be 46. In 1959 the first chromosomal disease in humans, trisomy 21, was discovered by Lejeune and colleagues and by 1970 over 20 different human chromosomal disorders were known. The development of chromosomal banding in 1970 markedly increased the ability to resolve small chromosomal aberrations, and so by 1990 more than 600 different chromosome abnormalities had been described, in addition to many normal variants.

Mitochondrial disorders

Mitochondria have their own chromosomes and these are inherited from a mother to all of her children. Mutations in genes on these mitochondrial chromosomes can cause disease and this was first shown in 1988 for a maternally inherited type of blindness (Leber optic neuropathy).

Single gene disorders

In 1902 Garrod presented his studies on alkaptonuria, a rare condition in which patients have arthritis and urine which darkens on standing. He found three of 11 sets of parents of affected patients to be blood relatives and, in collaboration with Bateson, proposed that this was a Mendelian recessive trait with affected persons homozygous for the underactive gene. This was the first disease to be interpreted as a single gene trait. Garrod also conceived the idea that patients with alkaptonuria and other inborn errors of metabolism really represented one extreme of human biochemical variation and that other less clinically significant variations were to be expected.

There followed numerous descriptions of distinct human single gene traits and at the present time more than 6600 human single gene traits are known (Table 1.1).

Table 1.1 Human single gene traits (adapted from McKusick, 1994).

	1966	1975	1986	1994
Autosomal dominant	837	1218	2201	4458
Autosomal recessive	531	947	1420	1730
X-linked	119	171	286	412
Y-linked	—	—	—	19
Mitochondrial	—	—	—	59
Total	1487	2336	3907	6678

Pauling in 1949 suspected an abnormal haemoglobin to be the cause of sickle cell anaemia, and this was confirmed by Ingram in 1956 who found an altered haemoglobin polypeptide sequence. This was the first demonstration in any organism that a mutation in a structural gene could produce an altered amino acid sequence. In 1959 only two abnormal haemoglobins were known; now the number exceeds 450. In 1948, Gibson demonstrated the first enzyme defect in an autosomal recessive condition (NADH-dependent methaemoglobin reductase in methaemoglobinaemia). The specific biochemical abnormalities in over 400 inborn errors of metabolism have now been determined but the polypeptide product is, however, still unknown in about 90% of human single gene disorders. Study of these rare, and not so rare, single gene disorders has provided valuable insight into normal physiological mechanisms; for example, our knowledge of the normal metabolic pathways has been largely derived from the study of inborn errors of metabolism.

Progress has also been made in the assignment of genes to individual chromosomes. Wilson identified the X-linked trait for colour blindness in 1911 and assigned the gene to the X chromosome, so making the first human gene assignment. Other X-linked traits rapidly followed and the first autosomal gene to be assigned was thymidine kinase to chromosome 17 in 1967. By 1987 a complete linkage map of all human chromosomes had been developed and this was followed in 1993 by the first physical map. These were essential steps towards the final goal of the human genome project which seeks to identify and sequence all human genes by 2007. The first human gene (chorionic somatomammotrophin) was cloned in 1977 and by late 1994 disease-producing mutations had been identified in almost 350 cloned genes.

Multifactorial (part-genetic) disorders

Galton studied continuous human characteristics such as intelligence and physique, which did not seem to conform to Mendel's laws of inheritance, and an intense debate ensued, with the supporters of Mendel on the one hand and those of Galton on the other. Finally, a statistician, Fisher, reconciled the two sides by showing that such inheritance could be explained by multiple pairs of genes, each with a small but additive effect. Discontinuous traits with multifactorial inheritance, such as congenital malformations, were explained by introducing the concept of a threshold effect for the disorder: expression only occurred when the combined genetic and environmental liability passed the threshold. Many human characteristics are determined in this fashion and usually factors in the environment interact with the genetic background.

Although the genetic contribution to multifactorial disorders is now well accepted the number and nature of the genes involved and their mechanisms of interaction among each other and environmental factors are largely unknown. This is the current focus of a great deal of research and progress has been made in identifying the genetic contribution for several of these conditions including insulin-dependent diabetes mellitus, rheumatoid arthritis, dementia due to Alzheimer's disease and premature vascular disease.

Somatic cell genetic (cumulative genetic) disorders

All cancers result from a cumulation of genetic mutations. Usually these mutations only occur after conception and are thus confined to certain somatic cells but in a small but clinically important proportion, an initial key mutation is inherited. Boveri had first advanced the idea that chromosomal changes caused cancer and early support for this idea came from the demonstration in 1973 of a specific chromosomal translocation (the Philadelphia chromosome, p. 167) in a type of leukaemia. Subsequently a large number of both specific and non-specific chromosomal changes have been found in a wide variety of cancers (p. 166). In turn these changes were clues to specific genes which were key determinants of progression to cancer. Many of these genes have now been cloned (p. 162) and this has resulted in an improved understanding of the molecular basis of cancer and provided the clinician with a means of detection of presymptomatic carriers of cancer predisposing genes.

CLINICAL APPLICATIONS OF MEDICAL GENETICS

Genetically determined disease has become an increasingly important part of ill health in the community now

Table 1.2 Some important landmarks in the development of medical genetics.

Year	Landmark	Key figure(s)
1839	Cell theory	Schleiden and Schwann
1859	Theory of evolution	Darwin
1865	Particulate inheritance	Mendel
1882	Chromosomes observed	Flemming
1902	Biochemical variation	Garrod
1903	Chromosomes carry genes	Sutton, Boveri
1910	First US genetic clinic	Davenport
1911	First human gene assignment	Wilson
1944	Role of DNA	Avery
1953	DNA structure	Watson and Crick
1956	Amino acid sequence of HbS	Ingram
1956	46 chromosomes in humans	Tjio and Levan
1959	First human chromosomal abnormality	Lejeune
1960	Prenatal sexing	Riis and Fuchs
1960	Chromosome analysis on blood	Moorhead
1961	Biochemical screening	Guthrie
1961	X inactivation	Lyon
1961	Genetic code	Nirenberg
1964	Antenatal ultrasound	Donald
1966	First prenatal chromosomal analysis	Breg and Steel
1967	First autosomal assignment	Weiss and Green
1970	Prevention of Rhesus isoimmunization	Clarke
1970	Chromosome banding	Caspersson
1975	DNA sequencing	Sanger, Gilbert
1976	First DNA diagnosis	Kan
1977	First human gene cloned	Shine
1977	Somatostatin made by genetic engineering	Itakura
1979	*In vitro* fertilization	Edwards and Steptoe
1979	Insulin produced by genetic engineering	Goeddel
1982	First product of genetic engineering marketed	
1985	DNA fingerprinting	Jeffreys
1986	Polymerase chain reaction	Mullis
1987	Linkage map of human chromosomes developed	Many contributors
1990	First treatment by supplementation gene therapy	Rosenberg, Anderson, Blaese
1993	First physical map of the human genome	Many contributors

that most infections can be controlled, and now that modern medical and nursing care can save many affected infants who previously would have succumbed shortly after birth. This has led to an increased demand for informed genetic counselling and for screening tests both for carrier detection and to identify pregnancies at risk.

Genetic assessment and counselling

Davenport began to give genetic advice as early as 1910 in the USA and the first British genetic counselling clinic was established in 1946 at Great Ormond Street, London. Public demand has since caused a proliferation of genetic counselling centres so that there are now more than 40 in the UK and more than 450 in the USA.

In addition to an accurate assessment of the risks in a family the clinical geneticist also needs to discuss reproductive options. Important advances in this respect have been made with regard to prenatal diagnosis with the option of selective termination, and this has been a major factor in increasing the demand for genetic counselling. Prenatal diagnosis offers reassurance for couples at high risk of serious genetic disorders and allows many couples, who were previously deterred by the risk, the possibility of having healthy children.

Prenatal diagnosis

Genetic amniocentesis was first attempted in 1966 and the first prenatally detected chromosome abnormality was trisomy 21 in 1969. Chromosome analysis following amniocentesis is now a routine component of obstetric care and over 200 different types of abnormality have been detected. Amniocentesis or earlier chorionic villus sampling can also be used to detect biochemical alterations in inborn errors of metabolism. This was first used in 1968 for a pregnancy at risk of Lesch–Nyhan syndrome and has since been used for successful prenatal diagnosis in over 150 inborn errors of metabolism. Prenatal diagnosis can also be performed by DNA analysis of fetal samples. This approach was first used in 1976 for a pregnancy at risk of alpha-thalassaemia and has now been used in over 200 single gene disorders and for many of these, including cystic fibrosis, the fragile X syndrome and Duchenne muscular dystrophy, it has become the main method of prenatal diagnosis.

These prenatal tests which detect chromosomal, biochemical or DNA alterations cannot detect many of the major congenital malformations. The alternative approach of fetal visualization has been necessary for these. High resolution ultrasound scanning was first used to make a diagnosis of fetal abnormality (anencephaly) in 1972 and since then over 400 different types of abnormality have been detected.

Treatment and prevention of genetic disease

There has also been an increasing possibility for effective treatment of genetic diseases and in 1990 the first attempts at human supplementation gene therapy for a single gene disorder (adenosine deaminase deficiency) were performed. Research interest in this field is particularly active and by the end of 1994 over 100 clinical trial protocols had been approved (60% relating to treatment of cancer, 25% to single gene disorders and 10% to acquired immune deficiency syndrome (AIDS)).

The majority of couples are not aware that they are at risk until they have an affected child. This has led to an increased emphasis on prenatal screening, for example by measurement of maternal serum alphafetoprotein and other analytes to detect pregnancies at increased risk of neural tube defects and chromosomal abnormalities. Neonatal screening was introduced in 1961 for phenylketonuria and several other conditions where early diagnosis and therapy will permit normal development, and it is likely that in the future there will be continued development of population screening, prenatal, neonatal and preconceptional. This should lead to a reduced frequency of many genetic diseases with consequent benefits for individual families and society in general.

Nucleic Acid Structure and Function

NUCLEIC ACID STRUCTURE	9		**MUTATION**		17
NUCLEIC ACID FUNCTION	12		Length mutations		17
Gene regulation	14		Point mutations		20
DNA REPLICATION	14		Molecular pathology of single gene disorders		23

NUCLEIC ACID STRUCTURE

In humans, as in the other organisms, nucleic acid is the carrier of genetic information and has a structure which is ideally suited to this function. There are two main types of nucleic acid, DNA (deoxyribonucleic acid) and RNA (ribonucleic acid), which each consist of a sugar–phosphate backbone with projecting nitrogenous bases (Fig. 2.1). The nitrogenous bases are of two types, purines and pyrimidines. In DNA there are two purine bases, adenine (A) and guanine (G), and two pyrimidine bases, thymine (T) and cytosine (C). RNA also contains A, G and C, but has uracil (U) in place of T. In DNA the sugar is deoxyribose, whereas in RNA it is ribose (Fig. 2.2). The nitrogenous bases are attached to the 1' (one prime) position of each sugar, and the phosphate links 3' and 5' hydroxyl groups. Each unit of purine or pyrimidine base together with the attached sugar and phosphate group(s) is called a nucleotide.

A molecule of DNA is composed of two nucleotide chains which are coiled clockwise around one another to form a double helix with 10-nucleotides per complete turn of DNA (Fig. 2.3). The two chains run in opposite directions (i.e. 5' to 3' for one and 3' to 5' for the other) and are held together by hydrogen bonds between A in one chain and T in the other or between G and C. This base pairing is very specific, although rarely erroneous combinations may occur. Since A : T and G : C pairing is obligatory the parallel strands must be complementary to one another. Thus if one strand reads 5'-ATGC-3' the com-

plementary strand must read 5'-GCAT-3' (not 5'-TACG-3'). Hence the ratio of A to T is 1 to 1 and of G to C is likewise 1 to 1 (Chargaff's rule). Wide variation exists in the $(A + T)/(G + C)$ ratio. Higher plants and animals tend to have an excess of $(A + T)$ and in humans the ratio is 1.4 to 1.

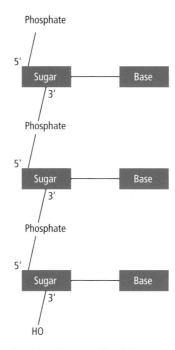

Fig. 2.1 Diagram of nucleic acid structure. The 5' phosphate end is at the top and the 3' hydroxyl group is at the bottom of the molecule.

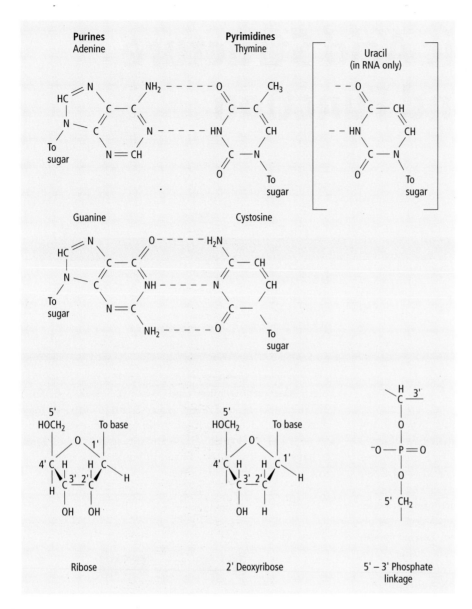

Fig. 2.2 Chemical structure of purines, pyrimidines, ribose, deoxyribose and the 5′ to 3′ phosphate linkage. The hydrogen bonds between adenine and thymine (or uracil) and guanine and cytosine are indicated.

The unit of length of DNA is the base pair (bp) with 1000 bp in a kilobase (kb) and 1 000 000 bp in a megabase (Mb). The total length of DNA in a half (haploid) set of human chromosomes is 3000 Mb (3×10^9 bp) and as the distance between base pairs in the DNA helix is 0.34 nm (Fig. 2.3), the total length of haploid DNA if extended would be one metre.

There are an estimated 60 000–70 000 structural genes encoded in human DNA. Each structural gene usually has only one copy in the haploid genome and these single copy genes and their related regulatory sequences account for 70% of the total DNA (which would predict an average gene size of 30 kb). The remaining 30% of DNA is repetitive and has no proven function. Repetitive DNA is subdivided into tandem repeats (satellite DNA) and interspersed repeats (Table 2.1).

Tandem repeats are subdivided according to their length. Microsatellite repeats are under 1 kb and the most common repeat motifs are A, AC, AAAN (where N is any nucleotide), AAN and AG. AC repeats commonly have 10–60 repeats (with corresponding lengths of 20–120 bp) and are found approximately every 30 kb (Fig. 2.4). The repeat number for corresponding chromosomes commonly differs and these common genetic differences or polymorphisms can be used to track the inheritance of that region of each chromosome (p. 24).

Minisatellite repeats are usually 1–30 kb in length and have longer repeat motifs than the microsatellite repeats. They again show marked variation in repeat number and the single copy minisatellites are thus useful for gene tracking and the multilocus minisatellites provide an individual-specific pattern of bands

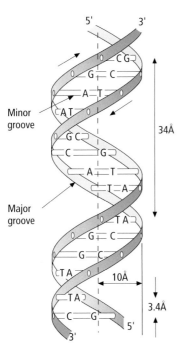

Fig. 2.3 Diagram of DNA double helix.

Table 2.1 Proportions of different types of nuclear DNA.

Type of DNA	Percentage of total DNA
Single copy	70
Repetitive DNA	30
Tandem repeats	(10)
Microsatellites	
Minisatellites	
Macrosatellites	
Interspersed repeats	(20)
Short interspersed repeats (SINES)	
Long interspersed repeats (LINES)	

which can be used for forensic identification (e.g. see Fig. 3.7).

Macrosatellite repeats are larger still and may be many megabases in length. They are found at the ends (telomeres) of the chromosomal arms and in the central chromosomal constriction (the centromere, p. 36). Length variation is common and accounts for visible differences in the size of chromosomal centromeric regions (e.g. Fig. 4.11).

In contrast, interspersed repeats usually occur as single copies and these are subdivided according to length. Short interspersed repeats (SINES) are under 500 bp and the commonest type is the Alu repeat. Alu repeats are about 300 bp long and contain a cutting site for the restriction enzyme *Alu*I (p. 24). They are very common (6% of all

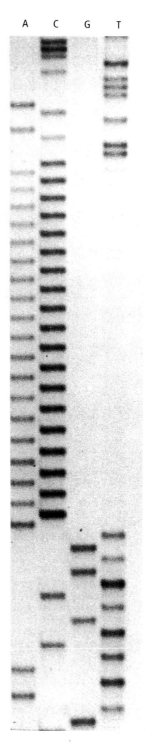

Fig. 2.4 DNA sequence of an AC repeat (the sequence is read from the bottom and the columns correspond to the bases thymine (T), cytosine (C), guanine (G) and adenine (A).

Table 2.2 Types of RNA.

Type	Location	Comments
Messenger RNA (mRNA)	Nucleus and cytoplasm	Variable size, base sequence complementary to transcribed DNA, about 4% of total cellular RNA, half-life 7–24 h
Transfer RNA (tRNA)	Cytoplasm	Hairpin-loop shape, 40 types, amino acid-specific, about 10% of total cellular RNA with tens to hundreds of copies of the genes for each tRNA species
Ribosomal RNA (rRNA)	Ribosomes and nucleoli	40–50% total cellular RNA, synthesized and stored in the nucleolus
Heterogeneous RNA (hnRNA)	Nucleus	High molecular weight mRNA precursors; 40–50% of total cellular RNA
Small nuclear RNA (smRNA)	Nucleus	Six types (U1–U6) involved in RNA splicing

DNA) and occur every 5–10 kb. Alu repeats are specific to humans and other higher primates and this is useful in forensic testing. Long interspersed repeats (LINES) are often 1.5–5 kb in length and include the Kpn LINE family. Kpn repeats vary in size from 500 bp to 10 kb and contain a cutting site for the restriction enzyme *Kpn*I. Kpn repeats have some structural similarities to retroviruses and some may have the capacity to replicate themselves and insert a copy at a new location in the genome. This new location may disrupt a gene and cause a genetic disorder (e.g. some patients with haemophilia).

Single copy and repeat DNA are double-stranded whereas RNA is single-stranded and subdivided into five main types (Table 2.2).

Ribosomal RNAs (rRNAs) are synthesized directly on DNA templates which occur as multiple clustered copies (the nucleolus organizer regions on the short arms of chromosomes 13–15, 21 and 22, and on chromosome 1). The rRNAs are synthesized as large precursors in the nucleolus and then enzymically cleaved.

Transfer RNAs (tRNAs) are also synthesized directly on a DNA template and although 61 different types may be expected (Table 2.3) only 40 are found as some tRNAs can bind to more than one codon. The DNA templates for tRNAs tend to occur as multiple copies which may be clustered or dispersed.

NUCLEIC ACID FUNCTION

Nucleic acids have two major functions: the direction of protein synthesis and transmission of this information from one generation to the next. Proteins, whether structural components, enzymes, carrier molecules, hormones or receptors, are all composed of a series of amino acids. Twenty amino acids are known, and the sequence of these

determines the form and function of the resulting protein. All proteins are encoded in DNA, and the unit of DNA which codes for a protein is, by definition, its gene. Genes vary greatly in size from small genes like the globins to medium sized genes of 15–45 kb to enormous genes such as dystrophin (Table 2.4).

Each set of three DNA base pairs (called a triplet) codes for an amino acid. As each base in the triplet may be any of the four types of nucleotide (A, G, C, T) this results in 4^3 or 64 possible combinations or codons. The codons for each amino acid are given in Table 2.3, and it is important to note that, by convention, each codon is shown in terms of the messenger RNA (mRNA), and so the corresponding DNA codon will be complementary. For example, the mRNA sequence 5'-AUG-3' is the codon for methionine and is transcribed from a complementary DNA template 5'-CAT-3'.

All amino acids except methionine and tryptophan are coded by more than one codon: hence the code is said to be degenerate. Three of the 64 codons designate the termination of a message and these are called stop codons (UAA, UGA, UAG), and one codon, AUG (which also codes for methionine), acts as a start signal for protein synthesis. With a few possible exceptions this code is identical in all species.

The first stage in protein synthesis is transcription. The two strands of DNA separate in the area of the gene to be transcribed. One strand (the template strand—this strand is consistent for a given gene but varies from one gene to another) functions as a template and is read 5' to 3', and mRNA is synthesized in the 5' to 3' direction with a complementary sequence under the influence of the enzyme RNA polymerase II (Fig. 2.5) (by convention the mRNA sequence is referred to as a *sense* strand and the complementary DNA sequence which serves as the transcriptional template is referred to as an *antisense* strand).

Table 2.3 The genetic code with codons shown as messenger RNA 5′ to 3′. The corresponding DNA codons are complementary.

First base	Second base				Third base
	U	C	A	G	
U	UUU Phe	UCU Ser	UAU Tyr	UGU Cys	U
	UUC Phe	UCC Ser	UAC Tyr	UGC Cys	C
	UUA Leu	UCA Ser	UAA STOP	UGA STOP	A
	UUG Leu	UCG Ser	UAG STOP	UGG Trp	G
C	CUU Leu	CCU Pro	CAU His	CGU Arg	U
	CUC Leu	CCC Pro	CAC His	CGC Arg	C
	CUA Leu	CCA Pro	CAA Gln	CGA Arg	A
	CUG Leu	CCG Pro	CAG Gln	CGG Arg	G
A	AUU Ile	ACU Thr	AAU Asn	AGU Ser	U
	AUC Ile	ACC Thr	AAC Asn	AGC Ser	C
	AUA Ile	ACA Thr	AAA Lys	AGA Arg	A
	*AUG Met	ACG Thr	AAG Lys	AGG Arg	G
G	GUU Val	GCU Ala	GAU Asp	GGU Gly	U
	GUC Val	GCC Ala	GAC Asp	GGC Gly	C
	GUA Val	GCA Ala	GAA Glu	GGA Gly	A
	GUG Val	GCG Ala	GAG Glu	GGG Gly	G

Abbreviations for amino acids (short code):

Ala	Alanine (A)	Leu	Leucine (L)
Arg	Arginine (R)	Lys	Lysine (K)
Asn	Asparagine (N)	Met	Methionine (M)
Asp	Aspartic acid (D)	Phe	Phenylalanine (F)
Cys	Cysteine (C)	Pro	Proline (P)
Gln	Glutamine (Q)	Ser	Serine (S)
Glu	Glutamic acid (E)	Thr	Threonine (T)
Gly	Glycine (G)	Trp	Tryptophan (W)
His	Histidine (H)	Tyr	Tyrosine (Y)
Ile	Isoleucine (I)	Val	Valine (V)

Other abbreviation:

STOP Chain terminators (X).

* Start codon for protein synthesis.

Transcription proceeds at about 30 nucleotides per second until the transcription terminator is reached. After some processing and modification (which is described in detail in the next section) the mRNA molecule diffuses to the cytoplasm and the DNA strands reassociate.

The next stage of protein synthesis occurs in the cytoplasm and is called translation. Each mRNA molecule becomes attached to one or more ribosomes. As the ribosome moves along the mRNA from the 5′ to the 3′ end each

codon is recognized by a matching complementary tRNA which contributes its amino acid to the end of a new growing protein chain until a stop codon (UAA, UGA or UAG) is reached.

The average protein contains about 300 amino acids which could be coded by 900 bp of DNA. Human genes, however, tend to be much larger than expected (Table 2.4). This excess is mainly due to the presence of intervening sequences and post-translational modification of the initial protein product.

The vast majority of genes consist of alternating coding segments for mature mRNA, or exons, and non-coding segments of 50 to over 10 000 bp, called intervening sequences or introns, whose function is unknown (Fig. 2.5). The initial mRNA (heterogeneous RNA, hnRNA) is a complete transcript of the gene (including exons, intervening sequences and flanking sequences), but prior to its entry to the cytoplasm the segments corresponding to the intervening sequences are removed by splicing (Fig. 2.6). Thus the initial mRNA may be 2–3 times the length of the definitive mRNA. The sequences around the intron/exon junctions serve as recognition sites for splicing enzymes, and characteristically an intron begins GT (the 5′ donor site) and ends AG (the 3′ acceptor site). Mutations in the bases adjacent to the exon/intron boundaries interfere with mRNA splicing and can cause genetic disease.

The mRNA 5′ end is blocked or capped (with a methyl guanylate residue) and the 5′ untranslated region or leader extends from this cap site to the beginning of the protein-coding sequence. At the other end, the 3′ untranslated region or trailer extends from the protein translation stop codon to the polyadenylic tail. This tail of 100–200 As is not coded in the DNA but is added enzymatically to aid cytoplasmic transport.

Many proteins are not in their final form after ribosomal translation and post-translational alterations include the formation of disulphide bonds, hydroxylation, glycosylation, proteolytic cleavage and phosphorylation (Fig. 2.7). Each step in the production of the final protein is important, as many proteins are highly dependent for function upon their exact three-dimensional shape, which in turn is determined by their amino acid sequence and post-translational modifications. In general acidic (e.g. Asp, Glu) and basic (e.g. Lys, Arg, His) amnio acids are found on the surface of a folded protein with hydrophobic amino acids (e.g. Ala, Val, Leu) internally orientated. The effect of an amino acid substitution thus not only depends upon its relationship to the active site of the protein but also upon the change in charge and hence disruption to the protein's tertiary structure.

Table 2.4 Examples of genes and their protein products.

Protein	Number of amino acids in final protein	Approximate gene size (bp)	Number of coding regions in each gene
Alpha-globin	141	850	3
Alpha$_1$ antitrypsin	394	10 000	5
Beta-globin	146	1600	3
Coagulation factor VIII	2332	189 000	26
Cystic fibrosis transmembrane regulator protein	1480	230 000	27
Dystrophin	3700	2 400 000	80
Glucose-6-phosphate dehydrogenase	515	18 000	13
Hypoxanthine-guanine phosphoribosyl transferase	217	44 000	9
Insulin	51	1430	3
Low density lipoprotein receptor	839	45 000	18
Phenylalanine hydroxylase	451	90 000	13

Gene regulation

All nucleated cells of an individual have an identical genome, yet at any one time in a cell only a small fraction of the total is being expressed and the relative pattern of expression needs to vary widely, not only for the initial differentiation of cells and tissues, but also to meet fluctuating demands for the synthesis of different proteins in each cell. Areas of DNA flanking each gene play an important role in regulating transcription and hence synthesis of each protein (Fig. 2.8). Immediately upstream of the gene is the promoter which is involved in the attachment of RNA polymerase II to the DNA template strand. Promoters for RNA polymerase II are usually several hundred nucleotides long and often contain a consensus sequence 5'-TATA-3' (the TATA box). This sequence binds a series of *general transcription factors* (e.g. TFIIB, TFIID, TFIIE, TFIIF, TFIIH) which are relatively abundant proteins used to initiate the transcription of nearly all mRNAs.

The activity of many promoters is modulated (increased or decreased) by one or more enhancers. Enhancers are generally short (less than 20–30 bp) sequences that bind *specific transcription factors*. Most enhancers function whether on the coding or non-coding strand of DNA and can be located up to several kilobases from their target promoter. Most enhancers are active only in specific cell types and thus play a central role in regulating tissue specificity of gene expression. Further, the large number of specific transcription factors and their interaction at individual enhancers allows for complex patterns of gene activation in response to particular circumstances.

About 80% of genes are only expressed at specific times and places (e.g. insulin in the pancreatic islet beta cells). The other 20%, which are called housekeeping genes, are expressed in all tissues, generally fulfill basic metabolic needs and account for 90% or more of the genes expressed in any particular cell type. The majority of housekeeping genes and about 40% of tissue-specific genes have CpG islands near their 5' ends. The CpG islands are about 1 kb in length and contain a high proportion of 5'-CG-3' dinucleotide pairs (indicated as C, p for phosphate, G to distinguish them from G hydrogen bonded to C in opposite DNA strands). Generally, cytosine residues in CpG dinucleotides are methylated but in CpG islands associated with active neighbouring gene expression, there is usually a lack of methylation.

Although the bulk of regulation probably occurs at transcriptional level, regulation of a gene's activity may also occur later with, for example, alteration of either the rate of translation or alternative splicing of the mRNA to produce different gene products (e.g. calcitonin or calcitonin gene-related neuropeptide).

Mutations within a gene's regulatory sequences can occur and may result in no gene product (e.g. some patients with beta-thalassaemia), abnormal persistence of a fetal gene product (e.g. hereditary persistence of alphafetoprotein or haemoglobin F) or anomalous patterns of gene expression (e.g. ectopic expression of creatine kinase).

DNA REPLICATION

Accurate replication of DNA must occur with each cell division. The two strands separate at a number of points (up to 100 per chromosome) and each strand serves as a

cccctgtggagccacaccctagggttgg[ccaat]ctactcccaggagcagggagggcaggagccagggctggg[cataaaa]

gtcagggcagagccatctattgctt**ACATTTGCTTCTGACACAACTGTGTTCACTAGCAACCTCAAACAGACACC**[ATG]   5' leader

VaIHisLeuThrProGluGluLysSerAlaValThrAlaLeuTrpGlyLysValAsnValAspGluValGlyGlyGlu   Exon 1
GTGCACCTGACTCCTGAGGAGAAGTTGGCCTTACTCGCCCTGTGGGGCAAGGTGAACGTGGATGAAGTTGGTGGTGAG

AlaLeuGlyArg   Intron 1
GCCCTGGGCAGG**TTGGTATCAAGGTTACAAGACAGGTTTAAGGAGACCAATAGAAACTGGGCATGTGGAGACAGAGAAG**

ACTCTTGGGTTTCTGATAGGCACTGACTCTCTCTGCCTATTGGTCTATTTTCCCACCCTTAGG⌒ CTGCTGGTGGTCTAC LeuLeuValValTyr

ProTrpThrGlnArgPhePheGluSerPheGlyAspLeuSerThrProAspAlaValMetGlyAsnProLysValLys   Exon 2
CCTTGGACCCAGAGGTTCTTTGAGTTCTTTGGGGATCTGTCCACTCCTGATGCTGTTATGGGCAACCCTAAGGTGAAG

AlaHisGlyLysLysValLeuGlyAlaPheSerAspGlyLeuAlaHisLeuAspAsnLeuLysGlyThrPheAlaThr
GCTCATGGCAAGAAAGTGCTCGGTGCCTTTAGTGATGGCCTGGCCCACCTGGACAACCTCAAGGGCACCTTTGCCACA

LeuSerGluLeuHisCysAspLysLeuHisValAspProGluAsnPheArg⌒
CTGAGTGAGCTGCACTGTGACAAGCTGCACGTGGATCCTGAGAACTTCAGG**GTGAGTCTATGGGACCCTTGATGTTTT**

CTTTCCCCTTCTTTTCTATGGTTAAGTTCATGTCATAGGAAGGGGAGAAGTAACAGGGTACAGTTTAGAATGGGAAAC

AGACGAATGATTGCATCAGTGTGGAAGTCTCAGGATCGTTTTAGTTTCATTTTATTTGCTGTTCATAACAATTGTTTTC

TTTTGTTTAATTCTTGCTTTCTTTTTTTTTTCTTCTCCGCAATTTTTACTATTATACTTAATGCCTTAACATTGTGTAT   Intron 2

AACAAAAGGAAATATCTCTGAGATACATTAAGTAACTTAAAAAAAAAACTTTACACAGTCTGCCTAGTACATTACTATT

TGGAATATATGTGTGCTTATTTGCATATTCATAATCTCCCTACTTTATTTTCTTTTATTTTTTAATTGATACATAATCA

TTATACATATTTATGGGTTAAAGTGTAATGTTTTAATATGTGTACACATATTGACCAAATCAGGGTAATTTTGCATT

TGTAATTTTAAAAAATGCTTTCTTCTTTTAATATACTTTTTTGTTTATTTTATTTCTAATACTTTCCCTAATCTCTTT

CTTTCAGGGCAATAATGATACAATGTATCATGCCTCTTTGCACCATTCTAAAGAATAACAGTGATAATTTCTGGGTTA

AGGCAATAGCAATATTTCTGCATATAAATATTTCTGCATATAAATTGTAACTGATGTAAGAGGTTTCATATTGCTAA

TAGCAGCTACAATCCAGCTACCATTCTGCATTTATTTTATGGTTGGGATAAGGCTGGATTATTCTGAGTCCAAGCTAG

GCCCTTTTGCTAATCATGTTCATACCTCTTATCTTCCTCCCACAG⌒CCCCTGGGCAACGTGCTGGTCTGTGTGCTGGCC LeuLeuGlyAsnValLeuValCysValLeuAla

HisHisPheGlyLysGluPheThrProProValGlnAlaAlaTyrGlnLysValValAlaGlyValAlaAsnAlaLeu   Exon 3
CATCACTTTGGCAAAGAATTCACCCCACCAGTGCAGGCTGCCTATCAGAAAGTGGTGGCTGGTGTGGCTAATGCCCTG

AlaHisLysTyrHis   3' trailer
GCCCACAAGTATCAC[TAA]GCTCGCTTTCTTGCTGTCCAATTTCTATTAAAGGTTCCTTTGTTCCCTAAGTCC**AACTAC**

TAAACTGGGGGATATTATGAAGGGCCTTGTGCATCTGGATTCTGGCTAATAAAAAACATTTATTTTCATTGCaatgat

gtatttaaattatttctgaatatttttactaaaaagggaatgtgggaggtcagtgcatttaaaacataaagaaatgatg

agctgttcaaaccttgggaaaatacactatatcttaaactccatgaaagaaggtgaggccgcaaccagctaatgcaca

ttggcaacagccccctgatgcctatgccttattcatccctcagaaaaggattcttgtagaagcttgatttgcaggttaa

agttttgctatgctgtatttttacattacttattgttttagctgtcctcatgaatgtcttttccctacccatttgctta

tcctgcatctctctcagccttgact

Fig. 2.5 Nucleotide sequence of the human beta-globin gene. The nucleotide sequence of the mRNA strand is shown from the 5' to 3' direction (with T in place of U). Large and small capital letters represent sequences corresponding to mature mRNA and introns respectively (after Lawn *et al*, 1980).

Primary mRNA transcript

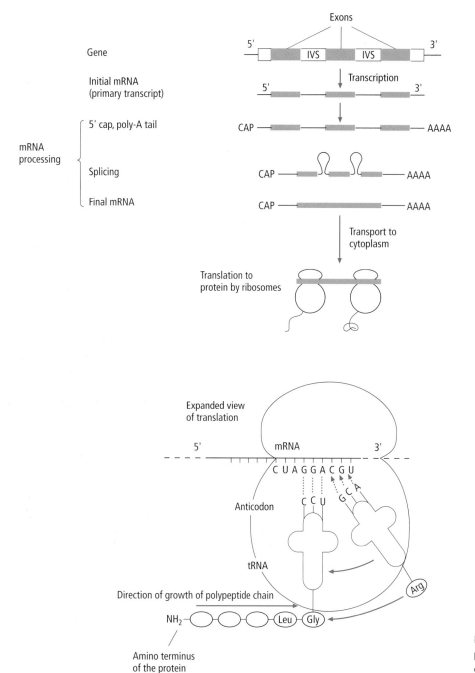

Fig. 2.6 Diagram of transcription, mRNA processing and translation. By convention the 5′ end of the mRNA molecule is placed to the left.

template upon which the missing partner can be reconstructed by base pairing with free nucleotides (Fig. 2.9). These nucleotides are bound together by the action of the enzyme DNA polymerase III and are hydrogen-bonded to the template strand. Replication proceeds in both directions from each initiation point until the two new strands of DNA are complete. This method of replication is called semiconservative, as one strand of each new DNA mole-

cule has been conserved (Fig. 2.10). This can be shown very effectively by growing cells through two cell divisions in culture medium containing bromodeoxyuridine (BrdU), an analogue of thymine. New growing strands incorporate BrdU, so that at the end of two divisions each chromosome has only one original strand lacking BrdU. This strand can be stained differentially to give the chromosome a harlequin appearance—one dark (con-

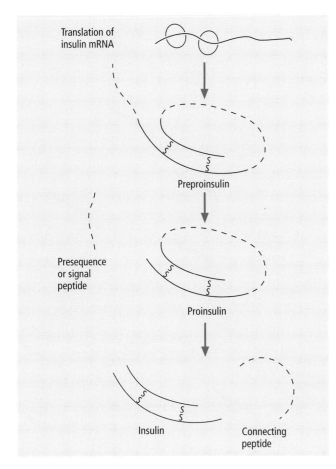

Fig. 2.7 Post-translational modification of insulin.

MUTATION

Mutations of DNA are broadly divisible into length mutations with gain or loss of genetic material and point mutations with alteration of the genetic code but no overall gain or loss of genetic material.

Length mutations

Length mutations include deletions, duplications, insertions and trinucleotide repeat amplifications. Deletions of DNA can range from a single nucleotide to many megabases (and then be visible as a chromosomal deletion, p. 62). Larger deletions can arise from chromosomal breakage, as a result of a parental chromosome rearrangement (p. 57) or from unequal crossing over. Small deletions (often 1–5 nucleotides) commonly result from slipped mispairing and this is favoured by the presence of direct repeats of two bases or more and by runs of the same nucleotide. The spontaneous rate of chromosomal breakage is markedly increased by ionizing radiation and by some mutagenic chemicals. Unequal crossing-over is especially likely to occur in areas with duplicated genes of similar sequence. This is exemplified by studies on the genes responsible for colour vision. There are three separate genes for each of the cone pigments blue (on chromosome 7), red and green (near the tip of the long arm of the X chromosome). There is a single red gene on each X chromosome and one to three copies of the green genes. The red and green genes have 96% sequence homology, and unequal crossing-over in the area can result in loss of gene function for one type or hybrid genes which produce pigments of altered function (Fig. 2.12).

taining the original strand) and one light chromatid (Fig. 2.11).

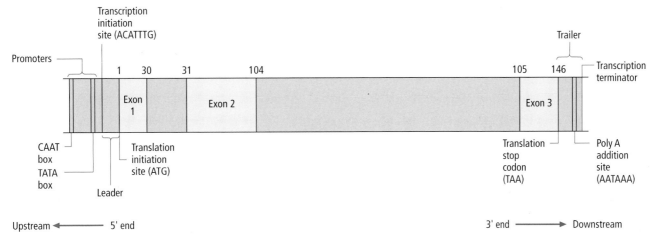

Fig. 2.8 The human beta-globin gene, indicating the sequences involved in the regulation of transcription.

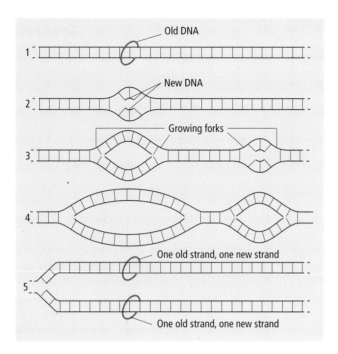

Fig. 2.9 Initiation of replication.

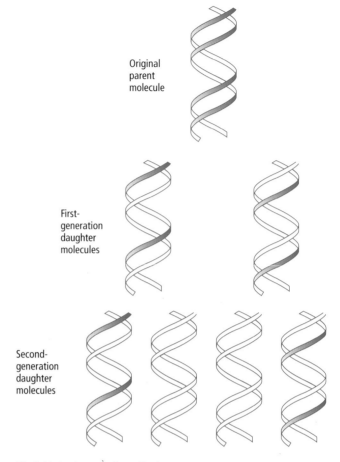

Fig. 2.10 Semiconservative replication.

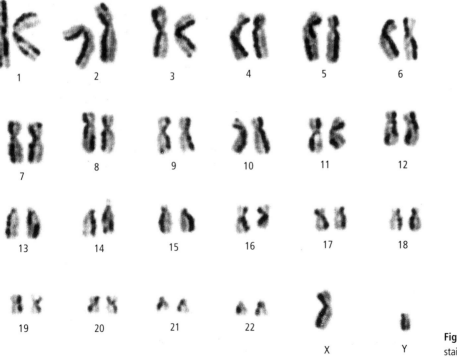

Fig. 2.11 Harlequin chromosomes (BrdU staining).

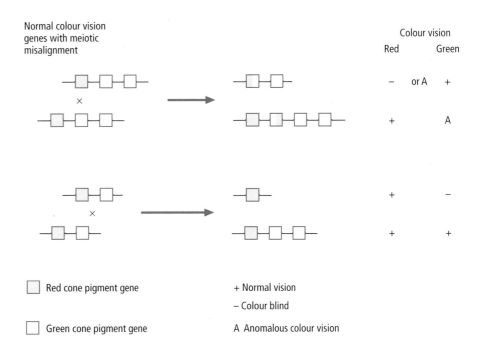

Fig. 2.12 Unequal recombination in the colour vision gene cluster resulting in loss of genes or creation of fused hybrid genes with altered action spectrums.

Large deletions remove many adjacent genes (contiguous gene disorders) and these should be suspected if a boy has several X-linked disorders or if a patient with a single-gene disorder has unexplained mental handicap and/or congenital malformations. Removal of all of a gene directly prevents transcription but smaller deletions of more or less than 3 (or a multiple of 3) bp can be equally serious by altering the reading frame of the mRNA (frameshift mutations, Table 2.5).

Duplications of a chromosomal region can also disrupt the reading frame and in some patients with single gene disorders the gene has been disrupted by insertion of a repeat element from a distant site (p. 11) or by a short insertion (often one nucleotide) after slipped mispairing.

Another mechanism of length (or point) mutation is gene conversion whereby one allele is converted to another. This may occur at mitosis or meiosis during the process of recombination. In normal recombination between chromosomes or chromatids (Chapter 5) the products contain all of the original sections of DNA but in an altered configuration. In contrast when gene conversion occurs the product lacks one of the original sections of chromosome and this results in a 3 : 1 allele ratio for the involved region in contrast to the expected 2 : 2 ratio (Fig. 2.13).

Another important mechanism of length mutation is trinucleotide repeat amplification. About 10% of the genome is composed of tandem repeats (p. 10) which are mostly stably inherited. These include repeats of trinucleotides which may occur within or between genes. Some of these trinucleotide repeats become unstable if longer than a critical number of repeat elements and if associated with a gene, this can result in a single gene disorder. The faulty gene is identified by a trinucleotide repeat which is longer than normal and the instability of long repeats means that different members of the same family can show different repeat lengths and corresponding clinical variation in disease severity. This is exemplified by

Table 2.5 Examples of DNA mutation.

DNA base sequence	mRNA sequence	Amino acid sequence	Comment
CAA TTC CGA CGA	GUU AAG GCU GCU	Val-Lys-Ala-Ala	Normal sequence
CAA TTT CGA CGA	GUU AAA GCU GCU	Val-Lys-Ala-Ala	Point mutation with unchanged AA sequence
CAA CTC CGA CGA	GUU GAG GCU GCU	Val-Glu-Ala-Ala	Point mutation with AA substitution (missense mutation)
CAA ATC CGA CGA	GUU UAG GCU GCU	Val-stop	Point mutation with premature chain termination (nonsense mutation)
CAA—TCG GAC GA	GUU AGG CUG CU	Val-Arg-Leu	Base deletion with frameshift (nonsense mutation)
CAA TTT CCG ACG A	GUU AAA GGC UGC	Val-Lys-Gly-Cys	Base insertion with frameshift (nonsense mutation)

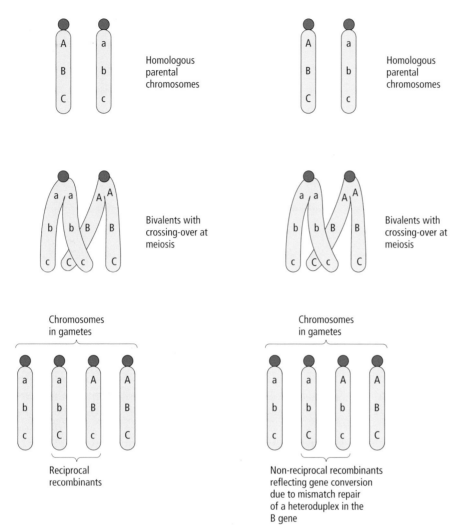

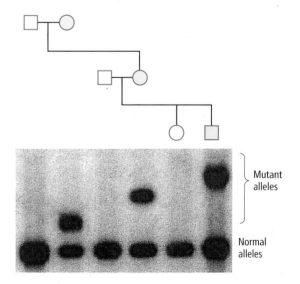

Fig. 2.13 Diagram to compare normal recombination (left) with gene conversion (right).

myotonic dystrophy which is an adult onset type of muscular dystrophy. The CTG repeat normally occurs 5–35 times but in affected patients there is an expansion from 50 to over 1000 repeats (Fig. 2.14).

Point mutations

In a point mutation, a single nucleotide base is replaced by a different nucleotide base (transitions if purine to purine or pyrimidine to pyrimidine, A ↔ G, or T ↔ C; transversions if purine to pyrimidine or vice versa, G ↔ C or A ↔ T). This may lead to no change in the amino acid coded for that triplet (25%, silent mutations) due to degeneracy of the code (Table 2.3) or may result in the substitution of a different amino acid (70%, missense mutations) or alteration to a chain terminator (5%, nonsense mutations).

Single nucleotide substitutions are a common type of human mutation and their frequency reflects the fidelity

Fig. 2.14 DNA analysis of a family with myotonic dystrophy. (Note the instability of the larger mutant allele.)

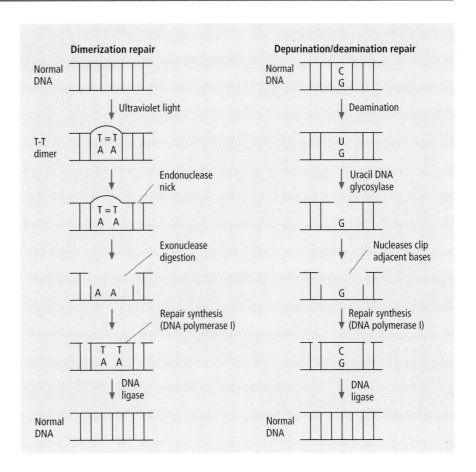

Fig. 2.15 Examples of DNA repair mechanisms.

of DNA replication and the efficiency of subsequent error correction mechanisms. Most are spontaneous and unexplained with a mutation rate in the order of one base substitution for every 10^9 to 10^{10} bases replicated. This rate is markedly increased by exposure to mutagenic chemicals (e.g. deamination by hydroxylamine or alkylation by nitrogen mustard) in proportion to the concentration of the chemical and the duration of exposure. Ultraviolet light can also cause mutations including pyrimidine dimers in which pairs of adjacent pyrimidine bases become linked. Defence mechanisms exist to identify and repair such damage (Fig. 2.15) and patients with inherited deficiencies of key components of these pathways rapidly accumulate mutations and develop premature cancer (Plate 1). A separate multistep DNA mismatch repair process is involved in error correction at the time of DNA replication and patients with inherited deficiencies of components of this pathway are also prone to premature cancer, particularly of the colon (p. 165).

These repair mechanisms cannot recognize one particular type of point mutation and in consequence this mutation is overrepresented amongst point mutations which cause single gene disorders (e.g. accounts for nearly one half of all point mutations in unrelated patients with haemophilia). Deamination of cytosine produces uracil which is recognized and removed by the depurination/deamination repair pathway (Fig. 2.15). However, cytosine when it occurs in conjunction with guanine as a 5′-CpG-3′ dinucleotide is generally methylated at the 5′ position and deamination of methylated cytosine results in thymine (Fig. 2.2). In turn, this substitution of T for C results in substitution of A for G on the complementary strand and neither of these changes can be recognized by the repair mechanisms. This results in an overall tendency to lose methylated CpG dinucleotides (their frequency is 1 in 50–100 as compared with a random dinucleotide frequency of 1 in 16) and an overrepresentation of C to T transitions amongst point mutations (they account for 35–50% of all point mutations). Non-methylated cytosine residues are spared and hence CpG dinucleotides have a relatively high frequency in non-methylated CpG islands which are associated with the 5′ ends of many genes (p. 14). These C to T transitions most commonly occur in male germ cells (sevenfold higher frequency than in females) and this

Possible faults

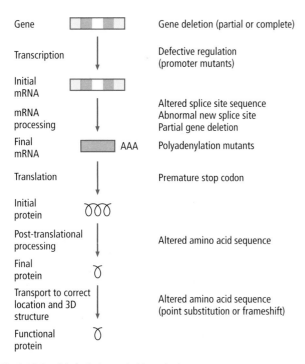

Gene	Gene deletion (partial or complete)
Transcription	Defective regulation (promoter mutants)
Initial mRNA	
mRNA processing	Altered splice site sequence Abnormal new splice site Partial gene deletion
Final mRNA	Polyadenylation mutants
Translation	Premature stop codon
Initial protein	
Post-translational processing	Altered amino acid sequence
Final protein	
Transport to correct location and 3D structure	Altered amino acid sequence (point substitution or frameshift)
Functional protein	

Fig. 2.16 Possible faults in protein biosynthesis.

Table 2.6 Examples of mutations causing cystic fibrosis.

Mutation	Nomenclature	Consequence
3 bp deletion nt 1652–1655	ΔF508	In-frame deletion of codon for phenylalanine at aa position 508
G → T at nt 1756	G542X	Nonsense mutation with substitution of a chain terminator for glycine at aa position 542
G → A at nt 1784	G551D	Missense mutation with substitution of aspartic acid for glycine at aa 551
Insertion of a T after nt 3905	3905insT	Frameshift due to a one-base insertion
Deletion of 22 bp from nt 852	852del22	Frameshift due to a 22 bp deletion
G → A at nt 1 from 5′ junction of intron starting after nt 621	621 + 1G → T	Splice junction mutation
G → A at nt 1 from 3′ junction of intron ending before nt 1717	1717 − 1G → A	Splice junction mutation
G or A at nt 1716	1716G/A	Silent mutation which leaves the amino acid unaltered (Glu at 528)

nt, nucleotide; aa, amino acid.

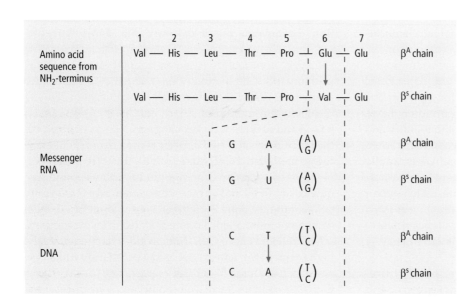

Fig. 2.17 Point mutation in beta-globin at amino acid 6 causing sickle cell disease (β^s chain homozygote).

might reflect the heavy methylation of sperm DNA as compared with oocyte DNA which tends to be undermethylated.

Molecular pathology of single gene disorders

For most single gene disorders a diversity of molecular lesions (occurring at any stage in the protein biosynthetic pathway) are found (Fig. 2.16). Generally with length mutations (frameshifts, insertions, deletions), nonsense point mutations (chain terminators) and point mutations adjacent to the intron/exon boundaries which interfere with splicing (p. 13), the biological activity of the protein product is reduced in proportion to the reduction in amount of the protein. In this situation commonly little, none of, or a truncated protein is produced and the mutation is termed null, protein° or cross-reacting material (CRM) negative. In contrast, with missense mutations (amino acid substitutions) there is often a relatively normal amount of protein produced but its function is impaired to some extent (also referred to as leaky, protein⁺ or cross-reacting material positive mutations).

Most single gene disorders can be caused by either length or point mutations but for several one particular type of pathology predominates. For example, length mutations due to trinucleotide repeat amplifications are the major pathology found in myotonic dystrophy, the fragile X syndrome (a cause of mental handicap) and Huntington disease (a cause of dementia). Rarely, all patients have the same point mutation; for example, in sickle cell anaemia all patients have a point mutation which results in substitution of valine for glutamic acid at amino acid position 6 in beta-globin (Fig. 2.17). Where there is a range in the type of molecular pathology, geographical differences may be observed which reflect factors operating at a population genetic level. Thus, for example, two-thirds of Caucasian patients in the UK and USA with cystic fibrosis have a three-base deletion at amino acid position 508 whereas this mutation is found in less than one-third of Turkish or Arab patients with cystic fibrosis.

Mutations can be described using a standardized nomenclature which is based upon the type of mutation, the amino acid short code (Table 2.3) and the amino acid position within the protein (Table 2.6). For missense and nonsense point mutations, the amino acid position is indicated by its number in the protein sequence preceded by the letter denoting the normal residue followed by the letter of the mutant. For insertions and deletions, the nucleotide position within the coding sequence is indicated followed by ins or del and the number or actual nucleotides which are altered.

Splicing mutations are generally point mutations within introns close to the intron/exon boundary. They are numbered fom the closest exon with the convention of plus when counting 5′ to 3′ and minus when counting 3′ to 5′.

C H A P T E R   3

DNA Analysis

C O N T E N T S

INDIRECT MUTANT GENE TRACKING 24
Techniques for demonstration of DNA polymorphisms 26

DIRECT MUTANT GENE ANALYSIS 27

Medical genetics utilizes a wide range of DNA analysis techniques for both research and genetic counselling. This chapter will focus on the basic techniques and applications of most relevance to clinical practice and further reading is provided for those needing wider or more detailed coverage. The clinical applications can be broadly divided into *indirect mutant gene tracking* and *direct mutant gene analysis*. These techniques all start with DNA from the key family members which can be extracted from any nucleated tissue. The lymphocytes from a 10 ml anticoagulated venous blood sample yield about 300 µg of DNA which is sufficient for multiple DNA analyses.

INDIRECT MUTANT GENE TRACKING

Gene tracking utilizes DNA sequence variations to follow the inheritance of mutant (and normal) genes within a family. In order to be useful for distinguishing the mutant gene from its partner, the sequence variations at a site are ideally multiple and frequent. By definition frequent (involving >2% of the population) discontinuous genetic variations are called polymorphisms and hence these markers are usually referred to as DNA polymorphisms (Table 3.1).

Site polymorphisms occur every 200–500 bp in the genome and the majority are of no clinical significance as they occur in non-coding DNA or do not result in amino acid substitutions within coding DNA (silent mutations, p. 20). About one in six site polymorphisms may be identified by using DNA cleavage enzymes which will only cut at specific DNA sequences. These sequence-specific

enzymes are called restriction enzymes and they are found naturally in bacteria where they function as a defence mechanism against the incorporation of foreign DNA. More than 400 different restriction enzymes have been described, which have over 100 different recognition sites for DNA cleavage. Each is named after the organism from which it was first isolated (e.g. *Eco*RI was found in *Escherichia coli*). The recognition site is commonly 4 or 6 bp in length and the cleavage may produce flush (blunt) or staggered (sticky) ends (Fig. 3.1). By convention, each recognition site is written 5′ to 3′ using the symbols N for any nucleotide, R for either purine (A or G), Y for either pyrimidine (T or C) and A, T, C, G for specific bases.

The enzyme *Taq*I will cut DNA at each point where the sequence 5′-TCGA-3′ occurs. Human DNA contains about 1 m *Taq*I recognition sites and so cleavage (digestion) with this enzyme results in about 1 m fragments of DNA. These fragments would be of variable length but each would have the same base order at their staggered ends. Gel electrophoresis can be used to order these fragments according to size but in order to identify particular fragments relating to one site polymorphism amongst a large number of fragments, a specific DNA probe is required. DNA probes are labelled (radioactive or non-radioactive) sections of DNA from tens of base pairs to several kilobases in size which are used to identify complementary (p. 10) base sequences. The probe and its target sequences are rendered single-stranded (denatured) and upon recognition of its complementary sequence(s) the single-stranded probe and target DNA molecule hybridize to form a labelled double-stranded molecule which can then be visualized.

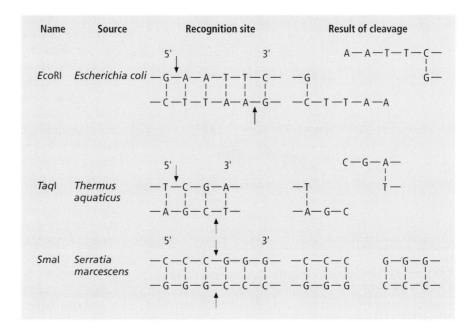

Fig. 3.1 Examples of restriction enzymes and their recognition sites.

Table 3.1 DNA polymorphisms useful for indirect mutant gene tracking.

Site polymorphisms
DNA point variations (restriction fragment length polymorphisms, RFLPs)

Length polymorphisms (variable number of tandem repeats, VNTRs)
Microsatellites
Minisatellites

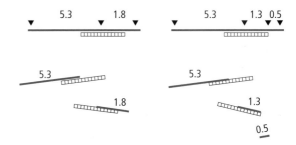

Fig. 3.2 Diagram of a coagulation factor IX intragenic RFLP. Arrows indicate restriction enzyme (*Taq*I) recognition sites, and the hatched segments represent the DNA probe. Fragment sizes are in kilobases.

A specific example is illustrated in Fig. 3.2. This shows portions of the clotting factor IX gene from two different X chromosomes. The gene on the right has four *Taq*I recognition sites whereas the gene on the left has only three as a DNA point variation has abolished one recognition site. The probe shown is a 2.5 kb fragment from within the factor IX gene and its area of complementarity is indicated. Thus after digestion it will hybridize to a constant 5.3 kb fragment from each gene and to a 1.8 kb fragment from the gene on the left and a 1.3 kb fragment from the gene on the right. Thus these two factor IX genes can be distinguished by the different pattern of fragments produced after *Taq*I digestion.

A female with two X chromosomes will generate one of three patterns: 1.8 kb fragments from each X chromosome (1.8 kb/1.8 kb), 1.3 kb fragments from each X chromosome (1.3 kb/1.3 kb) or a 1.8 kb fragment from one X chromosome and a 1.3 kb fragment from the other (1.8 kb/1.3 kb). Males with only a single X chromosome will generate only 1.8 kb or 1.3 kb fragments.

Figure 3.3 illustrates the use of gene tracking with this RFLP in a family with haemophilia B due to deficiency of clotting factor IX. The affected son (shaded square, lane 4) has inherited the disease and the 1.8 kb fragment from his mother who is known to be a carrier on the basis of her family history. The unaffected son (lane 2) has inherited the mother's normal factor IX gene and her 1.3 kb fragment. The daughter at risk (lane 5) has inherited the 1.3 kb fragment from both her father (lane 1) and her mother (lane 3). As the 1.3 kb fragment in the mother is the marker of the normal gene the daughter is predicted not to be a carrier for haemophilia B. This is a very reliable prediction as the RFLP is within the gene of interest (an intragenic RFLP). If an RFLP outside the gene of interest had been used (an extragenic RFLP) then there would have been a chance of error due to recombination between the marker RFLP and the mutant gene (see Fig. 2.13).

Site polymorphisms due to DNA point variations show only two forms (presence or absence of the recognition site) and hence at most only one-half of the population

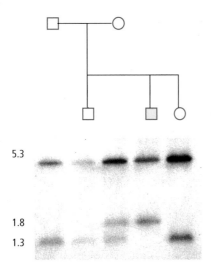

Fig. 3.3 Pedigree and results of DNA analysis in a family with haemophilia B studied with the intragenic factor IX RFLP shown in Fig. 3.2. Fragment sizes are in kilobases (kb), squares represent males, circles represent females. Each DNA lane corresponds to the individual above it.

will be heterozygous at a site. In practice, this is an important limitation, as if key individuals in a family are homozygous for the marker RFLP, it can no longer be used for genetic prediction. This limitation can be avoided by the use of length polymorphisms which often have multiple alleles and correspondingly high heterozygosity frequencies.

Length polymorphisms due to variable number of tandem repeats are subdivided according to length into microsatellite repeats and minisatellite repeats (p. 10). Microsatellite repeats are under 1 kb and the most common repeat motifs are A, AC, AAN (where N is any nucleotide), AAN and AG. AC repeats commonly have 10–60 repeats (with corresponding lengths of 20–120 bp) and are found every 30 kb (see Fig. 2.4). In about 70% of repeats the number of repeats differs between corre-

sponding chromosomes and thus the length of a DNA fragment generated by restriction enzyme digestion which carries the repeat will vary in length (Fig. 3.4).

Minisatellite repeats are usually 1–3 kb in length and have longer repeat motifs than the microsatellite repeats. They again show marked variation in repeat number so that about 70% of individuals are heterozygous for each polymorphism. Figure 3.5 illustrates the use of a minisatellite DNA polymorphism for gene tracking in a family with adult onset polycystic kidney disease (PKD). Three alleles (and some fainter shadow bands) are evident and the affected mother has handed the mutant gene and allele 2 to the affected daughter (lane 4) and affected son (lane 5). The mother has handed on her normal gene and allele 3 to each unaffected child. Figure 3.6 shows DNA analysis of a minisatellite repeat in a family where nonpaternity was suspected. The sons have inherited the father's lower band but the daughter has not inherited a paternal band thus confirming the suspicion of nonpaternity.

A further development of minisatellite polymorphism analysis is to use probes which simultaneously detect multiple minisatellite loci. The result, known as a DNA fingerprint, consists of multiple bands of different sizes which are specific to an individual. Half of the bands are inherited from each parent and thus DNA fingerprinting has been widely used for disputed paternity cases, resolving family relationships in immigration disputes and for forensic identification of tissue samples at crime scenes (Fig. 3.7).

Techniques for demonstration of DNA polymorphisms

Two approaches are widely used for identification of DNA polymorphisms for indirect gene tracking: Southern analysis and the polymerase chain reaction (PCR). Figure

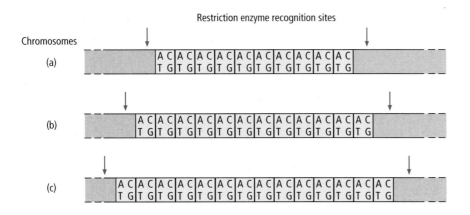

Fig. 3.4 Diagram of an AC microsatellite DNA polymorphism with 10, 12 and 14 repeats between the two restriction enzyme recognition sites in chromosomes (a)–(c) respectively.

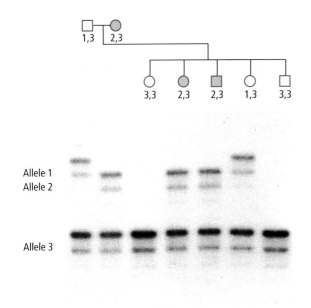

Fig. 3.5 Pedigree of a family with adult onset polycystic kidney disease showing results of DNA analysis for a microsatellite polymorphism.

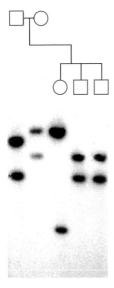

Fig. 3.6 Pedigree and results of DNA analysis using an autosomal minisatellite polymorphism in a family where non-paternity was suspected.

3.8 illustrates the steps involved in Southern analysis (named after its inventor). The DNA is cleaved into fragments using a specific restriction enzyme and the fragments are then separated according to size by gel electrophoresis (with the smallest fragments migrating furthest in the gel). At this stage the multitude of fragments can be visualized as a continuous smear (Fig. 3.8a). These fragments are then transferred to a DNA binding

filter and the complementary fragments are identified by autoradiography with a radiolabelled specific probe. This type of analysis relies on starting with sufficient copies of the DNA target and in practice needs 5–10 µg of DNA and takes 5–7 days to produce a result.

DNA polymorphism analysis using PCR has advantages in terms of speed and sensitivity (producing a result in under a day from 50 ng of DNA target). Figure 3.9 illustrates the steps involved in PCR. Two oligonucleotide primers are required which are complementary to the flanking sequences of the target segment of DNA which is to be amplified (commonly up to 1 kb in length, occasionally up to 5 kb). The primers direct repeated rounds of localized DNA replication to produce an exponential increase in the number of copies of the target sequence. After 20–30 rounds (which takes 2–3 h in an automated procedure) the target DNA will have been amplified 10^5-fold and will constitute the bulk of all DNA present. The amplified DNA fragment can then be digested with an appropriate restriction enzyme and the resulting fragments separated by gel electrophoresis and directly visualized under ultraviolet light when stained with ethidium bromide.

DIRECT MUTANT GENE ANALYSIS

Indirect mutant gene tracking needs DNA samples from multiple family members and relies on an accurate clinical diagnosis for selection of appropriate markers. It also has an error rate if markers are at some distance from the mutant gene and non-paternity can interfere with the analysis. Direct mutant gene analysis needs fewer samples and by demonstration of a mutation confirms the clinical diagnosis. It is not susceptible to errors due to recombination or non-paternity and hence is likely to become the procedure of first choice for DNA analysis for genetic counselling applications. Its drawbacks are that at present not all genes have been cloned and the underlying molecular pathology needs to be defined for each family. This is complicated by the diversity of molecular pathology which is evident for most single gene disorders and the technical challenge of finding point mutations and small length mutations in large genes.

Length mutations may be demonstrated by Southern analysis or PCR depending upon the length of the target DNA sequence. Deletions will be evident as shortened or missing bands (Fig. 3.10) and trinucleotide repeat amplifications as bands of increased size (e.g. see Fig. 2.14).

Specific point mutations may be demonstrated by loss or gain of a particular RFLP, by allele specific oligonucleotide probes and by DNA sequencing. Sickle cell

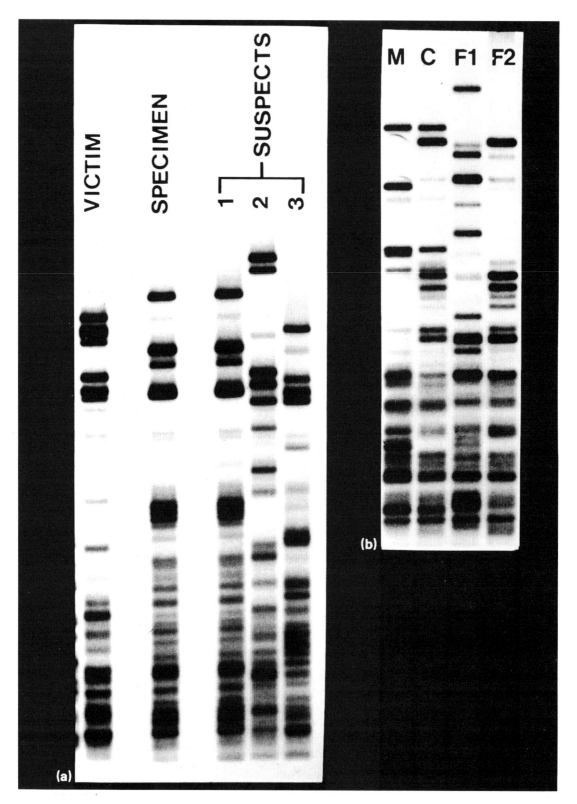

Fig. 3.7 DNA fingerprints. (a) From a rape victim, the semen specimen and three suspects. Which suspect matches the specimen? (Answer p. 215). (b) From a family where paternity was disputed: M, mother; C, child; F1, F2 are the potential fathers. Which is the father of the child? (Answer p. 215).

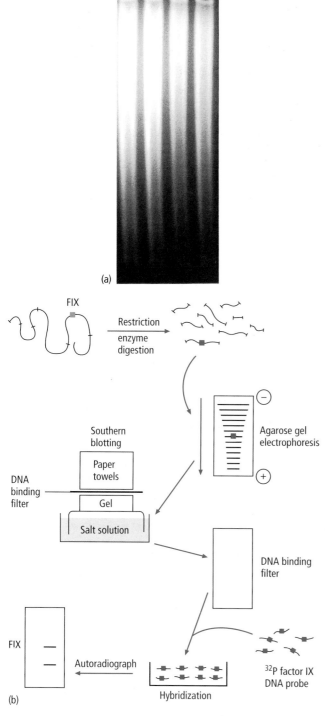

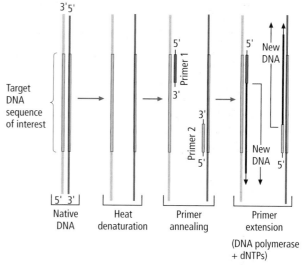

First round of the PCR

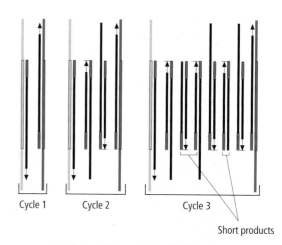

Products at the ends of early PCR cycles

Fig. 3.9 Steps involved in amplification of a DNA segment using the polymerase chain reaction (PCR). After several cycles the target short products predominate.

Fig. 3.8 (a) Smear of DNA fragments of various sizes after digestion of four DNA samples and gel electrophoresis (visualized under ultraviolet light after staining with ethidium bromide). (b) Diagram of the steps involved in Southern analysis.

disease (an inherited cause of anaemia) is most unusual amongst single gene disorders in that there is a single molecular pathology (Fig. 2.17). When this mutation is present, a recognition site for *Mst*II is lost and a fragment of 424 bp is produced rather than two fragments of 223 bp and 201 bp (Fig. 3.11).

Allele-specific oligonucleotide (ASO) probes are short (17–30 nucleotide) probes which have the complementary sequence to either the normal DNA or the mutant DNA sequence. Under appropriate experimental conditions the presence or absence of hybridization with these probes will distinguish normals from heterozygotes and homozygous affected individuals (Fig. 3.12).

DNA sequencing utilizes a single-stranded DNA template to generate a series of oligonucleotide fragments of

Lanes

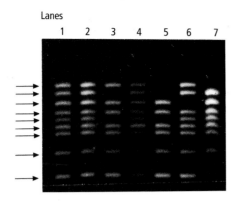

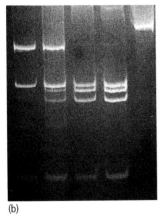

Fig. 3.10 Simultaneous PCR amplification of nine segments (arrowed) of the gene for Duchenne muscular dystrophy in seven patients (lanes 1–7). Note missing bands corresponding to deletions in lanes 3, 5, 6 and 7.

increasing length, each one nucleotide longer than the last. The fragments are radioactively or chemically labelled and separated on the basis of length by gel electrophoresis and identified according to their position on the gel (Fig. 3.13). With radioactive labelling, four parallel reactions are set up which each contain the DNA template, the four nucleotide substrates (dATP, dCTP, dGTP and dTTP of which at least one is radiolabelled) and DNA polymerase but with a small amount of ddATP (dideoxyadenosine triphosphate), ddCTP, ddGTP or ddTTP depending on the base at which chain termination is to occur. Once a dideoxy molecule is incorporated, further elongation of that chain is halted and the result is a series of partially completed product chains each with a particular dideoxynucleotide at its 3′ end. For radiolabelled products, these are identified by autoradiography

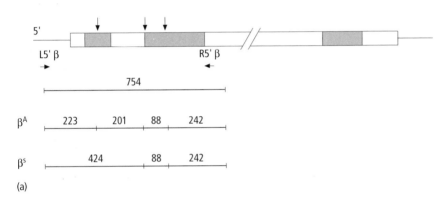

(a)

(b)

Fig. 3.11 Diagram (a) and results (b) of PCR amplification of a portion of the beta-globin gene and digestion with *Mst*II in a sickle cell disease homozygote (lane 1), a sickle cell heterozygote (lane 2) and two normal homozygotes (lanes 3 and 4). Lane 5 is a control containing amplified but undigested DNA.

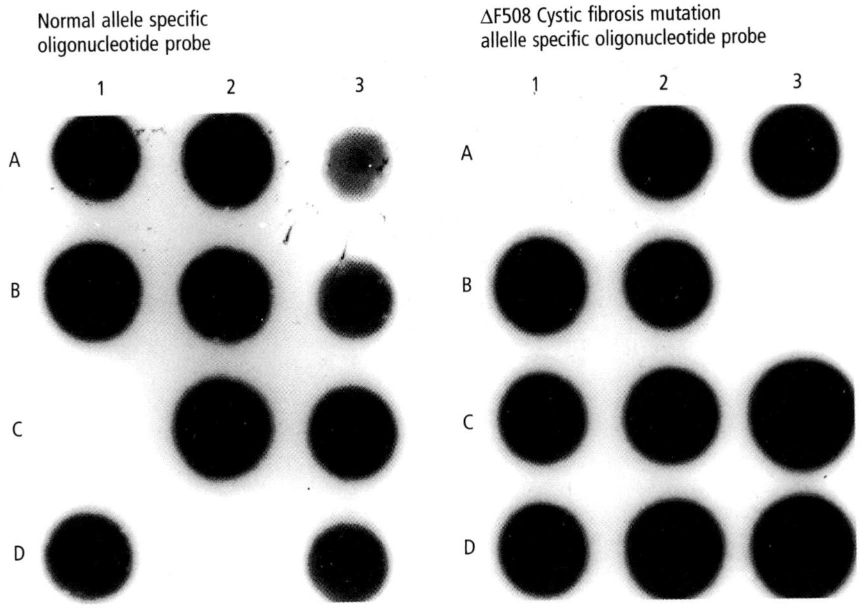

Normal allele specific
oligonucleotide probe

ΔF508 Cystic fibrosis mutation
allelle specific oligonucleotide probe

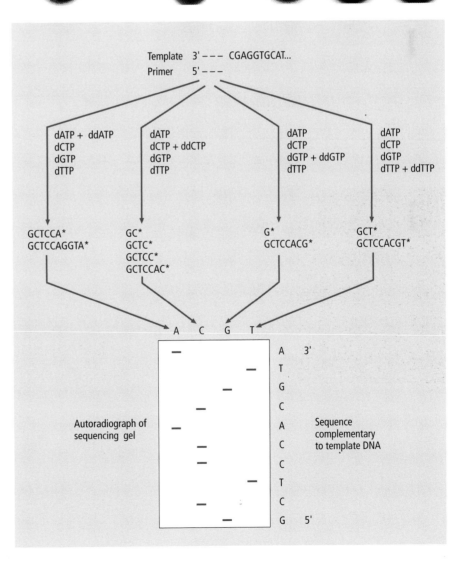

Fig. 3.12 Dot-blot analysis using radiolabelled allelle-specific oligonucleotide probes. Each DNA sample is dotted twice and hybridized with either the normal probe or the probe for the common cystic fibrosis mutation (ΔF508). Column 1 shows controls which are homozygous normal (A1), heterozygous (B1 and D1) and homozygous mutant (C1). Column 2 shows a family, A2 = mother, B2 = father, C2 = normal sib and D2 = child with cystic fibrosis. Column 3 shows miscellaneous samples. Which are carriers for the mutant gene? (Answers p. 215).

Fig. 3.13 Diagram of DNA sequencing (Sanger dideoxy method). (A* = ddATP).

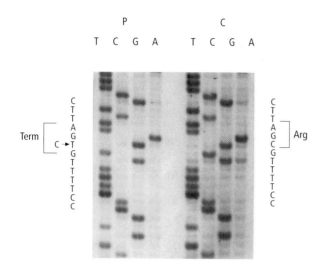

Fig. 3.14 DNA sequencing in a patient (P) with haemophilia A and a normal male control (C). The sequence is read from the bottom and the columns correspond to the bases thymine (T), cytosine (C), guanine (G) and adenine (A). A C → T point mutation results in replacement of arginine with a stop codon.

after separation from the template DNA and gel electrophoresis of the four reaction mixtures (Fig. 3.14). The sequence is read from the bottom and in Fig. 3.14 is thus CTGTGCC, etc. This process can be automated and examples are illustrated in Plate 2.

Chromosomes

CONTENTS

CHROMOSOME ANALYSIS (KARYOTYPING) 33
The normal human karyotype 34
Flow karyotyping 37
CHROMOSOME HETEROMORPHISMS 37

CHROMOSOMES IN OTHER SPECIES 42
MITOCHONDRIAL CHROMOSOMES 43
MITOSIS 43

Chromosomes are named for their ability to take up certain stains (Greek: *chromos* = coloured; *soma* = body). They are present in all nucleated cells and contain DNA with associated acidic and basic proteins in an imperfectly understood arrangement. The basic structure is the elementary fibre, 110 Å in diameter, composed of repeating units called nucleosomes each made up of eight histone molecules, around which the DNA molecule is coiled almost two times (Fig. 4.1). The elementary fibre of linked nucleosomes (which appears under the electron microscope as a string of 10 nm 'beads') is in turn coiled into a chromatin fibre of 360 Å diameter.

The metaphase chromosome has a central scaffold formed of acidic protein to which the chromatin fibre is attached at repeated sequences, so that loops of fibre (Laemli loops — each containing 30–150 kb of DNA) radiate out from the scaffold to form the body of the chromatid, some 0.6 μm in diameter. While the details are unclear, this method of compaction allows approximately 2 m of double-stranded DNA to be packaged for cell division into metaphase chromosomes which range in size from 10 μm (chromosome 1 containing 200 Mb of DNA) to 2 μm (chromosome 21 containing 40 Mb of DNA).

Individual Laemli loops appear to be fundamental functional units as each appears to contain only active euchromatin or inactive heterochromatin and the latter are associated with histone H_1 which blocks transcription. In contrast to areas of euchromatin, areas of heterochromatin contain few active genes and replicate late during S phase. Heterochromatic areas are commonly located close to the telomeres (tips) and centromeres (central chromosomal constrictions) and often contain macrosatellite DNA repeats (p. 9). Certain macrosatellite repeats are found close to the centromeres of all chromosomes whilst others are specific for one or a small number of chromosomes.

CHROMOSOME ANALYSIS (KARYOTYPING)

Chromosomes are most conveniently studied in peripheral blood lymphocytes, but almost any growing tissue including bone marrow, cultivated skin fibroblasts or cells from amniotic fluid or chorionic villi can also be used.

Five to ten millilitres of heparinized venous blood is required. The heparin prevents coagulation which would interfere with the later separation of the lymphocytes. Samples need to be delivered without delay, but a karyotype can still usually be obtained on a blood sample delivered by first-class post.

In the cytogenetics laboratory phytohaemagglutinin is added to cultures set up from each blood sample and this stimulates the T-lymphocytes to transform and divide. After 48–72 h incubation, cell division is arrested at metaphase by the addition of colchicine (which interferes with production of spindle microtubules), and a hypotonic solution is added to swell the cells and separate the individual chromosomes before fixation. The fixed cell suspension is dropped onto microscope slides and air-dried to spread the chromosomes out in one optical plane.

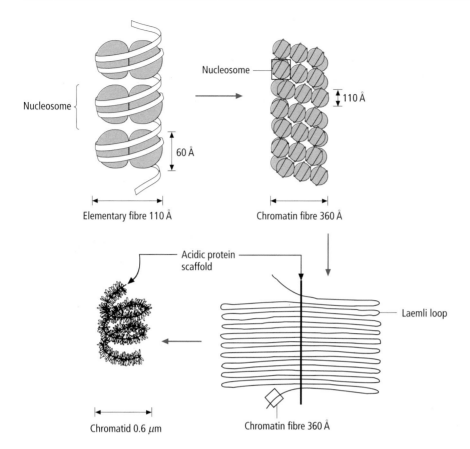

Fig. 4.1 A possible arrangement of DNA and its associated protein in the nucleosome, chromatin fibre and chromatid.

The chromosomes may be stained with numerous stains, but for routine karyotyping G-banding (Giemsa banding) is usually preferred. This produces 300–400 alternating light and dark bands which are characteristic for each chromosome pair (Figs 4.2 & 4.3), and which reflect differential chromosomal condensation. With G-banding the dark bands appear to contain relatively few active genes, to be A + T rich and to replicate late in S phase whereas light bands contain about 80% of the active genes, including all housekeeping genes (p. 14), are relatively G + C rich and replicate early in S phase. Alternatively, a similar banding pattern can be produced by staining in quinacrine and examining under ultraviolet light (Q-banding). Modern banding allows precise identification of each chromosome and missing or additional material of 4000 kb (4 Mb) or greater can be visualized on routine chromosome analysis. Improved resolution of smaller defects is possible by earlier arrest of the dividing cell (prometaphase banding, Fig. 4.3) or by flow cytometry (see Fig. 4.7).

The chromosomes can also be treated in a number of different ways to show features such as: highly repetitive macrosatellite repeat DNA in heterochromatin at the centromeres, especially of chromosomes 1, 9 and 16, and the long arm of Y (C-banding, Fig. 4.4); active nucleolus or-ganizer regions which contain the ribosomal RNA genes in the satellite stalks of the acrocentrics (silver NOR stain, Fig. 4.5); the late-replicating X chromosome (5-bromodeoxyuridine, BrdU incorporation towards the end of DNA synthesis); or the centromeric heterochromatin of 1, 9 and 16 together with distal Yq and proximal 15p (DAPI + distamycin A). Some laboratories routinely use R-banding (reverse banding), in which the bands stain in the opposite fashion from that seen with G-banding; this is achieved by heating the chromosomes in a saline buffer before staining with Giemsa and may be useful if the telomeres are involved in aberrations.

The normal human karyotype

Figure 4.3 shows a normal human female karyotype. In total there are 46 chromosomes which are arranged in order of decreasing size as 23 matching or homologous pairs. They are divided into the autosomes (numbers 1–22 inclusive) and the sex chromosomes, which are two X chromosomes in a normal female. One of each pair of the autosomes and one X is of maternal origin and the other 23 are of paternal origin. In a normal male there are again 46 chromosomes with 22 pairs of autosomes, but a different

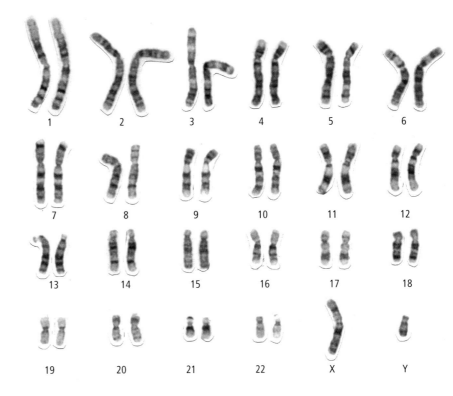

Fig. 4.2 Normal human male karyotype
(G-banding, 300 bands).

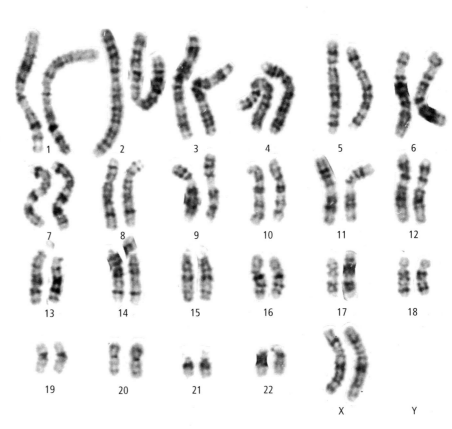

Fig. 4.3 Normal human female karyotype
(G-banding, 800–1000 bands).

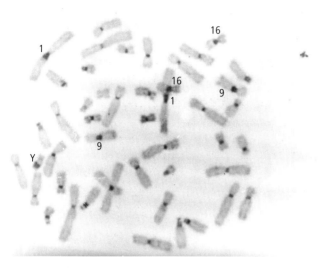

Fig. 4.4 Normal male karyotype (C-banding).

fibres by which the two chromatids are drawn to opposite poles of the spindle during cell division. The position of the centromere is constant for a given chromosome, and three subgroups are identified on the basis of the position of the centromere: metacentric—centromere in the middle; acrocentric—centromere close to one end; and submetacentric—intermediate position of centromere. Each chromosome has a long and a short arm. The short arm is labelled p (from French: *petit*) and the long arm q. The tip of each arm is the telomere.

Chromosomes 1, 3, 16, 19 and 20 are metacentric or nearly so. Chromosomes 13, 14, 15, 21, 22 and the Y are acrocentric, and the remainder are submetacentric. Metaphase chromosomes often show lack of condensation in the nucleolus organizer regions of the short arms of chromosomes 13–15 and 21 and 22 due to activation of their clustered ribosomal genes (p. 12) in the formation of the nucleoli. Thus ends of the short arms appear as 'satellites', separated from the rest of the chromosome arm by narrow stalks, also known as secondary constrictions (Fig. 4.5).

Karyotypes may be described using a shorthand system of symbols (Paris nomenclature). In general this has the order: total number of chromosomes; sex chromosome constitution; and description of abnormality.

Thus a normal female karyotype is 46,XX whereas that of a normal male is 46,XY. Table 4.1 lists the other com-

pattern of sex chromosomes, namely one X chromosome together with a smaller Y chromosome (Fig. 4.2). One of each pair of autosomes and the X are of maternal origin, whilst the father contributes the Y and the remaining autosomes.

Each chromosome has a narrow waist called the centromere, which is the site of attachment of the spindle

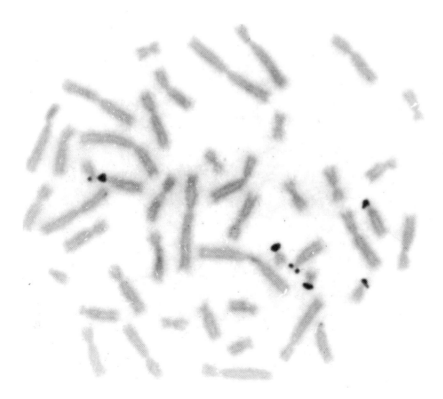

Fig. 4.5 Normal male karyotype (silver NOR stain). Note that not all acrocentrics may be stained—this reflects NOR activity.

Table 4.1 Symbols used for karyotype description.

p	Short arm
q	Long arm
pter	Tip of short arm
qter	Tip of long arm
cen	Centromere
h	Heteromorphism
del	Deletion
der	Derivative of a chromosome rearrangement
dic	Dicentric
dup	Duplication
i	Isochromosome
ins	Insertion
inv	Inversion
mat	Maternal origin
pat	Paternal origin
r	Ring chromosome
t	Translocation
::	Breakage with reunion
/	Mosaicism
+/–	Before a chromosome number indicates gain or loss of that whole chromosome
+/–	After a chromosome number indicates gain or loss of part of that chromosome
upd	Uniparental isodisomy
h	Heterodisomy
i	Isodisomy

monly used symbols. A standardized numbering system is used for the bands seen with G-banding and this is shown diagrammatically in the human idiogram (Fig. 4.6). This permits accurate description of break points in chromosome rearrangements and is useful for describing the location of genes in the chromosomal map. Each chromosome in this idiogram is divided into a number of chromosome regions using the ends, centromere and most prominent G-bands as landmarks. The centromere divides the chromosome into short (p) and long (q) arms. Most arms are divided into two or more regions by prominent bands, and each region is further subdivided according to the number of visible bands. Thus, band Xp21.2 is to be found in the short arm (p) of the X chromosome, in region 2, band 1, sub-band 2.

Flow karyotyping

It is possible to harness the technique of flow cytometry to measure the DNA content of individual chromosomes as they pass in a fluid stream through the laser beam of a fluorescence-activated cell sorter (FACS) at a speed of 2000 chromosomes s^{-1}. The suspension of chromosomes is first stained by a fluorescent dye (usually ethidium bromide), and the fluorescence generated by the laser beam in each chromosome is collected in a photomultiplier and stored in a computer. After several minutes, sufficient individual measurements have been collected to generate a histogram or flow karyotype (Fig. 4.7), which groups the chromosome measurements according to increasing DNA content. Many chromosomes form separate peaks, and the median of each peak provides an accurate and reproducible measure of the relative DNA content of a particular pair of chromosomes. The area under each peak represents the relative number of chromosomes in each group. As shown in Fig. 4.7, male and female flow karyotypes are clearly distinguished by the size of the X chromosome peak, females having twice the size of the male peak. The technique is useful for assessing variation in individual chromosomes (see Fig. 4.12) and for identifying chromosome aberrations, in particular microdeletions, as its lower limit of resolution is 1–2 Mb compared with 4 Mb for the light microscope. As the FACS can also sort chromosomes according to their DNA content, sufficient individual chromosomes or groups of chromosomes can be collected for the preparation of chromosome-specific DNA libraries.

The technique of dual laser flow cytometry allows chromosomes to be resolved not only by their DNA content but also by their AT:GC ratio. The chromosomes are stained by a mixture of two dyes (Hoechst 33258, which has an affinity for AT-rich DNA, and chromomycin A3, which has an affinity for GC-rich DNA) and pass sequentially through the laser beams, which allows the fluorescence generated by each dye to be analysed separately. Figure 4.8 shows bivariate flow karyotypes which not only resolve each chromosome more efficiently than the univariate karyotype but also demonstrate separation of individual homologues.

CHROMOSOME HETEROMORPHISMS

Detailed DNA measurements by flow cytometry or microdensitometry reveal that all chromosomes show interindividual variation in DNA content, which is heritable. The Y chromosome shows most variation, whilst the X chromosome is least variable. The most obvious differences in the appearance of the chromosomes can be seen under the oil immersion lens in at least 30% of the population. Such differences are called heteromorphisms and are examples of genetic polymorphisms (discontinuous genetic variants present in 2% or more of the population). The size polymorphisms usually involve repetitive DNA, and the degree of variation shows a normal distribution. Four main groups of chromosome heteromorphisms are

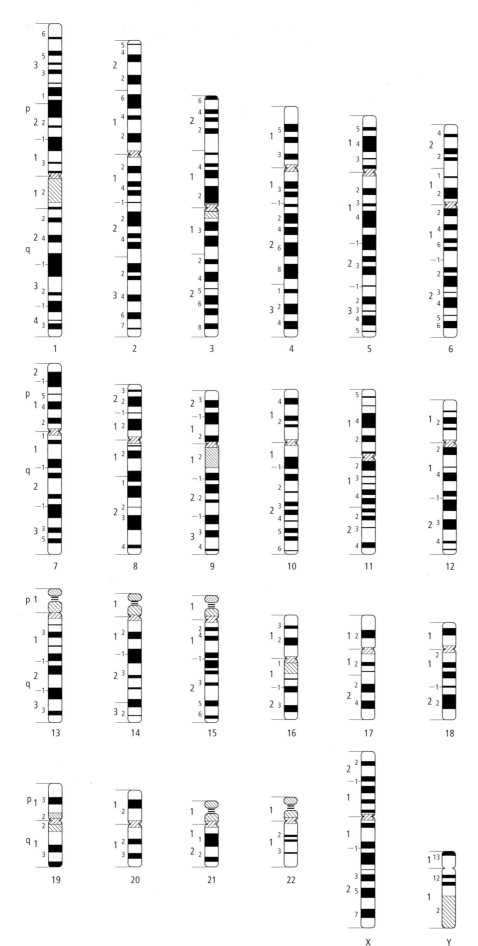

Fig. 4.6 Human idiogram (only the more prominent bands are numbered).

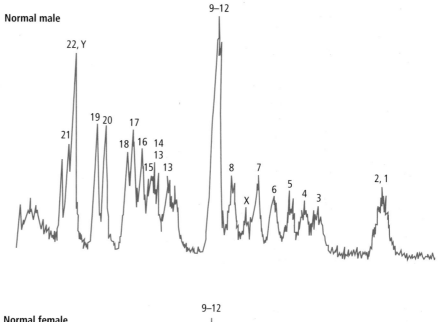

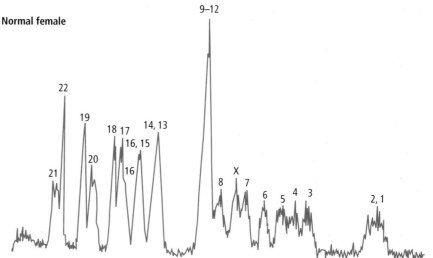

Fig. 4.7 Flow karyotypes of a normal male and a normal female. The peaks correspond to individual chromosome pairs or groups of chromosomes as indicated.

known: size of Yq; size of centromeric heterochromatin; satellite polymorphisms; and fragile sites.

Size of Yq

The commonest chromosomal polymorphism relates to the length of the long arm of the Y chromosome. About 10% of clinically normal males have a Y which is obviously longer or shorter than usual (Fig. 4.9). The long arm of the Y contains non-transcribed repetitive DNA and fluoresces intensely under ultraviolet light with dyes such as quinacrine (Q-banding). This fluorescence may be visible in an interphase nucleus and is referred to as the Y-chromatin (Fig. 4.10).

Size of centromeric heterochromatin

Variations in the size of the centromeric heterochromatin are relatively frequent for chromosomes 1, 9 and 16. Figure 4.11 shows a large chromosome 16 due to excess centromeric heterochromatin which was present in several healthy family members. Figure 4.12 shows the flow karyotype of an individual with this heteromorphism.

Satellite polymorphisms

Variation in size of the satellites and in the degree of intensity with which they stain by Q-banding may be seen for the acrocentric chromosomes 13, 14, 15, 21 and 22.

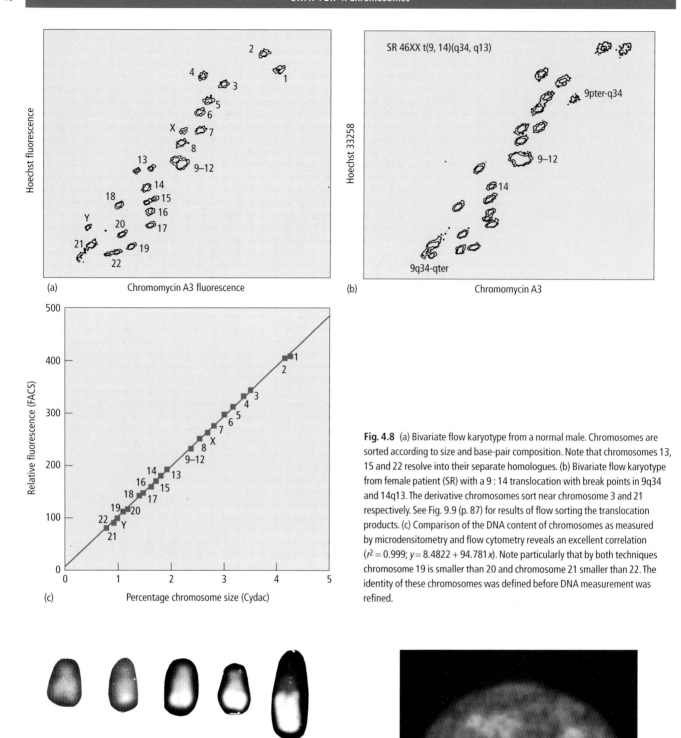

(a)   Chromomycin A3 fluorescence

(b)   Chromomycin A3

SR 46XX t(9, 14)(q34, q13)

9pter-q34

9–12

14

9q34-qter

(c)   Percentage chromosome size (Cydac)

Fig. 4.8 (a) Bivariate flow karyotype from a normal male. Chromosomes are sorted according to size and base-pair composition. Note that chromosomes 13, 15 and 22 resolve into their separate homologues. (b) Bivariate flow karyotype from female patient (SR) with a 9 : 14 translocation with break points in 9q34 and 14q13. The derivative chromosomes sort near chromosome 3 and 21 respectively. See Fig. 9.9 (p. 87) for results of flow sorting the translocation products. (c) Comparison of the DNA content of chromosomes as measured by microdensitometry and flow cytometry reveals an excellent correlation ($r^2 = 0.999$; $y = 8.4822 + 94.781x$). Note particularly that by both techniques chromosome 19 is smaller than 20 and chromosome 21 smaller than 22. The identity of these chromosomes was defined before DNA measurement was refined.

Fig. 4.9 Yq polymorphisms.

Fig. 4.10 Fluorescent Y-chromatin.

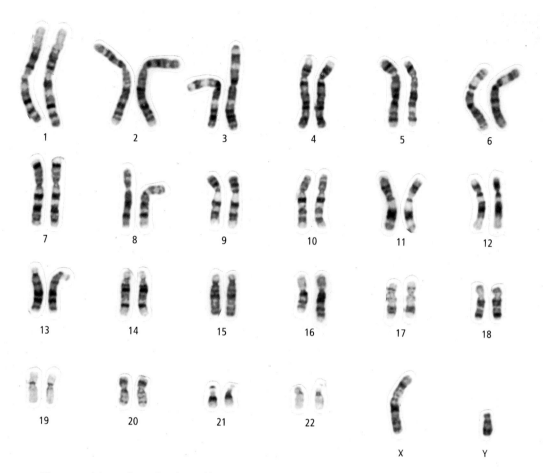

Fig. 4.11 Chromosome 16 centromeric heterochromatin polymorphism (16qh+).

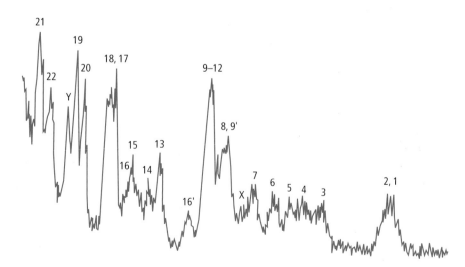

Fig. 4.12 Flow karyotype of 16qh+.

Much of the variation is due to repetitive DNA, but variation in the number of ribosomal genes also occurs. Size variation, due to differences in DNA content, may occur as a result of mispairing during meiosis at sites of repetitive DNA. This is often termed unequal crossing-over (see Fig. 2.12), and an example of tandem duplication involving a nucleolus organizer region on chromosome 15 is shown in Fig. 4.13.

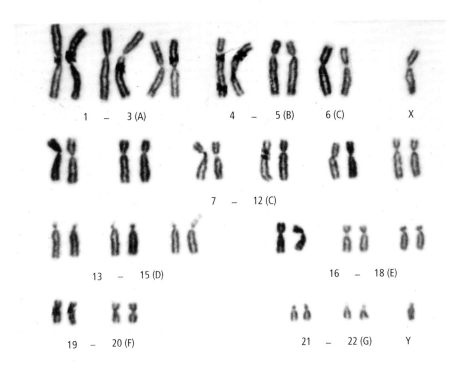

1 – 3 (A)   4 – 5 (B)   6 (C)   X

7 – 12 (C)

13 – 15 (D)   16 – 18 (E)

19 – 20 (F)   21 – 22 (G)   Y

Fig. 4.13 Tandem duplication involving a nucleolus organizer region on chromosome 15 (aceto-orcein).

Fragile sites

Constrictions at sites other than the centromere may be seen and these secondary constrictions may be particularly liable to chromatid breaks. There are at least 80 common fragile sites which can be induced at low levels in everybody by aphidicolin and which usually involve both homologues. In addition, 26 rare fragile sites have been described which collectively occur in about 5% of the population. Most of these are induced by antifolate agents in culture and almost all are autosomal (e.g. at 2q13, Fig. 4.14). These rare autosomal fragile sites usually involve only one homologue, show Mendelian inheritance. Most are not associated with any clinical abnormality (except for the X chromosomal fragile site at Xq27.3 which is associated with mental handicap; see p. 136). The molecular basis of these fragile sites appears to involve tracts of trinucleotide repeats which have been amplified beyond a critical threshold.

CHROMOSOMES IN OTHER SPECIES

The chromosomes appear essentially similar in all races of man, and the X chromosome is remarkably constant in size and banding pattern amongst primates. Other chromosomes are more variable and the variation in chromosome number and appearance is in proportion to the timing of evolutionary separation of the species (Table 4.2). The gorilla, chimpanzee and orang-utan have 48

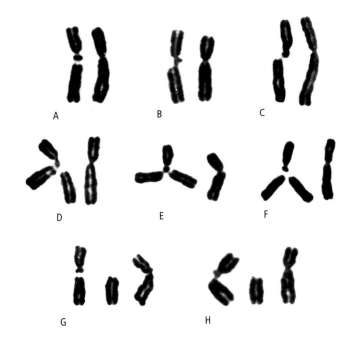

A   B   C

D   E   F

G   H

Fig. 4.14 Fragile site on chromosome 2 (at 2q13). A, Site shown as a gap. B, C, Site shown as chromatid break at gap. D–F, Triradial produced by chromatid breaks in previous division followed by non-disjunction of distal fragment. G, H, Acentric fragments generated by chromatid breaks.

Table 4.2 Chromosomes in different species.

Species	Chromosome number	Estimated number of structural genes
Man	46	60 000–70 000
Gorilla	48	–
Mouse	40	30 000
Dog	78	–
Goldfish	94	–
Drosophila	8	5000
Escherichia coli	1	3600

chromosomes, and the autosomes are similar to those in humans, with the exception of human chromosome 2, which appears to have been derived from two ape acrocentrics after separation of the species (Fig. 4.15). Interestingly, the fragile site on human chromosome 2 seems to mark the site of this ancient fusion (see Fig. 4.14).

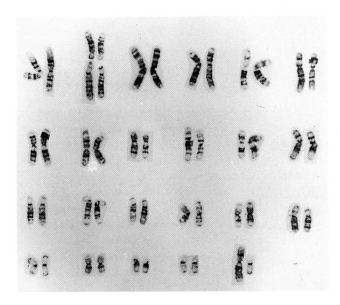

Fig. 4.15 Normal gorilla karyotype.

MITOCHONDRIAL CHROMOSOMES

Human mitochondria are cytoplasmic organelles which have their own chromosomes in the form of about 10 single circular double helices of DNA. These are self-replicating and contain, in their 16 569 bp, genes for 22 mitochondrial transfer RNAs and the two types of ribosomal RNA required for mitochrondrial protein synthesis in addition to 13 peptides which are subunits of the various steps involved in cellular oxidative phosphorylation.

Human mitochondrial DNA is different from nuclear DNA with respect to the codon recognition pattern for several amino acids (e.g. UGA codes for tryptophan rather than chain termination). Further it has no introns and both strands are transcribed and translated. Each cell has hundreds of mitochondria and as they are found in the cytoplasm they are transmitted in the egg from a mother to all of her children (i.e. maternal inheritance).

MITOSIS

Mitosis is the type of division in somatic cells whereby one cell produces two identical daughter cells. Mitotic cell division occurs in all embryonic tissues and continues at a lower rate in most adult tissues other than end cells, e.g. neurones. Thus mitosis is vital for both tissue formation and maintenance. In cultured mammalian cells the cycle varies but is usually about 24 h. Mitosis itself occupies only 20 min to 1 h of the total, whereas DNA synthesis for replication takes 6–8 h (Fig. 4.16).

Five arbitrary stages are apparent in mitosis (Fig. 4.17): interphase; prophase; metaphase; anaphase; and telophase. A cell which is not actively dividing is in interphase. This phase thus includes gap 1, S (DNA synthesis) and gap 2 periods of the cell cycle and during this phase the nuclear material appears relatively homogeneous. Replication of DNA occurs during the S phase, so that the nucleus in G2 has twice the diploid amount of DNA present in G1. Each chromosome has its own pattern of DNA synthesis, and some segments (e.g. housekeeping genes and expressed tissue-specific genes) replicate early and some late (e.g. centromeric heterochromatin and non-expressed tissue-specific genes). The inactive X is always the last chromosome to complete replication. As the cell prepares to divide the chromosomes condense and become visible. At this stage it can be seen that each

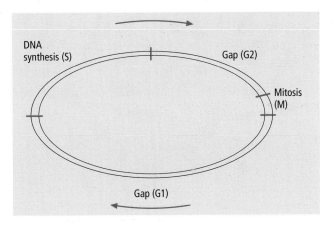

Fig. 4.16 Diagram of the cell cycle.

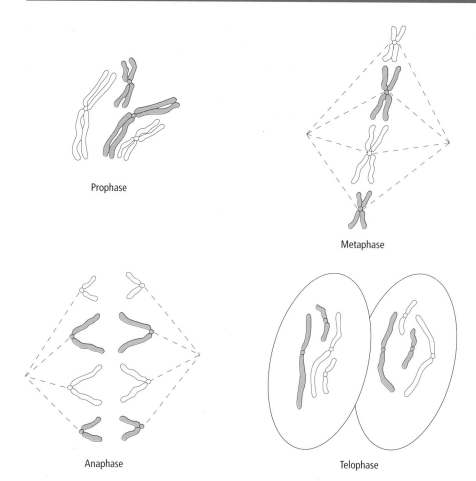

Prophase

Metaphase

Anaphase

Telophase

Fig. 4.17 Mitosis. Only two chromosome pairs are shown; the chromosomes from one parent are in outline, those from the other are coloured.

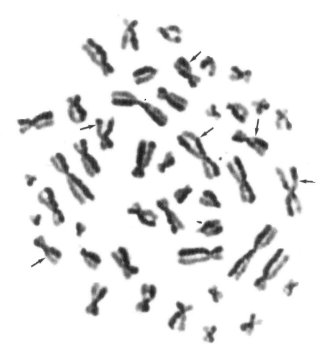

Fig. 4.18 Sister chromatid exchanges (some arrowed).

chromosome consists of a pair of long thin parallel strands, or sister chromatids, which are held together at the centromere. Cross-overs, with exchange of material between sister chromatids, may occur at this stage. BrdU may be used to demonstrate these sister chromatid exchanges or SCEs (Fig. 4.18). The nuclear membrane disappears and the nucleolus becomes undetectable as its component particles disperse. The centriole divides and its two products migrate towards opposite poles of the cell.

Metaphase begins when the chromosomes have reached their maximal contraction. They move to the equatorial plate of the cell and the spindle forms. The acrocentrics are often clustered at this stage (satellite association). Anaphase begins when the centromeres divide and the paired chromatids separate, each to become a daughter chromosome. The spindle fibres contract and draw the daughter chromosomes, centromere first, to the poles of the cell. Telophase starts when the daughter chromosomes reach each pole of the cell. The cytoplasm divides, the cell plate forms, and the chromosomes start to unwind. The nuclear membrane re-forms at this stage.

Thus mitosis results in two daughter cells, each with an

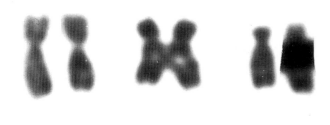

16   17   18

Fig. 4.19 Chiasma formation in a somatic cell.

identical genetic constitution. Rarely, somatic recombination may occur during mitosis with transfer of segments between homologous chromosomes, resulting in homozygosity at gene loci for which the rest of the body cells are heterozygous (Fig. 4.19). This can be an important step in the genesis of some cancers (see Fig. 17.2).

C H A P T E R   5

Gametogenesis

C O N T E N T S

MEIOSIS 46
First meiotic division (reduction division) 46
Second meiotic division 47
SPERMATOGENESIS 48
OOGENESIS 48

FERTILIZATION 50
LYONIZATION 50
SEX DETERMINATION AND DIFFERENTIATION 53
GENOMIC IMPRINTING (PARENTAL IMPRINTING) . . . 54

Gametogenesis (the production of gametes) occurs in the gonads. The somatic diploid chromosomal complement is halved to the haploid number of a mature gamete in such a way as to ensure that each gamete contains one member of each pair of chromosomes. This reduction is achieved by meiotic cell division. Fusion of the sperm and egg restores the diploid number in the fertilized egg. Meiotic cell division is found only in the gonads and is thus less readily studied than mitosis and as the testis is more accessible than the ovary for biopsy most human information relates to male meiosis. Furthermore, much of the prophase of female meiosis is completed during embryonic development and can thus only be studied in the fetus.

MEIOSIS

Meiosis consists of two successive divisions, the first and the second meiotic divisions (Fig. 5.1), in which the DNA replicates only once—before the first division.

First meiotic division (reduction division)

Prophase of the first meiotic division is complex, and five stages can be recognized: leptotene (threadlike); zygotene (pairing); pachytene (thickening); diplotene (appearing double); and diakinesis (moving apart).

Leptotene starts with the first appearance of the chromosomes (Fig. 5.2). At this stage each chromosome consists of a pair of sister chromatids (replication having occurred during the S phase of premeiotic interphase). Homologous chromosomes pair (starting at the telomeres and proceeding towards the centromere) during zygotene to form bivalents which are bound closely together by the synaptonemal complex (Fig. 5.3). The mechanism by which homologous chromosomes pair is unclear but dispersed blocks of repetitive DNA are suspected to be involved in the initial alignment. The X and Y chromosomes undergo synapsis only at the distal end of both short arms (the pairing or pseudoautosomal segments), and form a sex bivalent, which is out of phase with the others and is condensed early in pachytene as the sex vesicle. This early condensation may be important in preventing crossing-over between the non-pairing regions of the X and Y chromosomes. Pachytene is the main stage of chromosomal thickening, and the pattern of chromosome condensation appears to correspond to the banding pattern seen at mitosis (Fig. 5.4). Each chromosome is now seen to consist of two chromatids; hence each bivalent is a tetrad of four strands (Fig. 5.5). Satellite association of the acrocentrics also occurs at pachytene, perhaps due to the synapsis of homologous repetitive sequences on non-homologous chromosomes, or to their involvement in nucleolus organization. Diplotene, which follows, is very short and difficult to study in humans. During diplotene the bivalents start to separate. Although the two chromo-

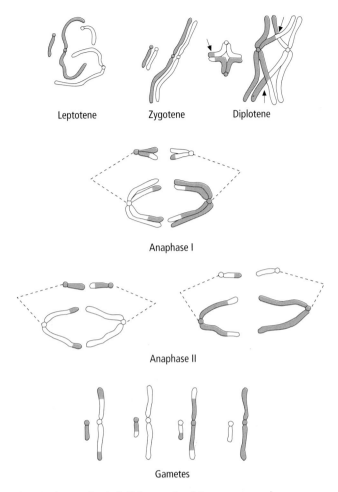

Leptotene   Zygotene   Diplotene

Anaphase I

Anaphase II

Gametes

Fig. 5.1 Diagram of meiosis. Only two pairs of chromosomes are shown; chromosomes from one parent are in outline, those from the other are coloured (cross-overs are arrowed).

somes of each bivalent separate, the centromere of each remains intact, so the two chromatids of each chromosome remain together. During longitudinal separation the two members of each bivalent are seen to be in contact at several places, called chiasmata (Fig. 5.6). These mark the location of cross-overs, where the chromatids of homologous chromosomes have exchanged material in late pachytene (Fig. 5.7). On average, there are about 52 chiasmata per human male cell with at least one chiasma per chromosome arm (with the exception of the short arms of the acrocentrics and chromosome 18). Short chromosomes with a single chiasma appear as a rod or cross, longer chromosomes with two chiasmata appear as a ring and those with three have a figure-of-eight appearance. At diplotene the sex bivalent opens out and the X and Y can be seen attached to one another by tiny pairing segments at the ends of their short arms indicating homology of these regions. This pairing region at the tip of the

short arms is called the pseudoautosomal segment as, in contrast to the remainder of the X and Y in the male, crossing-over is usual in this area during male meiosis, and sequences mapping to this region appear to show autosomal rather than sex-linked inheritance. The X–Y pairing region is particularly well demonstrated in electron microscopy (EM) preparations of the synaptonemal complex stained by silver nitrate (Fig. 5.8). Diakinesis is the final stage of prophase, during which the chromosomes coil more tightly and so stain more deeply.

Metaphase begins when the nuclear membrane disappears and the chromosomes move to the equatorial plane. At anaphase the two members of each bivalent disjoin, one going to each pole. These bivalents are assorted independently to each pole. The cytoplasm divides, and each cell now has 23 chromosomes, each of which is a pair of chromatids, differing from one another only as a result of crossing-over.

Second meiotic division

The second meiotic division follows the first without an interphase. It resembles mitosis, in that the centromeres now divide and sister chromatids pass to opposite poles. However, the second meiotic division chromosomes are rather more coiled than mitotic ones and show splaying of the chromatids. The X and Y chromosomes in the male are exceptions, and this may be related to the fact that, except for the tips of their short arms, they were not involved in recombination (Fig. 5.9). Thus meiosis differs from mitosis in several respects as outlined in Table 5.1.

Since the chromosomes assort independently during meiosis, this results in 2^{23} or 8 388 608 different possible combinations of chromosomes in the gametes from each parent. Hence there are 2^{46} possible combinations in the zygote. There is still further scope for variation provided by crossing-over during meiosis. If there is, on average, only one cross-over per chromosome and a 10% paternal/maternal allele difference, then the number of possible zygotes exceeds 6×10^{43}. This number is greater than the number of human beings

Table 5.1 Comparison of mitosis and meiosis.

	Mitosis	Meiosis
Site	All tissues	Gonads
Timing	All of life	Post-puberty in male, suspended until puberty in female
Result	Diploid daughter cells	Haploid gametes

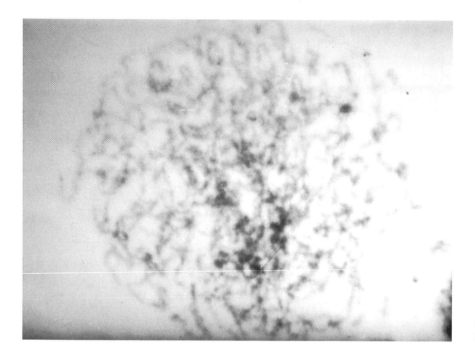

Fig. 5.2 Human primary spermatocyte in leptotene.

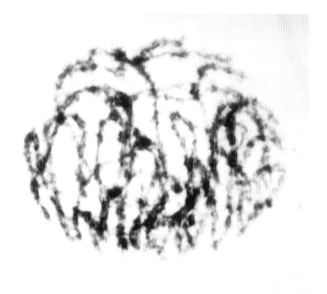

Fig. 5.3 Zygotene.

who have so far existed and so emphasizes our genetic uniqueness.

Meiosis thus has three important consequences:

1 gametes contain only one representative of each homologous pair of chromosomes;

2 there is random assortment of paternal and maternal homologues;

3 crossing-over ensures uniqueness by further increasing genetic variation.

SPERMATOGENESIS

Spermatogenesis occurs in the seminiferous tubules of the male from the time of sexual maturity onward (Fig. 5.10). At the periphery of the tubule are spermatogonia, of which some are self-renewing stem cells and others are already committed to sperm formation. The primary spermatocyte is derived from a committed spermatogonium. The primary spermatocyte undergoes the first meiotic division to produce two secondary spermatocytes, each with 23 chromosomes. These cells rapidly undergo the second meiotic division, each forming two spermatids which mature without further division into sperm. This process of production of a mature sperm from a committed spermatogonium takes about 61 days.

Normally semen contains $50–100 \times 10^6$ sperms per ml. Sperm production continues, albeit at a reduced rate, into old age, and the total lifetime production of a male exceeds 10^{12}. The numerous replications increase the chance for mutation, and the risk for several single gene mutations has already been shown to be increased in the offspring of older men.

OOGENESIS

In contrast to spermatogenesis the process of oogenesis is largely complete at birth. Oogonia are derived from the primordial germ cells, and each oogonium is the central cell in a developing follicle. By about the third month of fetal life, the oogonia have become primary oocytes and

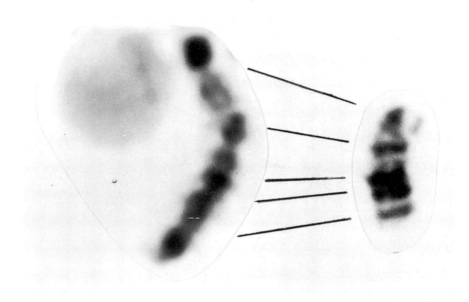

Fig. 5.4 Homology of banding pattern from meiotic (left) and mitotic chromosomes (chromosome 13 shown). Note nucleolus arising from short arm (top) of bivalent.

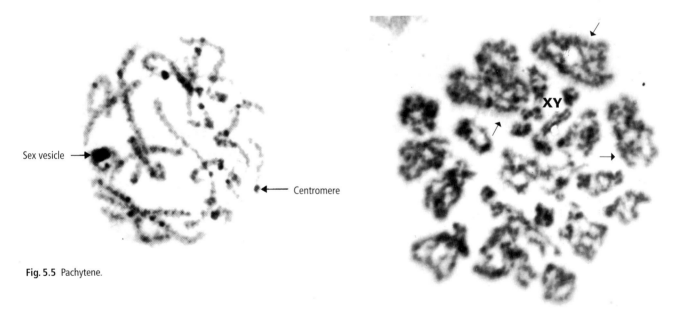

Fig. 5.5 Pachytene.

Fig. 5.6 Early diakinesis. Note multiple chiasmata (some arrowed).

some of these have already entered the prophase of first meiosis. The primary oocytes remain in suspended prophase (dictyotene) until sexual maturity. Then as each individual follicle matures and releases its oocyte into the Fallopian tube, the first meiotic division is completed. Hence completion of the first meiotic division in the female may take over 40 years.

The first meiotic division results in an unequal division of the cytoplasm, with the secondary oocyte receiving the great majority in contrast to the first polar body (Fig. 5.11).

The second meiotic division is not completed until after fertilization in the Fallopian tube and results in the mature ovum and a second polar body. The first polar body may also divide at this stage. Thus, whereas spermatogenesis produces four viable sperm per meiotic division, oogenesis produces only one ovum.

The maximum number of germ cells in the female fetus is 6.8×10^6 at 5 months. By birth the number is 2×10^6, and by puberty is less than 200 000. Of this number only about 400 will ovulate.

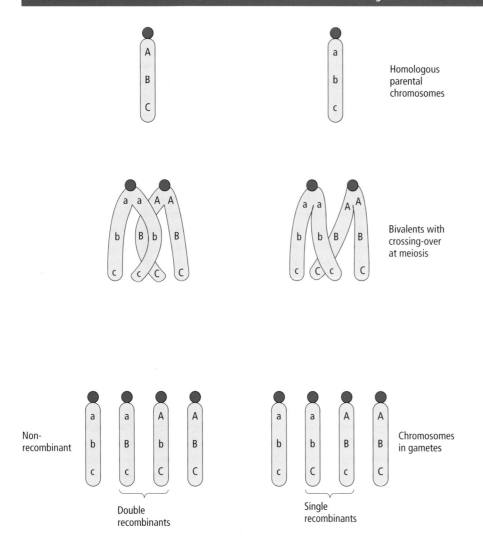

Fig. 5.7 Diagram of crossing-over.

The long resting phase during the first meiotic division may be a factor in the increased risk of failure of homologous chromosomes to separate during meiosis (nondisjunction) in the older mother.

FERTILIZATION

Fertilization usually occurs in the Fallopian tube. As the sperm penetrates the ovum a chemical change occurs which normally prevents the entry of other sperm. After entry the sperm rounds up as a male pronucleus. The ovum now completes the second meiotic division and produces the female pronucleus. These fuse to form the zygote and embryogenesis commences.

By a series of mitotic divisions the zygote produces the estimated 2×10^{12} cells found in the neonate and subsequently the 5×10^{12} cells found in the adult. Table 5.2 summarizes the major milestones in embryonic and fetal life of medical genetic importance.

LYONIZATION

Lyonization is the process of inactivation of one member of the pair of X chromosomes in every female cell. It applies to all mammals, and in humans, as evidenced by the appearance of the Barr body, occurs in trophoblast on the 12th day after fertilization and on the 16th day in the embryo proper which then consists of about 5000 cells (at this stage there are estimated to be 3–5 haemopoietic stem cells). Inactivation only occurs in somatic cells, since in the germ line both X chromosomes need to remain active. For each somatic cell it is random whether the paternal X or the maternal X is inactivated, but the choice is fixed for all subsequent descendants of that cell (Fig. 5.12). As only one X is active in the female the product levels for most genes on the X chromosome are similar in females and males where the single X always remains active, except in primary spermatocytes where it becomes part of the condensed sex vesicle.

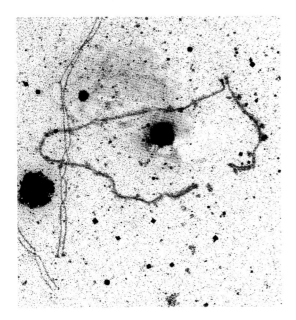

Fig. 5.8 EM photomicrograph of the sex bivalent at pachytene showing the X chromosome (left) and the Y chromosome (right) attached by their pairing segments (top).

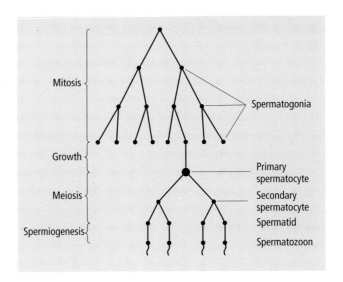

Fig. 5.10 Spermatogenesis.

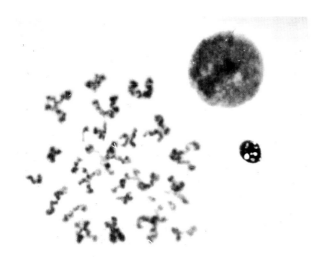

Fig. 5.9 Second meiotic metaphase showing single condensed X.

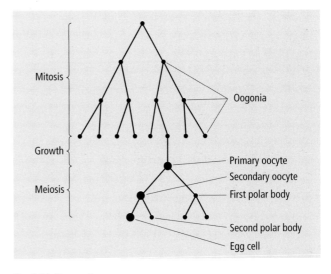

Fig. 5.11 Oogenesis.

X inactivation affects most genes carried on the human X chromosome but there are interesting exceptions. These are genes which have homologues on the Y chromosome including steroid sulphatase, amelogenin and ZFX (a zinc finger protein, possibly involved in germ cell development). Other loci involved in stature and the prevention of malformations found in Turner's syndrome (p. 121), which have yet to be characterized, are also presumed to belong to the class of active X–Y homologous loci, as are genes carried on the X–Y pairing segment. In contrast the locus XIST, which maps to Xq, is only active on the inactive X and this locus is believed to have an important role in regulating the inactivation process itself.

The inactive X completes its replication later in mitosis than any of the other chromosomes, and is thus out of phase with the active X. In females with loss of material from one X chromosome the structurally abnormal X is preferentially inactivated. In contrast, females with an

Table 5.2 Embryonic and fetal milestones.

Stage	Gestation from LMP	Crown–rump length	Comment
Embryo	Conception (2 weeks)		
	4 weeks	1 mm	Lyonization, first missed period, implantation complete, chorionic villi develop, primitive streak appears
	5 weeks	2 mm	Neural tube starts to fuse, organ primordia form
	6 weeks	4 mm	Neural tube closed, limb buds appear, heart starts to contract, pregnancy test positive, membranes apparent on ultrasound
	8 weeks	3 cm	Major organogenesis completed, fetal movements seen on ultrasound
Fetus	12 weeks	8 cm	External genitalia recognizable, chorionic villus sampling possible
	16 weeks	14 cm	Usual time for amniocentesis
	18 weeks	16 cm	Usual time for fetal blood sampling and detailed ultrasound scanning
	40 weeks	36 cm	Term pregnancy

LMP, last menstrual period.

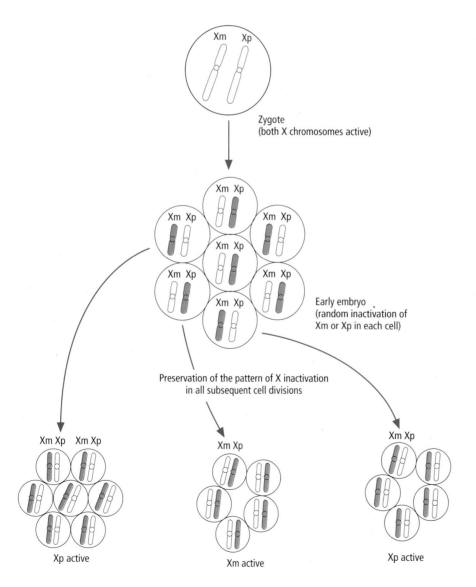

Fig. 5.12 Diagram of X inactivation (Lyonization). Xm = maternal X chromosome, Xp = paternal X chromosome, inactive X chromosomes are shaded.

X–autosome translocation preferentially inactivate the normal X, otherwise the inactivation could spread from the inactivation centre in Xq 13 into the autosomal genes, leading to autosomal monosomy.

The inactive X remains condensed during most of interphase and is visible in a variable proportion of the nuclei in most tissues as a densely stained mass of chromatin known as the Barr body or X chromatin (Fig. 5.13). Only about 30% of cells from a buccal smear of a normal female show X chromatin, as this depends upon the stage each cell is at in the cell cycle. If a cell has more than two X chromosomes then the extra ones are also inactivated and more than one Barr body will be seen in some cells. Thus the maximum number of Barr bodies per cell will be one less than the total number of X chromosomes in the karyotype. The sex chromatin may also be seen in 1–10% of female neutrophils as a small drumstick (Fig. 5.14).

The CpG islands (p. 14) of housekeeping genes on the inactive X are hypermethylated while the reverse is true of the active X. At other methylation sites limited evidence indicates that the active X is hypermethylated whereas the inactive X is hypomethylated. The mechanism of this differential methylation and its role in the maintenance of activity or inactivity is not understood.

Thus a female has a mixture of cells, some of which have

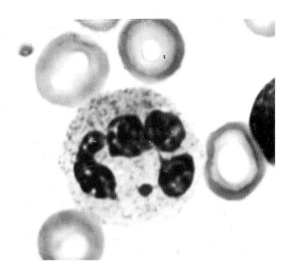

Fig. 5.14 Neutrophil drumstick.

an active paternal X chromosome and some of which have an active maternal X chromosome. The relative proportions vary from female to female (even in identical twins) due to the randomness of the inactivation process. This accounts for the patchy expression of mutant X-linked genes in carrier females.

SEX DETERMINATION AND DIFFERENTIATION

Studies of structural aberrations of the human Y chromosome reveal that maleness is determined by testis-determining factors (TDFs) located on the short arm of the Y chromosome. If this region is absent the undifferentiated gonad becomes an ovary and sex differentiation occurs along female lines. If the TDF region is present a testis forms, which produces two hormones which act locally. The Sertoli cells of the seminiferous tubules secrete a Mullerian duct inhibitor, which causes regression of the primitive uterus and Fallopian tubes, and the interstitial cells of the testis secrete testosterone, which both stimulates the Wolffian ducts to differentiate into epididymis, vas deferens and seminal vesicles, and also masculinizes the external genitalia. The gene SRY (sex-determining region of the Y) has been proposed as a possible candidate for TDF. The gene maps within the sex-determining region, is expressed in the undifferentiated gonad at an appropriate time in development and, in the mouse, causes sex reversal when introduced into female pre-embryos.

The normal pairing of the X and Y chromosomes in first meiosis and their regular segregation into different sec-

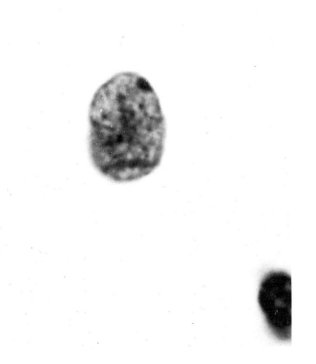

Fig. 5.13 Barr body.

ondary spermatocytes achieves approximately equal numbers of male and female conceptions. The location of the TDF region outside the pairing segment on the short arm of the Y normally ensures that recombination does not transfer the TDF to the X chromosome and thus separate it from other determinants carried on the long arm of the Y which are necessary for spermatogenesis.

Rare exceptions to the rule that sex determination depends on the presence or absence of the Y chromosome occur in *XY females*, some of which may have deletions or mutations affecting TDF, and *XX males*, in whom the TDF has been transferred from the Y to the X by accidental recombination (see p. 121).

GENOMIC IMPRINTING (PARENTAL IMPRINTING)

At most autosomal loci, both alleles are either active or inactive but in a small number only one allele is active and the allele chosen for inactivation depends upon the parental origin. Thus, for example, only the paternally inherited allele of the insulin growth factor 2 (*IGF2*) gene on 11p is active. This imprint is established during gametogenesis and seems to involve methylation differences at specific sites adjacent to the gene. The reason for such imprinting is unknown but one consequence is the difference in the clinical appearance for particular chromosomal disorders depending upon the parent of origin. Thus, for example, a deletion of the proximal long arm of chromosome 15 on a maternal chromosome results in mental handicap and clinical features of Angelman syndrome (p. 126) whereas a similar deletion on a paternal chromosome results in a clinically distinct condition called Prader–Willi syndrome (p. 126). The most extreme imbalance of maternal and paternal contributions occurs in hydatidiform moles which have a double paternal contribution and no maternal contribution. The chromosomes look normal but no fetus develops and the placenta is grossly abnormal.

C H A P T E R 6

Chromosome Aberrations

C O N T E N T S	

NUMERICAL ABERRATIONS 55
Aneuploidy 55
Polyploidy 56
STRUCTURAL ABERRATIONS 57
**IDENTIFICATION OF THE CHROMOSOMAL ORIGIN
    OF COMPLEX STRUCTURAL REARRANGEMENTS** . . . 65

OTHER ABERRATIONS 67
Mosaic 67
Chimaera 67
Uniparental disomy and isodisomy 68

Mutations sometimes involve very large parts of the chromosome, and when these are large enough to be visible under the light microscope they are termed chromosome aberrations. With routine light microscopy the smallest visible addition or deletion from a chromosome is about 4 Mb. Using the distance from London to New York as the length of the haploid DNA, this would be equivalent to a distance of about 8 km, and on this scale the average gene would be about 30 m in length. Thus, any visible abnormality usually involves many contiguous genes.

Abnormalities of the chromosomes are usually classified into numerical abnormalities, where the somatic cells contain an abnormal number of normal chromosomes, and structural aberrations, where the somatic cells contain one or more abnormal chromosomes. They may involve either the sex chromosomes or the autosomes and may occur either as a result of a germ cell mutation in the parent or more remote ancestor, or as a result of somatic mutation, in which case only a proportion of cells will be affected.

NUMERICAL ABERRATIONS

Normally somatic cells contain 46 chromosomes and are termed diploid (as the number is twice the haploid number of 23 as found in gametes). A chromosome number which is an exact multiple of the haploid number and exceeds the diploid number is called polyploidy, and one which is not an exact multiple is called aneuploidy (Table 6.1).

Aneuploidy

Aneuploidy usually arises from the failure of paired chromosomes or sister chromatids to disjoin at anaphase (non-disjunction). Alternatively, aneuploidy may be due to delayed movement of a chromosome at anaphase (anaphase lag). Thus by either of these mechanisms two cells are produced, one with an extra copy of a chromosome (trisomy) and one with a missing copy of that chromosome (monosomy). The cause of meiotic non-disjunction is not known, but it occurs at increased frequency with increasing maternal age, with maternal hypothyroidism, and possibly after irradiation or viral infection or as a familial tendency. The cause of mitotic non-disjunction is also unknown and no predisposing factors have been identified.

Aneuploidy can arise during either meiosis or mitosis, and meiotic non-disjunction may occur at either the first or the second meiotic divisions (Fig. 6.1). If the non-disjunction is at the first division then the gamete with the extra chromosome will contain both parental homologues of that chromosome, whereas if at the second division then both the normal and the extra copy of that

Table 6.1 Examples of numerical chromosomal aberrations.

Karyotype	Comment
92,XXYY	Tetraploidy
69,XXY	Triploidy
47,XX,+21	Trisomy 21
47,XY,+18	Trisomy 18
47,XX,+13	Trisomy 13
47,XX,+16	Trisomy 16
47,XXY	Klinefelter syndrome
47,XXX	Trisomy X
45,X	Turner syndrome
49,XXXXY	Variant of Klinefelter syndrome

chromosome will be either maternal or paternal in origin. Sometimes the origin of the non-disjunctional event can be determined from the knowledge that two alleles at one locus are contributed by one parent, or from the inheritance of chromosomal or DNA polymorphisms (Fig. 6.2).

Aneuploidy at a mitotic cell division may result in a mosaic, i.e. an individual with cell lines of two or more different chromosomal complements derived from a single zygote.

Polyploidy

A complete extra set of chromosomes will raise the total number to 69, and this is called triploidy (Fig. 6.3). This usually arises from fertilization by two sperms (dispermy), or from failure of one of the maturation divisions of either the egg or the sperm, so that a diploid gamete is produced. Thus the chromosomal formula for a triploid fetus (which will usually miscarry) would be 69,XXY (most common), 69,XXX or 69,XYY, depending upon the origin of the extra chromosomal set.

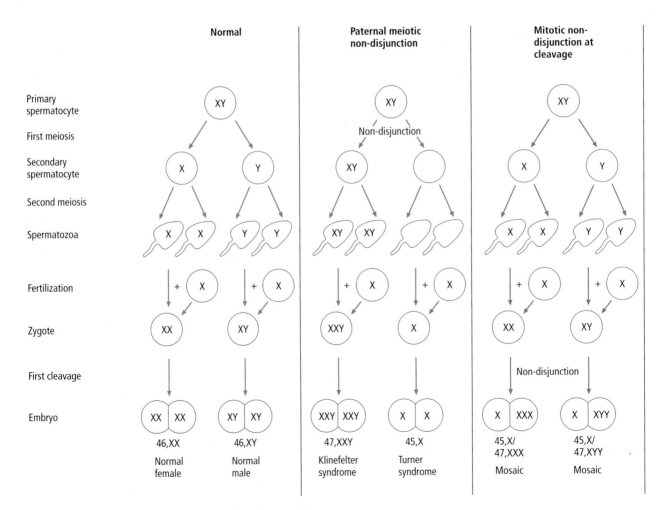

Fig. 6.1 Mitotic non-disjunction of sex chromosomes at first meiosis and early cleavage.

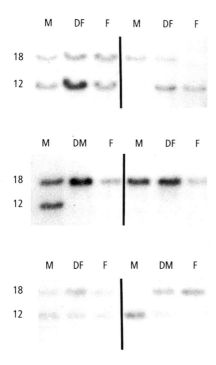

Fig. 6.2 Six families with, in each group of three, the parents (M = male, F = female) to either side of the child who has trisomy 21 showing the results of DNA analysis using a chromosome 21-specific DNA polymorphism which has allelic fragments of 18 and 12 kb. Try to identify the origin (parent and stage of meiosis) in each family. (Answers p. 215.)

Tetraploidy, or four times the haploid number, is usually due to failure to complete the first zygotic division. A proportion of polyploid cells occurs normally in human bone marrow, since megakaryocytes usually have 8–16 times the haploid number. Tetraploid cells are also a normal feature of regenerating liver and other tissues.

STRUCTURAL ABERRATIONS

Structural aberrations all result from chromosomal breakage. When a chromosome breaks two unstable sticky ends are produced. Generally, repair mechanisms rejoin these two ends without delay. However, if more than one break has occurred, then as the repair mechanisms cannot distinguish one sticky end from another there is the possibility of rejoining the wrong ends. The spontaneous rate of chromosomal breakage is markedly increased by exposure to ionizing radiation and is also increased in some rare inherited conditions (see pp. 171–2). X-rays produce double-stranded breaks at any stage of the cell cycle in a dose-dependent linear fashion, but without any increase in the number of sister chromatid exchanges. In contrast, chemical mutagens are S phase-dependent and induce sister chromatid exchanges rather than chromatid break and exchange abnormalities. Chromosomal breakage is not randomly distributed, and for all translocations the

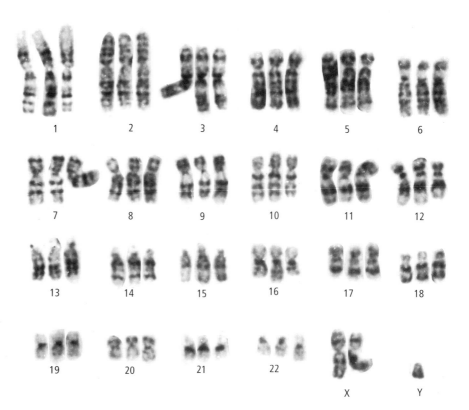

Fig. 6.3 Triploidy detected at amniocentesis.

Table 6.2 Examples of structural chromosomal aberrations.

Karyotype	Comment
46,XY,t(5;10)(p13;q25)	Balanced reciprocal translocation involving chromosomes 5 and 10 (break points indicated)
45,XX,t(13;14)(p11;q11)	Centric fusion translocation of chromosomes 13 and 14
46,XY,del(5)(p25)	Short arm deletion of 5, cri du chat syndrome
46,X,i(Xq)	Isochromosome of Xq
46,XX,dup(2)(p13p22)	Partial duplication of the short arm of chromosome 2 (p13 → p22)
46,XY,r(3)(p26 → q29)	Ring chromosome 3 (p26 → q29)
46,XY,inv(11)(p15q14)	Pericentric inversion of chromosome 11

spontaneous mutation rate is 1 in 1000 gametes (which is about 100-fold greater than the mutation rate for individual disease loci).

Structural aberrations are subdivided into translocations, deletion and ring chromosomes, duplications, inversions, isochromosomes and centric fragments (Table 6.2).

Translocations

A translocation is the transfer of chromosomal material between chromosomes. The process requires breakage of both chromosomes with repair in an abnormal arrangement, or accidental recombination between non-homologous chromosomes during meiosis. This exchange usually results in no loss of DNA and the individual is clinically normal and is said to have a balanced translocation. The medical significance is for future generations, because a balanced translocation carrier is at risk of producing chromosomally unbalanced offspring.

Three types of translocation are recognized: reciprocal; centric fusion (Robertsonian); and insertional.

Reciprocal translocations. In a reciprocal translocation, chromosomal material distal to breaks in two chromosomes is exchanged. Either the long or the short arm may break and any pair of chromosomes may be involved (either homologous or non-homologous). Thus in Fig. 6.4a breaks have occurred in the long arm of chromosome 10 and the long arm of chromosome 11 with reciprocal exchange, and Fig. 6.5 shows a balanced 5;10 reciprocal translocation. The carrier of either of these balanced translocations is healthy, but during gametogenesis unbalanced gametes may be produced. When these chro-

mosomes pair during meiosis a cross-shaped quadrivalent is formed, which allows homologous segments to be in contact (Fig. 6.4b–d). This later opens into a ring or chain held together by chiasmata (Fig. 6.5b,c). At anaphase these four chromosomes must segregate to the two daughter cells. Twelve possible gametes may be seen in each case. Figure 6.5d shows the six which result from a two to two segregation. Of these six possibilities only one gamete is normal and one is a balanced translocation. The other four result in various imbalances of the amounts of chromosomes 5 and 10. Such visible imbalance involves large numbers of genes, and affected conceptions may miscarry, or, if liveborn, mental handicap and multiple congenital malformations would be found. Three to one segregation results in a further six gametes, but the chromosomal imbalance in each of these is so gross that early spontaneous miscarriage would be invariable. Thus in the liveborn offspring of the carrier of either of these translocations one would expect a ratio of 1 normal to 1 balanced to 4 unbalanced. In practice, some of the unbalanced miscarry, and there may also be selection against the unbalanced gametes, so the actual risk of unbalanced offspring is always lower than expected (see p. 116).

For occasional translocations unbalanced offspring produced by a three to one segregation may be viable, e.g. with partial triplication of chromosome 22 (Fig. 6.6).

Centric fusion (Robertsonian) translocations. Centric fusion translocations arise from breaks at or near the centromere in two acrocentric chromosomes with cross-fusion of the products. In most cases the breaks are just above the centromere and so the products are a single chromosome with two centromeres (dicentric) and a fragment with no centromere (acentric) bearing both satellites. An acentric fragment cannot undergo mitosis and will usually be lost at a subsequent cell division. An alternative possibility is that at least some cases of centric fusion are due to accidental cross-overs between homologous sequences on non-homologous chromosomes during first meiosis (Fig. 6.7).

Centric fusion of chromosomes 13 and 14 is the single most frequent type of translocation in humans, and this is followed in frequency by centric fusion of 14 and 21. Figure 6.8 shows the partial karyotype of a balanced 14;21 centric fusion translocation. This combined chromosome is dicentric, and the acentric fragment has been lost, so leaving only 45 chromosomes in total. Again such an individual is healthy, but problems may arise at gametogenesis. When the chromosomes pair during meiosis a trivalent is formed, which allows homologous segments to be in contact (Fig. 6.9). At anaphase these three chromosomes must segregate to the gametes, and Fig. 6.10 shows the six possible gametes. Only one is normal; one is balanced and four are unbalanced. Again, in practice,

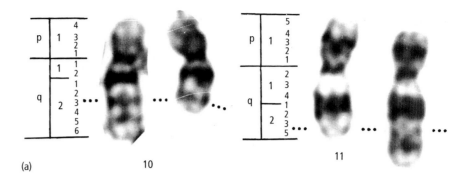

(a)   10   11

(b)

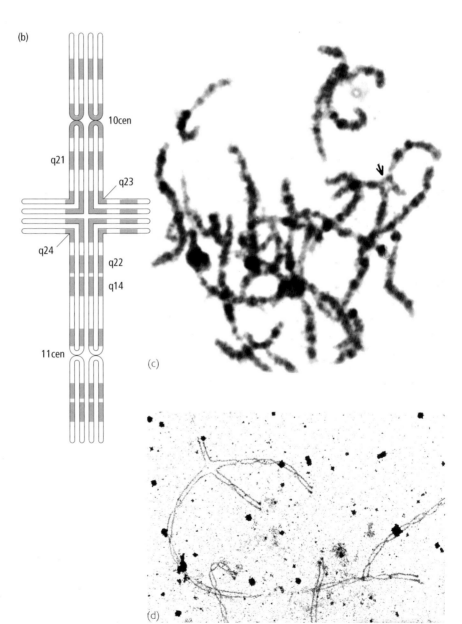

(c)

Fig. 6.4 (a) Reciprocal translocation between chromosomes 10 and 11. Normal chromosome on the left for each pair. (b) Meiotic quadrivalent configuration in a 10;11 translocation. (c) Meiotic quadrivalent at pachytene in a 10;11 translocation carrier (arrowed). (d) EM photomicrograph of the synaptonemal complex of a 9;20 translocation observed at pachytene in a translocation carrier (stained by silver nitrate).

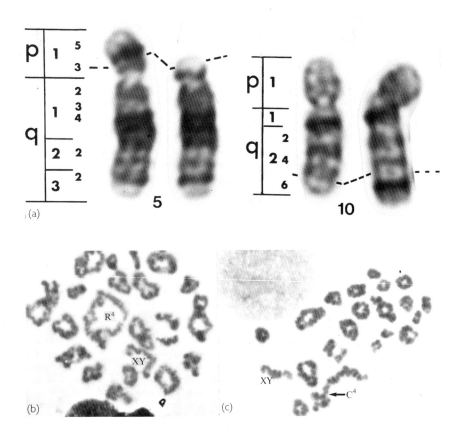

(a)

(b)   (c)

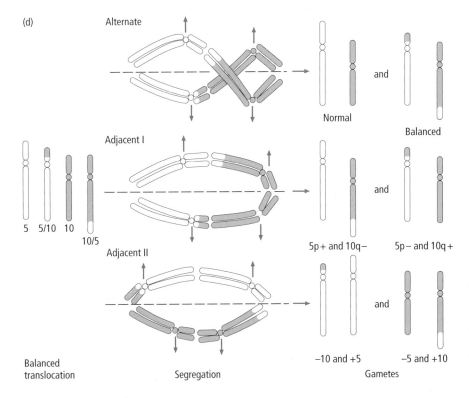

Fig. 6.5 (a) Reciprocal translocation between chromosomes 5 and 10. Normal chromosome placed on the left for each pair. (b) Meiotic quadrivalent for a balanced 5;10 reciprocal translocation at first meiosis. (c) Meiotic chain quadrivalent at diakinesis (arrowed). (d) Three types of segregation for a balanced 5;10 reciprocal translocation at first meiosis.

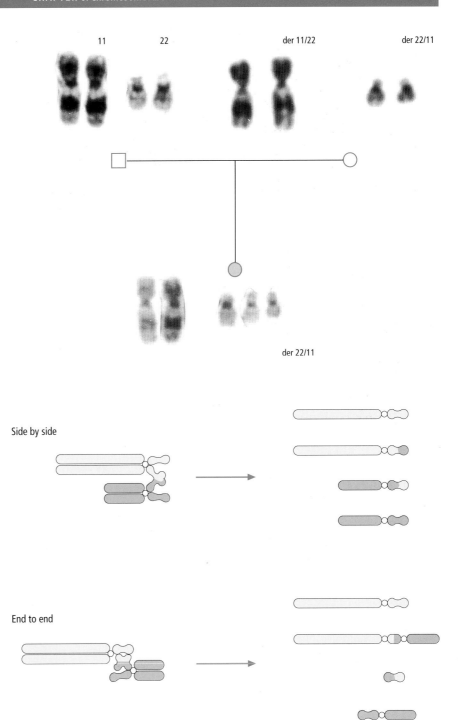

Fig. 6.6 Maternal reciprocal translocation between chromosomes 11 and 22 with 3 : 1 segregation to produce partial duplication of chromosome 22 in a mentally handicapped daughter.

Fig. 6.7 Accidental recombination between homologous regions of non-homologous chromosomes during meiosis as a cause of dicentric centric fusion chromosomes.

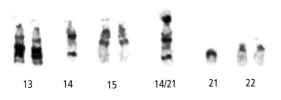

Fig. 6.8 Centric fusion translocation of chromosomes 14 and 21.

spontaneous abortion and gametic selection result in a lower observed frequency of unbalanced offspring than predicted (see p. 116).

Insertional translocations. For an insertional translocation three breaks are required in one or two chromosomes. If between two chromosomes, this results in an interstitial

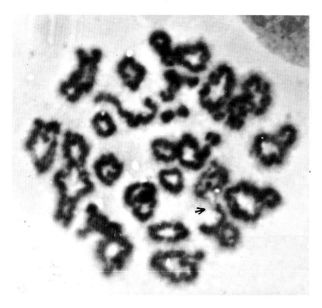

Fig. 6.9 Meiotic trivalent for a t(13;14) centric fusion translocation (arrowed).

arise from loss of a portion of the chromosome between two break points (interstitial deletions), as a result of unequal crossing-over, as a result of a parental translocation or as a terminal deletion. In the latter instance, the deletion continues proximally until a DNA region homologous to telamere sequences is reached when the enzyme telomerase is able to synthesize a new telomere and so arrest the deletion. The deleted portion lacks a centromere (an acentric fragment) and will be lost at a subsequent cell division. A ring chromosome arises from breaks in both arms of a chromosome: the terminal ends are lost and the two proximal sticky ends unite to form a ring. If the ring has a centromere then it may be able to pass through cell division. A sister chromatid exchange within a ring results in a dicentric ring of twice the size in subsequent divisions (Fig. 6.12).

As the smallest visible loss from a chromosome is about 4 Mb, individuals with visible deletions are rendered monosomic for large numbers of contiguous genes, and with autosomal deletions mental handicap and multiple congenital malformations are usual. Deletions of a size close to the limit of resolution with the light microscope are termed microdeletions and molecular techniques have been developed to aid their detection (p. 129).

deletion of a segment of one, which is inserted into the gap in the other (Fig. 6.11). Again the balanced carrier is healthy but may produce unbalanced offspring with *either* a duplication *or* a deletion but not both.

Deletions and ring chromosomes

A loss of any part of a chromosome is a deletion. Deletions

Duplications

In a duplication, an additional copy of a segment of a chromosome is present. It may originate by unequal crossing-over during meiosis, and the reciprocal product is a

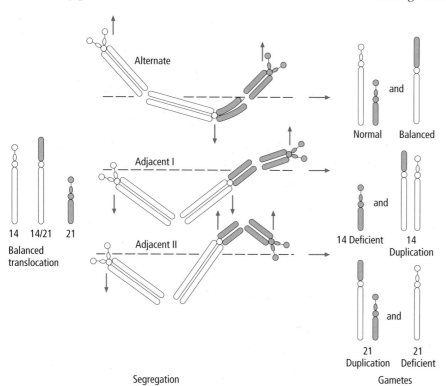

Fig. 6.10 Segregation of a centric fusion translocation at first meiosis.

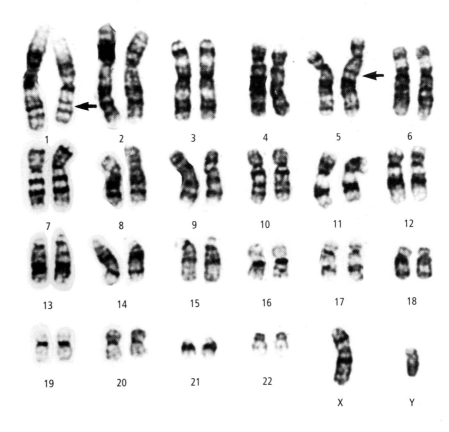

Fig. 6.11 Insertional translocation showing interstitial deletion of band 1q31 and insertion into band 5q13.

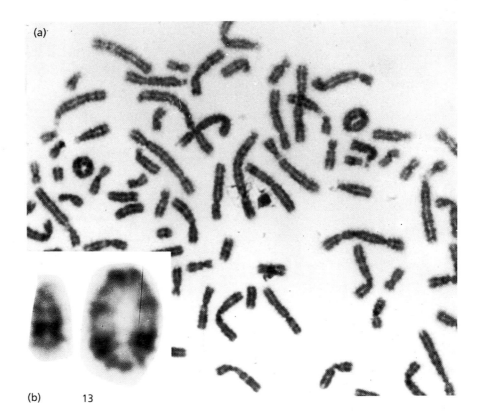

Fig. 6.12 (a) Ring chromosomes, dicentrics and acentric fragments following exposure to irradiation. (b) Double-ring chromosome 13.

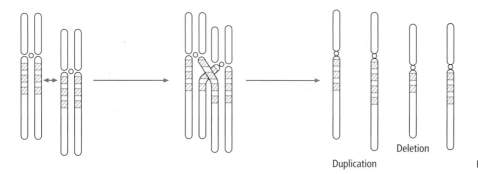

Duplication　　Deletion

Fig. 6.13 Results of unequal crossing-over.

deletion (Fig. 6.13). A duplication can also result from meiotic events in a parent with a translocation, inversion or isochromosome.

Duplications are more common than deletions and are generally less harmful. Indeed, tiny duplications at the molecular level (repeats) may play an important role in permitting gene diversification during evolution.

Inversions

Inversions arise from two chromosomal breaks with inversion through 180° of the segment between the breaks. If both breaks are in a single arm then the centromere is not included (paracentric inversion) (Fig. 6.14a) whereas if the breaks are on either side of the centromere it is included (pericentric inversion) (Fig. 6.14b). Generally

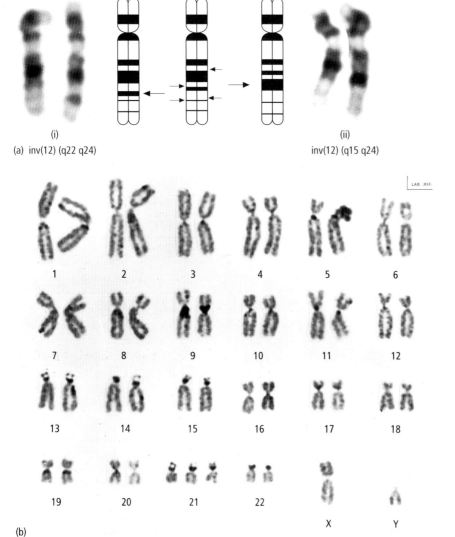

(i)

(a) inv(12) (q22 q24)

(ii)

inv(12) (q15 q24)

Fig. 6.14 (a) Two examples of paracentric inversions of chromosome 12. (b) Pericentric inversion of chromosome 9 which is present in 1% of the normal population (patient coincidentally has trisomy 21).

(b)

this change in gene order does not produce clinical abnormality. The medical significance lies with the increased risk of generating unbalanced gametes.

Inversions interfere with the pairing of homologous chromosomes during meiosis, and crossing-over tends to be suppressed within the inverted segment. For homologous chromosomes to pair, one member must form a loop in the region of the inversion (Fig. 6.15) or the chromosome arms distal to the inversion fail to pair. For a paracentric inversion, if a cross-over does occur within the loop then this will result in a dicentric chromatid and an acentric fragment. Both of these are unstable and rarely result in abnormal offspring. In contrast, for a pericentric inversion, if an uneven number of cross-overs occur within the loop then each of the two chromatids produced will have both a deletion and a duplication, and abnormal offspring may be produced (Figs 6.16 & 6.17). These unbalanced products always show a deletion of the segment distal to one of the break points and duplication of the segment distal to the other. The closer both break points are to the telomeres, the higher the likelihood of survival of the fetus to birth.

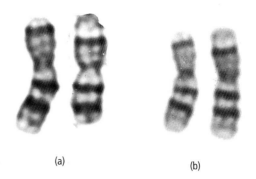

(a)   (b)

Fig. 6.16 Large pericentric inversion of chromosome 7. Normal chromosome in each case to the left. (a) Parent with balanced inversion. (b) Abnormal child with duplication (7q32-qter) and deficiency (7p22-pter) resulting from a cross-over within the paternal inversion.

Isochromosomes

An isochromosome is an abnormal chromosome which has deletion of one arm with duplication of the other. It may arise from transverse division of the centromere during cell division (Fig. 6.18a) or from an isochromatid break and fusion above the centromere (in which case it is dicentric). The commonest isochromosome in livebirths is an isochromosome of the long arm of X. This results in clinical abnormality (Turner syndrome, p. 121) due to short arm monosomy and long arm trisomy. Isochromosomes of Y are also seen in livebirths, but for other chromosomes an isochromosome usually results in an early spontaneous abortion; rare exceptions are isochromosomes of the short arms of chromosomes 9 and 12 (Fig. 6.18b). In many instances isochromosomes are dicentric, but one centromere becomes non-functional so that the chromosome segregates normally during cell division.

Centric fragments

Additional small, usually metacentric, fragments are sometimes detected during routine karyotyping. Some are familial and have resulted from a centric fusion translocation between satellited chromosomes (often involving the short arm of chromosome 15) arising in meiosis in a parent or ancestor. Provided the centric fragment contains only repetitive and ribosomal DNA, there will be no clinical consequences. Occasionally, transcribed genes are also included, in which case there may be associated disability.

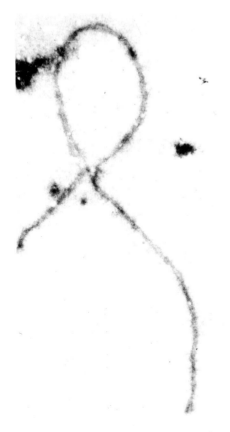

Fig. 6.15 EM photomicrograph of the synaptonemal complex of a 46,XY, inv(2) (p13;q25) carrier. Homologous pairing has been achieved by one homologue forming an inversion loop.

IDENTIFICATION OF THE CHROMOSOMAL ORIGIN OF COMPLEX STRUCTURAL REARRANGEMENTS

The identification of the chromosomes involved in numerical and gross structural rearrangements is usually

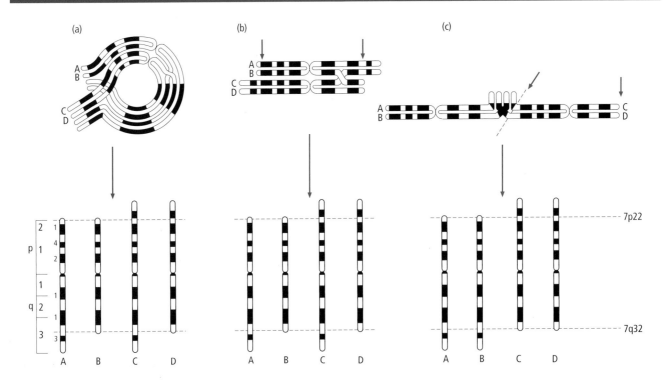

Fig. 6.17 The results of crossing-over at meiosis (a, b) within and (c) outside the pericentric inversion of chromosome 7 as shown in Fig. 6.16. A is the normal chromosome 7 and D has the pericentric inversion. In (a) and (b) two types of abnormal recombinant chromosomes are formed (B and C, each with a duplication deficiency). In (c) crossing-over outside the inversion produces no abnormal recombinant.

obvious using standard G-banding procedures. The origin of smaller duplications and deletions may be more difficult to determine particularly if the aberration is unbalanced and has arisen *de novo*. Complex rearrangements involving several chromosomes, for example as found in some malignant tissues, may prove impossible to resolve by chromosome banding alone. In these situations DNA probes may be used in molecular *in situ* hybridization procedures to label the specific components of an abnormal chromosome and so identify their origins. There are many types of chromosome-specific probes which can be used, including repetitive (alphoid) probes which are centromere-specific and cosmid or YAC probes which contain an insert large enough to provide a clear signal in the majority of metaphases. Non-isotopic detection systems which incorporate fluorescent molecules are most often used together with biotin or digoxigenin labelled DNA probes. Plate 4 shows alphoid repeat probes for the X chromosome (labelled with Texas red) and chromosome 18 (labelled with fluorescein-isothiocyanate, FITC) in a fluorescence *in situ* hybridization (FISH) procedure which clearly identifies both chromosomes in both metaphase and interphase. Chromosome-specific DNA probes can be made from an entire chromosome and used to 'paint' by FISH those parts of a structural aberration derived from that chromosome (Plate 3). Chromosome paints may be made from chromosome-specific genomic libraries, single chromosome somatic cell hybrids or polymerase chain reaction (PCR) amplified chromosomes sorted by a fluorescence activated cell sorter (FACS). All these probes require a pre-annealing step to suppress repetitive DNA sequences before application in FISH experiments.

Chromosome paints may also be made from *abnormal* chromosomes which are sorted by FACS, amplified by PCR and painted onto *normal* metaphases. As shown in Plate 5, the paint probe reveals the origin of each chromosome segment present in the abnormal chromosome and, at the same time, identifies the exact break point involved in each chromosome. This technique of 'reverse painting' has revealed that most *de novo* duplications are tandem duplications or other forms of intrachromosomal rearrangement.

Multicolour FISH is a recent development which enables several DNA probes to be used simultaneously. When applied to chromosome paints it is possible to give each chromosome a distinctive colour and this may have an application in the analysis of complex chromosome rearrangements (Plate 6). The coloured bar code technique has particular application in the analysis of intrachromosomal rearrangements (Plate 3e).

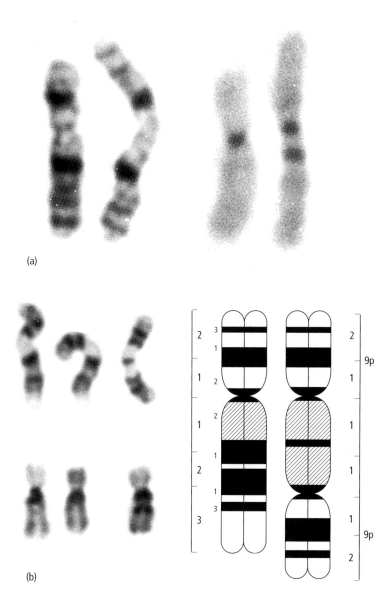

Fig. 6.18 (a) Dicentric isochromosome for the long arm of the X (stained by G- and C-banding). (b) Dicentric isochromosome for the short arm of chromosome 9 in a patient with the features of trisomy 9p syndrome. Only one centromere (the top one) is functional.

OTHER ABERRATIONS

Mosaic

A mosaic is an individual with two or more cell lines which were derived from a single zygote. For example, about 1% of patients with trisomy 21 are mosaics with normal and trisomic cell lines. This arises after fertilization. Usually the initial zygote has trisomy 21 and a normal cell line is produced at a subsequent mitosis by anaphase lag. Less frequently the initial zygote is normal and a trisomic cell line arises at a subsequent mitosis by non-disjunction. In this event a cell line with monosomy 21 will also be produced, which will tend to be lost. The presence of the normal cell line tends to ameliorate the clinical picture, and if the abnormal cell line is confined to the gonad (gonadal mosaic) then an outwardly normal parent may have a high risk of producing abnormal children.

Chimaera

A chimaera is an individual with two cell lines which were derived from two separate zygotes. This could arise by the early fusion of fraternal twin zygotes, by double fertilization of the egg and a polar body or, more commonly, by exchange of haemopoietic stem cells *in utero* by dizygotic twins. Chimaerism is confirmed if a double contribution of maternal and paternal alleles can be demonstrated in the two cell lines.

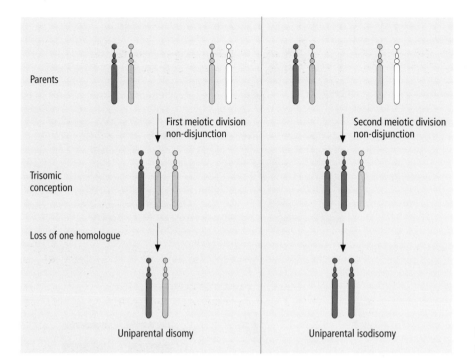

Fig. 6.19 Diagram of mechanism of origin of uniparental disomy and isodisomy.

Uniparental disomy and isodisomy

Normally each parent contributes one member of each pair of autosomes and one sex chromosome but occasionally both homologues of an autosome are from one parent with loss of the corresponding homologue from the other parent. This can arise if the conception is trisomic for the homologue and one homologue is lost by anaphase lag at an early cell division to leave the two copies of the homologue which came from the same parent (trisomic rescue). If the trisomy resulted from non-disjunction at the first meiotic division the gamete with the extra chromosome will contain both parental homologues of that chromosome and uniparental disomy will be found in the patient whereas if the trisomy resulted from non-disjunction at the second meiotic division then both the normal and the extra copy of that chromosome will be either maternal or paternal and uniparental isodisomy will be found in the patient (Fig. 6.19).

Uniparental disomy and isodisomy result in a normal karyotype but can be detected by DNA marker analysis. Their clinical consequences arise from genomic imprinting (p. 54) of certain chromosomal regions with consequent parent specific expression of alleles in these regions. For example, Prader–Willi syndrome (p. 126) is usually caused by a paternal deletion of the proximal long arm of chromosome 15 but occasional patients with the same clinical appearance have no deletion but maternal uniparental disomy for chromosome 15. Uniparental isodisomy can also result in homozygosity for mutant genes on the involved chromosome and so result in an autosomal recessive single gene disorder with only one parent a carrier.

C H A P T E R 7

Autosomal Inheritance

C O N T E N T S

AUTOSOMAL SINGLE GENE INHERITANCE 69
AUTOSOMAL DOMINANT INHERITANCE 69
AUTOSOMAL RECESSIVE INHERITANCE 71

AUTOSOMAL CODOMINANT INHERITANCE 74
SUMMARY OF AUTOSOMAL INHERITANCE 75

Single gene disorders (Mendelian disorders) are due to mutations in one or both members of a pair of autosomal genes or to mutations in genes on the X or Y chromosomes (sex-linked inheritance — Chapter 8). These disorders show characteristic patterns of inheritance in family pedigrees. Figure 7.1 shows some of the more commonly used symbols for constructing family trees (see Fig. 12.1, p. 104, for other symbols).

AUTOSOMAL SINGLE GENE INHERITANCE

The 44 autosomes comprise 22 homologous pairs of chromosomes. Within each chromosome the genes have a strict order, each gene occupying a specific location or locus. Thus the autosomal genes are present in pairs, one member of maternal and one member of paternal origin. Alternative forms of a gene are called alleles and these arise by mutation of the normal allele and may or may not have an altered function. If both members of a gene pair are identical then the individual is homozygous for that locus. If different, then the individual is heterozygous for that locus.

Any gene-determined characteristic is called a trait. If a trait is expressed in the heterozygote then the trait is dominant, whereas if only expressed in the homozygote it is recessive. In some instances the effects of both alleles may be seen in the heterozygote, and these are called codominant traits.

AUTOSOMAL DOMINANT INHERITANCE

Autosomal dominant inheritance is most easily demonstrated by considering an example. The patient in Fig. 7.2 has cholesterol deposits (xanthomata) over his extensor tendons and also has premature coronary artery disease.

His pedigree (Fig. 7.3) shows the typical features of autosomal dominant inheritance. Both males and females are affected in approximately equal numbers. Persons are affected in each generation and males can transmit the condition to males or females and vice versa. Unaffected persons do not transmit the condition. This condition, familial hypercholesterolaemia (FH), is due to a single mutant gene on the short arm of chromosome 19. Thus each of the affected persons in this family is a heterozygote, and as each has married an unaffected person (normal homozygote) the expected ratio of affected to unaffected offspring is as seen in Fig. 7.4.

It is equally likely for a child to receive the mutant or the normal allele from the affected parent, and so on average there is a 1 in 2 or 50% chance that each child of a heterozygous parent will be affected. Although each affected individual has the same mutant gene there is variation in the time of onset and severity of xanthomata and vascular disease. This variable expression (variable expressivity) is typical of an autosomal dominant trait but its basis is unclear.

The gene for FH has been cloned and over 200 different mutations identified. It produces a protein which acts as a receptor for circulating low density lipoproteins which

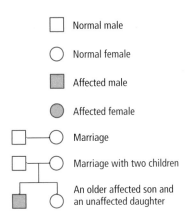

Fig. 7.1 Symbols used in pedigree construction.

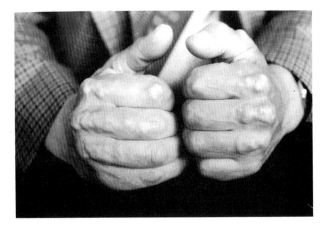

Fig. 7.2 Tendon xanthomata in familial hypercholesterolaemia.

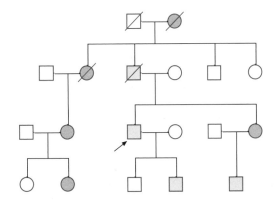

Fig. 7.3 Pedigree of a family with familial hypercholesterolaemia. Patient in Fig. 7.2 is indicated by an arrow.

can be bound and then internalized by a wide variety of cells. Defects in this receptor result in defective clearance and hence elevated levels of low density lipoproteins including cholesterol.

FH affects 1 in 500 individuals and marriages have occurred between affected heterozygotes. In such mar-

riages on average one-quarter of the offspring will be unaffected, one-half will be heterozygous affected and one-quarter will be homozygous affected. In the homozygous affected persons there are no normal low density lipoprotein receptors and the disease shows precocious onset and increased severity with death from coronary heart disease in late childhood.

Family members at risk can be counselled on the basis of plasma lipid profiles and by tracking the defective gene within a family using DNA analysis.

So far 4458 autosomal dominant traits are known in humans. Some of the commoner and more clinically important of these are shown in Table 7.1. The pedigree pattern for each is similar to FH. In general they tend to be less severe than recessive traits, and whereas recessive traits usually result in defective enzymes, dominants

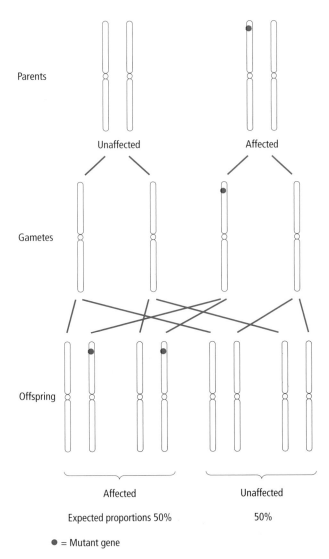

Fig. 7.4 Diagram of autosomal dominant inheritance.

Table 7.1 Autosomal dominant diseases.

Disease	Frequency/1000 births
Inherited colon cancer	?5
Inherited breast cancer	?5
Dominant otosclerosis	3
Familial hypercholesterolaemia	2
von Willebrand disease	1.0
Adult polycystic kidney disease	1.0
Multiple exostoses	0.5
Huntington disease	0.5
Neurofibromatosis	0.4
Myotonic dystrophy	0.2
Congenital spherocytosis	0.2
Tuberous sclerosis	0.1
Polyposis coli	0.1
Dominant blindness	0.1
Dominant congenital deafness	0.1
Others	0.8
Total	20/1000

often alter structural, carrier or receptor proteins. In some dominant traits, for example inherited colon cancer, an individual may have the mutant gene and yet have a normal phenotype. This is called non-penetrance and is an important exception to the rule that unaffected persons do not transmit an autosomal dominant trait. These individuals can pass the condition to descendants and so produce a skipped generation. In some other dominant traits, for example Huntington disease, the onset of symptoms (and hence the penetrance) is age-dependent and reassurance of family members at risk on the basis of clinical examination is not possible until they reach an advanced age. Variable expression and non-penetrance (total and age-related) are important factors when providing genetic counselling for families with autosomal dominant traits.

When a condition shows full penetrance then the recurrence risk for the clinically normal parents of an affected child is low but not negligible because of gonadal mosaicism. Such mutations confined to the gonad carry a high recurrence risk (of up to 1 in 2) and can only be proven when unaffected parents have a second affected child. This possibility thus needs to be considered when counselling a family with an apparently new mutation.

Counselling problems can also arise when the mutant gene is unstable. Myotonic dystrophy is a common adult-onset form of muscular dystrophy which is due to an unstable length mutation. Small length mutations may produce few or no symptoms but amplification in successive generations can result in increasing disease severity (p. 144).

Some autosomal dominant traits are so serious that they usually preclude reproduction (e.g. Apert syndrome and progressive myositis ossificans). In this situation neither parent will be affected and the child will be a new mutation. If the child fails to reproduce then the mutant gene goes no further and there will be but one affected individual in the family. For several autosomal dominant traits, including Apert syndrome, progressive myositis ossificans, Marfan syndrome and achondroplasia, the risk for a new mutation increases with increasing paternal age, and for some dominant traits (e.g. retinoblastoma and neurofibromatosis) DNA analysis has demonstrated a paternal excess of new mutations.

AUTOSOMAL RECESSIVE INHERITANCE

Sickle cell disease is an example of an autosomal recessive trait. Figure 7.5 shows the characteristic sickle-shaped red cells in an affected patient. These distorted red cells have a reduced survival time and this results in a severe chronic haemolytic anaemia with a need for repeated blood transfusions. The distorted red cells may also occlude vessels causing recurrent infarctions, especially of the lungs, bones and spleen.

The predominant haemoglobin in normal adults is haemoglobin A (HbA) which has two alpha-globin and two beta-globin polypeptide chains in each molecule. Sickle cell disease is caused by a point mutation in each beta-globin gene on chromosome 11 at the codon for the sixth amino acid. The resulting haemoglobin S has a substitution of valine for glutamic acid (see Fig. 2.17, p. 22) and this difference causes distortion of red cells especially at reduced oxygen tension and also alters the electrophoretic mobility in a starch gel (Fig. 7.6). Affected patients with sickle cell disease have two mutant haemoglobin S genes (HbS/HbS) which are inherited one from each parent.

The pedigree of a family with sickle cell disease is shown in Fig. 7.7. The parents in this family are clinically normal yet are heterozygotes (carriers) for the mutant beta-globin gene (HbA/HbS). Their normal beta-globin gene produces sufficient haemoglobin A to prevent symptoms. Apart from the two children, no other individuals are affected in the family but their carrier status can be resolved by haemoglobin electrophoresis.

Figure 7.8 shows the possible offspring for parents who are both carriers for sickle cell disease. On average, one-quarter of their children will be homozygous normal, one-half heterozygous and one-quarter homozygous affected. The observed segregation ratio can be compared with that predicted; however, two points must be borne in mind when using this approach for a suspected autosomal

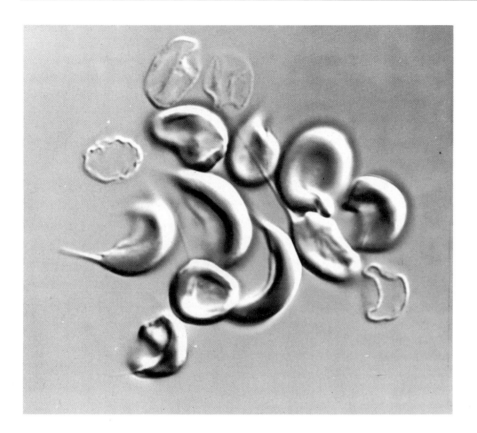

Fig. 7.5 Sickle-shaped red cells in an HbS homozygote.

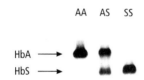

Fig. 7.6 Haemoglobin electrophoresis at alkaline pH to demonstrate individuals who are homozygous for HbS, heterozygous (HbS/HbA) or homozygous normal (HbA/HbA).

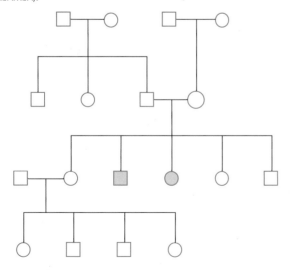

Fig. 7.7 Pedigree of a family with children affected with sickle cell disease.

recessive trait. First, it is unlikely that any single family will have produced sufficient children to give the ratio directly. Second, there is an automatic bias, since families only come to medical attention by virtue of an affected child, and those carrier parents who by chance produce only unaffected children will be missed. As shown in Fig. 7.9, when both parents are carriers for a recessive trait, if they have only two children then the proportions of none to one to both affected will be 9 : 6 : 1, and hence only seven of every 16 couples at risk will come to medical attention. A correction for this bias needs to be made by not counting the first affected child in each family when determining the segregation ratio.

For a parent with sickle cell disease, each child must receive a mutant allele but if married to a homozygous normal person (HbA/HbA) then only unaffected heterozygotes (HbA/HbS) will be produced. If by chance a person with sickle cell disease marries a heterozygote, then there will be a 1 in 2 chance on average that each child will be affected. If both parents have sickle cell disease then only children with sickle cell disease can be produced.

Family members at risk can be screened by haemoglobin electrophoresis and, where a pregnancy is at risk of homozygous sickle cell disease, prenatal diagnosis by DNA analysis may be offered.

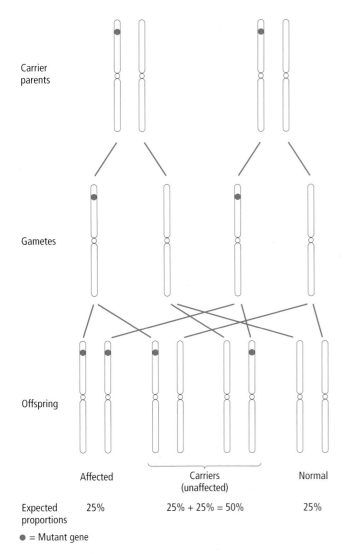

Carrier parents

Gametes

Offspring

| Affected | Carriers (unaffected) | Normal |

| Expected proportions | 25% | 25% + 25% = 50% | 25% |

● = Mutant gene

Fig. 7.8 Diagram of autosomal recessive inheritance.

The majority of parents of children with sickle cell disease are not blood relatives (consanguineous), but if they are there is an increased risk for this and other autosomal recessive disorders. The increased risk in this situation is caused by the parents sharing one set of grandparents and the chance that each has inherited the same mutant gene from one grandparent (Table 7.2). The proportion of shared genes (coefficient of relationship, r) decreases by one-half for each step apart on the pedigree. In highly inbred populations the affected person has a substantial risk of mating with a carrier, and this may result in a pedigree with apparent vertical transmission of an autosomal recessive trait (quasidominant inheritance). Hence parental consanguinity, whilst not a prerequisite, is an important clue that a condition in their child is an autosomal recessive trait.

Sickle cell disease affects 1 in 40 African Blacks who have a carrier frequency of 1 in 3. This high frequency is due to the selective advantage of these carriers with regard to malarial infection (Chapter 11). Ethnic associations may also arise from the founder effect (Chapter 11) in genetically isolated populations (Table 7.3). Hence the ethnic origin of a patient may be an important clue to an autosomal recessive disorder.

So far 1730 autosomal recessive traits are known in humans. Some of the commoner and more clinically important of these are shown in Table 7.4. In about 15% of autosomal recessive traits an enzyme defect has already been demonstrated and is to be expected in many of the remainder. For many traits not just one but multiple different mutant alleles may occur at the locus (*multiple allelism*). Some, but not all, of these result in sufficient reduction of enzyme activity to produce disease in the homozygous state. An individual who has two different mutant alleles at a locus is termed a genetic compound.

Many conditions which were believed to be single genetic entities are now known to be genetically heterogeneous (i.e. to have several different genetic causes). This should be suspected if different modes of inheritance are

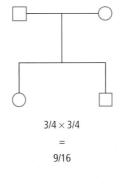

3/4 × 3/4
=
9/16

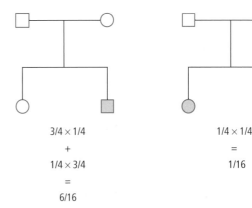

3/4 × 1/4
+
1/4 × 3/4
=
6/16

1/4 × 1/4
=
1/16

Fig. 7.9 Relative proportions of affected to unaffected offspring when both parents are carriers for an autosomal recessive trait.

Table 7.2 Proportions of genes in common in different relatives.

Degree of relationship	Examples	Proportion of genes in common (r)
First	Parents to child, sib to sib	1/2
Second	Uncles or aunts to nephews or nieces, grandparents to grandchildren	1/4
Third	First cousins, great grandparents to great grandchildren	1/8

Table 7.4 Autosomal recessive diseases.

Disease	Frequency/1000 births
Cystic fibrosis	0.5
Recessive mental retardation	0.5
Congenital deafness	0.2
Phenylketonuria	0.1
Spinal muscular atrophy	0.1
Recessive blindness	0.1
Adrenogenital syndrome	0.1
Mucopolysaccharidoses	0.1
Others	0.3
Total	2/1000

Table 7.3 Ethnic associations with autosomal recessive diseases.

Disease	Ethnic group(s)
Beta-thalassaemia	Mediterraneans, Thais, Blacks, Middle East populations, Indians, Chinese
Sickle cell disease	US and African Blacks, Asian Indians, Mediterraneans (especially Greeks) and Middle East populations
Tay–Sachs disease	Ashkenazi Jews
Gaucher disease	Ashkenazi Jews
Bloom syndrome	Ashkenazi Jews
Adrenogenital syndrome	Eskimos
Severe combined immunodeficiency	Apache Indians
Cystic fibrosis	Caucasians
Albinism	Hopi Indians

apparent in different families or if offspring of parents who are autosomal recessive homozygotes are not invariably affected. Genetic heterogeneity can be proven by demonstrating that different proteins or their respective genes are involved, or, by complementation studies. In complementation studies, cell lines from two affected individuals are mixed *in vitro* to determine if heterogeneous cross-correction of the phenotype can be demonstrated.

AUTOSOMAL CODOMINANT INHERITANCE

Autosomal codominant inheritance is illustrated by the inheritance of autosomal DNA polymorphism. An RFLP from the low density lipoprotein receptor gene on chromosome 19, is shown in Figs 7.10–7.12. The polymorphic fragments with this probe are 16.5 kb and 14 kb and as each individual has two copies of chromosome 19 each can be homozygous 16.5/16.5, heterozygous 16.5/14 or homozygous 14/14. Either fragment or both fragments can be identified in an individual and followed through a family. This ability to distinguish equally the presence of either allele is the hallmark of codominant inheritance.

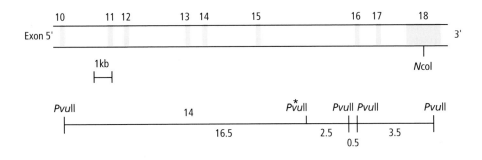

Fig. 7.10 An RFLP in the low density lipoprotein receptor gene. The probe (a cDNA probe) corresponds to the coding exons 10–18, and the polymorphic *Pvu*II site is indicated (*).

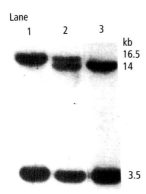

Lane
1   2   3
kb
16.5
14

3.5

Fig. 7.11 Autoradiograph showing the low density lipoprotein RFLP of Fig. 7.10. The 3.5 kb band (corresponding to exons 17 and 18) is constant. If the polymorphic *Pvu*II site is present a 14 kb fragment is produced whereas if absent a 16.5 kb fragment is produced. Lane 1 shows a 16.5/16.5 homozygote, lane 2 a l6.5/14 heterozygote and lane 3 a 14/14 homozygote.

Thus the pedigree pattern of human codominant traits resembles that of autosomal dominant inheritance, except that both alleles can be distinguished. Some of the commoner and more clinically important traits of this type are listed in Table 7.5. For many of these the rarest allele at the locus occurs with a frequency of more than 2%, and so these are examples of genetic polymorphisms (Chapter 11).

Table 7.5 Autosomal codominant traits.

Blood groups—ABO, Kell, MNS, Rhesus
Red cell enzymes—acid phosphatase, adenylate kinase
Serum proteins—haptoglobin
Cell surface antigens—human leucocyte antigen system (HLA)
Autosomal DNA polymorphisms

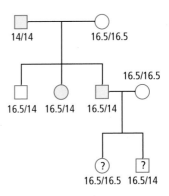

Fig. 7.12 Pedigree and results of DNA analysis using the low density lipoprotein receptor RFLP of Figs 7.10 and 7.11 in a family with familial hypercholesterolaemia. On the basis of these DNA results, identify whether the offspring in the third generation are carrying the mutant gene. (Answer p. 215).

SUMMARY OF AUTOSOMAL INHERITANCE

Table 7.6 summarizes the important distinguishing features of autosomal recessive and dominant inheritance.

Table 7.6 Comparison of autosomal dominant and recessive modes of inheritance.

Autosomal dominant	Autosomal recessive
Disease expressed in heterozygote	Disease expressed in homozygote
On average half of offspring affected	Low risk to offspring
Equal frequency and severity in each sex	Equal frequency and severity in each sex
Paternal age effect for new mutations	
Variable expressivity	Constant expressivity in a family
Vertical pedigree pattern	Horizontal pedigree pattern
	Importance of consanguinity

C H A P T E R 8

Sex-linked Inheritance

C O N T E N T S

Y-LINKED INHERITANCE
(HOLANDRIC INHERITANCE) 76
X-LINKED RECESSIVE INHERITANCE 77

Other X-linked recessive conditions 79
X-LINKED DOMINANT INHERITANCE 79
X-LINKED CODOMINANT INHERITANCE 81

A female has two X chromosomes: one of paternal and one of maternal origin. However, with the exception of several X–Y homologous genes (see p. 51), one of these X chromosomes is inactivated in each somatic cell (Lyonization, see p. 50). This mechanism ensures that the amount of most X-linked gene products produced in somatic cells of the female is equivalent to the amount produced in male cells. In the process of inactivation the choice between the maternal and paternal X homologues is random, although once established the same homologue is inactivated in each daughter cell. Thus the female is really a mosaic with a percentage of cells having the paternal X active, and the maternal X active in the remainder. Each son or daughter receives one or other X chromosome from their mother.

In contrast, a male has only one X chromosome and hence only one copy of each X-linked gene (and is sometimes called hemizygous). The X chromosome remains active in every somatic cell, and so any mutant X alleles will always be expressed in a male. (The X chromosome is inactivated in the male during the prophase of first meiosis as the autosomes are undergoing recombination.) Each daughter must receive her father's X chromosome, and each son must receive his father's Y chromosome. Hence fathers cannot transmit X-linked genes to their sons.

During meiosis (Chapter 5) the X and Y chromosomes undergo synapsis only within the small pairing (pseudo-autosomal) region at the distal ends of their short arms (see Fig. 5.8, p. 51). As this region is homologous, recombination can occur between genes in the pairing region and sex-determining genes on Yp. DNA sequences which

recognize polymorphisms have been cloned from the pairing region, and those sequences which are closest to the sex determinants show partial sex linkage, while those that are the most distal show 50% recombination and therefore appear to be transmitted as autosomal sequences.

The genes on the remainder of the sex chromosomes are distributed unequally to males and females within families. This inequality produces characteristic patterns of inheritance with marked discrepancies in the numbers of affected males and females.

The pedigree pattern depends upon which sex chromosome carries the mutant gene and whether the trait is recessive or dominant. Occasionally these pedigree patterns may be mimicked by autosomal traits which show sex limitation, and the distinguishing features are summarized in Table 8.1. If the affected males of an autosomal dominant trait with sex limitation are infertile then the pedigree pattern is identical to an X-linked recessive trait where males do not reproduce. In this event the demonstration of Lyonization in carrier females is an important clue to the correct mode of inheritance.

Y-LINKED INHERITANCE (HOLANDRIC INHERITANCE)

The inheritance of the TDF provides a human example of Y-linked inheritance. Males transmit TDF (and their Y chromosome) to all of their sons, but not to their daughters. So far, no human examples of Y-linked diseases have been established.

Table 8.1 Comparison of autosomal dominant with sex limitation to X-linked recessive and dominant inheritance.

	X-linked recessive	X-linked dominant	Autosomal dominant with sex limitation
Pedigree pattern	Knight's move	Vertical	Vertical
Sex ratio	M ≫ F	2F : 1M	M > F
Male-to-male transmission	Never	Never	50% of sons affected
Male-to-female transmission	All daughters carriers	All daughters affected	< 50% of daughters affected
Female-to-female transmission	50% of daughters carriers	50% of daughters affected	< 50% of daughters affected
Male severity	Uniform	Uniform	Variable
Female severity	Mild	Variable	Variable

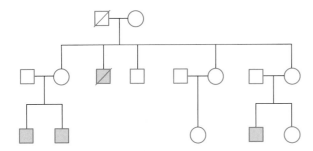

Fig. 8.1 Pedigree of a family with severe X-linked muscular dystrophy (Duchenne muscular dystrophy).

X-LINKED RECESSIVE INHERITANCE

Severe sex-linked muscular dystrophy (Duchenne muscular dystrophy) is an example of an X-linked recessive trait. This condition produces a progressive proximal muscle weakness with massive elevations of muscle enzymes in the serum including creatine kinase (CK). The onset is in early childhood, and most children are chairbound by 10 years of age and die of intercurrent infection by 20 years. Figure 8.1 shows a pedigree from an affected family. This pedigree illustrates the typical features of X-linked recessive inheritance. There is a marked discrepancy in the sex ratio, with only boys affected, and the affected boys have a similar disease course (no variation in expression). Heterozygous females are clinically unaffected (carriers) but transmit the condition to the next generation. This results in a 'knight's move' pedigree pattern of affected males. The condition is never transmitted by an unaffected male.

Figure 8.2 is a diagram of the expected proportions of affected to unaffected offspring when a carrier female marries a normal male. On average one-half of her daughters will be carriers and one-half of her sons will be affected.

The carrier female is usually clinically normal. However, because of Lyonization a proportion of her

muscle cells will have the mutant allele on the active X. These cells will release CK, and so in about two-thirds of female carriers the CK lies outside the normal range (Fig. 8.3). This is helpful in carrier detection, provided

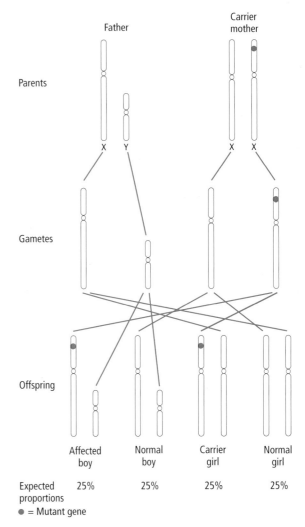

Fig. 8.2 Expected proportions of offspring for a female X-linked recessive heterozygote.

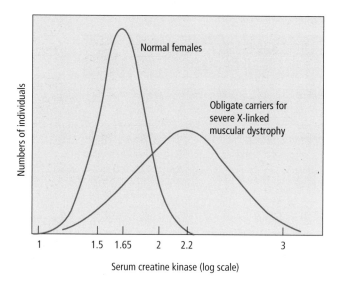

Fig. 8.3 Distribution of serum CK in normal females and obligate carriers for Duchenne muscular dystrophy.

precautions are taken to exclude other factors which can raise (exercise, intramuscular injections) or lower (pregnancy) this enzyme level. A woman with an affected child and an affected brother, or a woman with more than one affected child, is an obligate carrier, as the alternative explanation of multiple new mutations is so unlikely. For each daughter of an obligate carrier there is on average a 1 in 2 risk that she too is a carrier. CK testing may help to resolve this, and carrier detection using DNA analysis may also be helpful. Bayes' theorem is often used to combine this information about the carrier risk (Appendix 2).

Sometimes the child is the only affected individual in the family (Fig. 8.4). In this situation the mother is not an obligate carrier. In perhaps one-third of cases the child has a new mutation, whereas in the remainder the mother is a carrier (Chapter 11). CK testing may help to resolve these two possibilities, and the fact that in this example the mother has eight normal sons will diminish (but not obviate) her chance of being a carrier (Appendix 2).

Occasionally a female is affected with this X-linked form of muscular dystrophy. This might arise in a number of ways: atypical Lyonization (manifesting heterozygote); new mutation on the other X chromosome of a carrier female; a carrier with Turner syndrome (45,X); or an X–autosome translocation.

By far the commonest of these possibilities is atypical Lyonization. This arises in a female carrier when by chance inactivation of the normal X chromosome occurs in most of her muscle cells. Such a manifesting heterozygote is usually not affected to the same extent as an affected male. (This is also thought to be the mechanism for monozygotic female twins where one is affected and the other is asymptomatic.)

Theoretically a carrier female might also have a new mutation at the same locus on her other X chromosome, and she would then be as severely affected as a male. A woman with 45,X (Turner syndrome) cannot inactivate her normal X chromosome, which carries the mutant allele, and so she would be as severely affected as a male. Finally, a woman with an X–autosome translocation may be affected (Fig. 8.5). In X–autosome translocations the normal X is preferentially inactivated, as otherwise partial monosomy for the involved autosome might occur. This provided an important early clue to the localization of the gene for X-linked muscular dystrophy as in each female with muscular dystrophy due to an X–autosome translocation, the breakpoint was in the band Xp21. This resulted in damage to the gene for X-linked muscular dystrophy, with consequent expression of this abnormal gene when the normal X was inactivated.

This severe form of X-linked muscular dystrophy is called Duchenne muscular dystrophy. There is also a milder X-linked form of muscular dystrophy called Becker muscular dystrophy. These conditions are due to different mutant alleles in the gene for the protein dystrophin (multiple allelism). In about 65% of cases of X-linked muscular dystrophy, DNA analysis reveals a deletion of variable size (see Fig. 3.10, p. 30). Rarely such a deletion is visible using the light microscope (Fig. 8.6) and

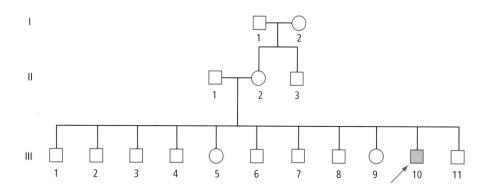

Fig. 8.4 Pedigree of a family with only one child affected by Duchenne muscular dystrophy.

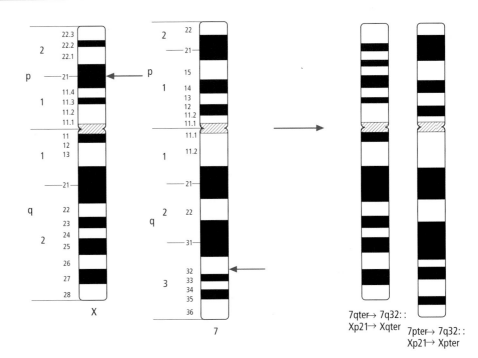

Fig. 8.5 An X–autosome translocation in a female with Duchenne muscular dystrophy [t(X;7)(p21;q32)].

occasionally other important contiguous structural genes may be included in the microdeletion. Before counselling a family with muscular dystrophy it is important to establish the precise type, as in addition to these X-linked forms, autosomal dominant and recessive forms of muscular dystrophy are known (genetic heterogeneity).

Other X-linked recessive conditions

So far 412 X-linked recessive traits are known in humans. Some of the commoner and more clinically important of these are listed in Table 8.2. The frequencies vary in different ethnic groups, for example colour blindness is rare in Eskimos, and in certain ethnic groups glucose-6-phosphate dehydrogenase deficiency is as frequent as colour blindness in the UK.

For some X-linked recessive disorders affected males may reproduce, and in this event all daughters will be carriers (obligate carriers) and all sons will be normal (Fig. 8.7).

The fragile X syndrome (p. 136) provides an important exception to the principle of consistent male severity within a family for an X-linked recessive trait. The fragile X syndrome is caused by an unstable length mutation; small length mutations may produce few or no symptoms in males or females but subsequent amplification to a larger length mutation results in mentally handicapped offspring.

Table 8.2 Human X-linked traits.

Trait	UK frequency/10 000 males
Red–green colour blindness	800
Fragile X syndrome	5
Non-specific X-linked mental retardation	5
Duchenne muscular dystrophy	3
Becker muscular dystrophy	0.5
Haemophilia A (factor VIII)	2
Haemophilia B (factor IX)	0.3
X-linked ichthyosis	2
X-linked agammaglobulinaemia	0.1

X-LINKED DOMINANT INHERITANCE

Vitamin D resistant rickets is inherited as an X-linked dominant trait and thus males and females can be affected. However, whereas in males the condition is uniformly severe, the female heterozygote is more variably affected because of Lyonization. The pedigree (Fig. 8.8) resembles that of an autosomal dominant trait but the key difference is the lack of male-to-male transmission with an X-linked dominant trait (Table 8.1).

The Xg blood group is also inherited as an X-linked dominant trait but the few other conditions which are inherited in this fashion are rare (Table 8.3). Two others deserve further mention, as in incontinentia pigmenti (p. 141) and Rett syndrome (p. 146) the affected males are

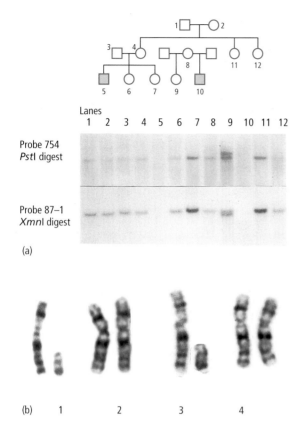

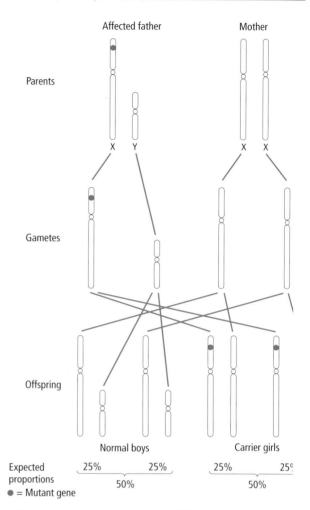

Fig. 8.6 (a) Pedigree and results of DNA analysis using an intragenic probe (87.1) for a family (GLA5099) with Duchenne muscular dystrophy. Both cousins are deleted for these probes and the obligate carriers have fragment dosage equivalent to a normal male (i.e. hemizygous). (b) Sex chromosomes from a normal male (1), a normal female (2), a deleted male (3) and a carrier mother (4) from the family shown in (a). Compare the relative intensity of the dark band Xp21 in each.

Fig. 8.7 Diagram of the expected proportions of offspring for an affected male with an X-linked recessive trait.

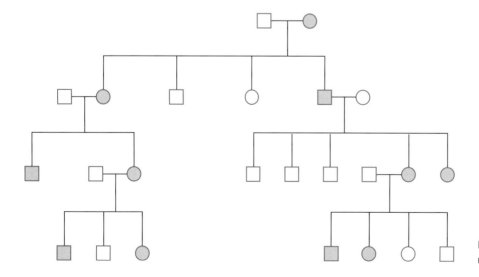

Fig. 8.8 Pedigree of a family with vitamin D resistant rickets.

Table 8.3 Examples of human X-linked dominant traits.

> Xg blood group
> Vitamin D resistant rickets
> Variant of hereditary motor and sensory neuropathy
> Incontinentia pigmenti*
> ? Rett syndrome*

* Lethal in hemizygous male.

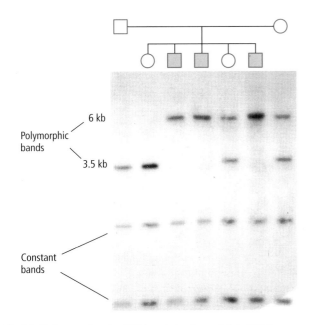

Fig. 8.9 Pedigree and results of DNA analysis using an X-linked RFLP (P20/*MspI*) in a family with X-linked congenital adrenal hypoplasia. In this and other families this marker cosegregates with the disease. Can this marker be used to clarify the carrier state of the daughters in this family? (Answer p. 215.)

believed to be so severely affected that spontaneous abortion is usual and hence only affected females are seen with these conditions.

X-LINKED CODOMINANT INHERITANCE

X-linked codominant inheritance is illustrated by the inheritance of X-linked DNA polymorphisms (Figs 3.2 & 3.3). Figure 8.9 illustrates a further example of a family studied with an X-chromosomal probe which has polymorphic fragments of 6 kb and 3.5 kb in addition to two constant bands. Males with a single X chromosome have either 6 kb (each son) or 3.5 kb (father). Females with two X chromosomes can be heterozygous 6 kb/3.5 kb (mother and one daughter), homozygous 6 kb/6 kb or homozygous 3.5 kb/3.5 kb (other daughter). This ability to distinguish equally the presence of either allele in an individual is the hallmark of codominant inheritance.

CHAPTER 9

Genomics

CONTENTS

FAMILY LINKAGE STUDIES 82
IN SITU HYBRIDIZATION 86
INTERSPECIFIC SOMATIC CELL HYBRIDIZATION 87

FLOW SORTED CHROMOSOME DOT-BLOT
   ANALYSES 90
STRUCTURE AND ORGANIZATION OF
   THE GENOME 90

Genomics includes gene mapping and nucleic acid sequencing which are complementary approaches for analysis of the structure and organization of the genome. Mapping determines the general location of genes on the chromosomes and their positions relative to each other and the full nucleotide sequence is the ultimate map. Sequencing is outlined elsewhere (p. 29) and this chapter will focus on the approaches to gene mapping and summarize the current gene map and knowledge about genomic organization.

Pedigree pattern analysis may confirm that a disorder is inherited as an autosomal or sex-linked trait and the next step is to map the gene locus to a chromosomal region. For single gene disorders with unknown pathophysiology, mapping is usually accomplished by family linkage studies.

FAMILY LINKAGE STUDIES

Two genes are linked if their loci are close together on the same chromosome. In this situation the alleles at these two loci tend to pass together rather than independently into each gamete. Thus disturbance of independent assortment (Mendel's second law, p. 4) is an important clue that the two genes are linked. If the chromosomal location of one of the genes is known, then by inference the other can be mapped to that area of the chromosome.

In a family linkage study two loci are considered, one for the disease or trait in question and another for the marker (Table 9.1). All family members are examined to determine whether or not they are affected and to assess their status with respect to the marker trait. If the disease and the marker loci are on separate chromosomes, then independent assortment will occur and the disease and marker should be found as often together as apart in the gametes and hence the offspring (Fig. 9.1). If, however, the disease and marker loci are close together on the same chromosome then independent assortment will not occur and the disease and marker will occur together in each child unless by chance they are separated by a cross-over at meiosis (Figs 9.2 & 9.3). If the disease and marker loci are far apart on the same chromosome, a cross-over between the loci is very likely: the disease and marker traits will occur separately in each recombinant but together in the non-recombinants (Fig. 9.4). So for a distant marker trait, the number of recombinants will equal the number of non-recombinants, and the recombination fraction or proportion of recombinants will be 50%, which mimics independent assortment. As the distance between the marker and disease loci *decreases*, the chance of crossing-over diminishes, the number of recombinants becomes fewer, the recombination fraction falls and the disturbance of independent assortment increases (Table 9.2). Thus the recombination fraction varies from zero (tight linkage) to 50% (equivalent to independent assortment).

Figure 9.5 shows two families affected by an autosomal dominant disorder and for each individual the result of DNA analysis for an autosomal DNA polymorphism is

Table 9.1 Polymorphic marker traits for family linkage studies.

DNA variants
Restriction fragment length polymorphisms (RFLPs)
Variable number of tandem repeats (VNTRs) (microsatellite and minisatellite repeats)

Protein variants
Blood groups, enzymes, etc.

Chromosomal variants

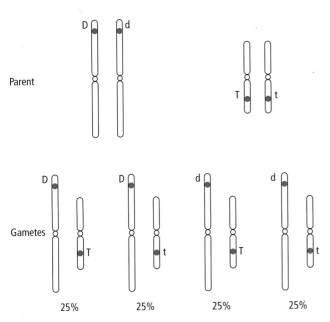

Fig. 9.1 Diagram of independent assortment at meiosis of the disease locus (disease allele D and normal allele d) and the marker locus (alleles T and t).

chance is the same as the probability of correctly calling heads or tails for nine consecutive tosses of a coin, that is $(0.5)^9 = 0.002$. However, if these two loci are linked with a recombination fraction of, say, 0.1 (10%) the probability of the disease segregating with allele 1 or the normal allele segregating with allele 2 is 0.9 for each child and the

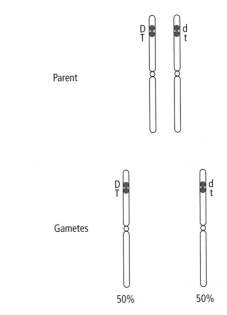

Fig. 9.2 Lack of independent assortment at meiosis for tightly linked disease locus alleles (D and d) and marker locus alleles (T and t).

shown. In family 1 the affected man in the second generation has received the disease allele together with the marker allele 1 from his father. Similarly, he has received the normal allele and the marker allele 2 from his mother. If these two loci are on the same chromosome then it follows that he must have one chromosome that carries the disease allele together with allele 1, while the other chromosome of the pair carries the normal allele and allele 2. Hence the arrangement of the disease and marker alleles (the phase) can be deduced with certainty in this individual. If the loci are linked, it should be apparent in the next generation as a tendency for the disease allele to segregate with allele 1 and the normal allele to segregate with allele 2 and this is what is observed since all four affected offspring are 1/2 while the five unaffected children are 2/2.

If the loci are not linked, the probability of such a striking departure from independent assortment occurring by

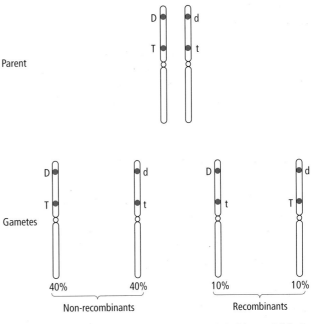

Fig. 9.3 Some independent assortment at meiosis with linked disease (alleles D and d) and marker (alleles T and t) loci.

Table 9.2 Dependence of the recombination fraction on the relative positions of two loci.

	Loci on the same chromosome			Loci on different chromosomes
	Very close	Nearby	Far apart	
Frequency of crossing-over between the two loci	Rare	Some	Frequent	—
Linkage	Present	Present	Absent	Absent
Recombination fraction	0%	1–49%	50%	50%

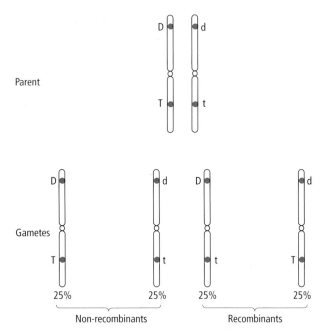

Fig. 9.4 Distant disease and marker loci on the same chromosome mimic independent assortment due to frequent cross-overs.

probability of not observing a single recombinant event in all nine children is $(0.9)^9 = 0.4$. It follows that linkage at 10% recombination is a more likely explanation for the family than no linkage: 200 times more likely, to be exact $(0.4/0.002 = 200)$. Similarly, for a recombination fraction of zero we would not expect any recombination and the probability of observing this family would be $(1.0/0.002 = 500)$. To proceed with the analysis, the logarithms of these probability ratios are calculated and referred to as lod (logarithm of odds or Z) scores. For family 1 at a recombination fraction of 10% the lod score is therefore $\log_{10}200 = 2.3$ and at a recombination fraction of zero the lod score is $\log_{10}500 = 2.7$. Proof that two loci are linked usually involves combining data from several families and before this can be done lod scores must be calculated in the same way for other possible values of the recombination fraction, as shown in Table 9.3.

Suppose a second family (family 2, Fig. 9.5) is studied, similar to the first but with only two generations. All four affected children are 1/2 and four of their five healthy siblings are 2/2. As in family 1, this signifies a marked disturbance of independent assortment and suggests linkage between the disease and marker loci, with allele 1 segregating with the disease allele. If this is the case, the youngest child must represent a recombinant since he has inherited allele 1 from his father but not the disease allele. Alternatively allele 1 could be linked to the disease allele and allele 2 with the corresponding normal gene, in which

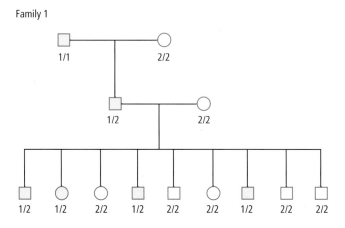

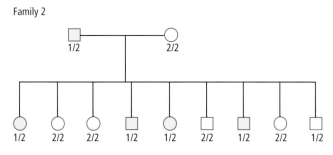

Fig. 9.5 Two families with an autosomal dominant trait showing results of DNA analysis for a DNA polymorphism with alleles 1 and 2.

Table 9.3 Lod scores at values of the recombination fraction from 0 to 40%. For the two families shown in Fig. 9.5.

Family	Recombination fraction				
	0%	10%	20%	30%	40%
Family 1	2.7	2.3	1.8	1.3	0.7
Family 2	$-\infty$	1.0	0.9	0.6	0.3
Both families	$-\infty$	3.3	2.7	1.9	1.0

case the youngest child is a non-recombinant and all his brothers and sisters represent recombinations. This is a less likely possibility but it cannot be excluded because without information about the grandparents the relationship between the disease and marker alleles in the father cannot be determined. In other words, the phase is unknown. Calculation of the lod scores for such a family is more complicated since the two possible phases must be taken into account. The results are given in Table 9.3. Whichever phase is considered, at least one recombination between disease and marker loci must have taken place, so that the possibility that the recombination fraction is zero is excluded by this family.

To combine the data from these two families, the lod scores at each recombination fraction (theta, θ) are simply added together (Table 9.3). The maximum value of the lod score ($\hat{Z}$) then corresponds to the most likely value for the recombination fraction ($\hat{\theta}$) between the two loci. In this example the maximum lod score is 3.3 at 10% recombination. The ease with which data from phase-known and phase-unknown families can be combined in this way is the reason why the use of lod scores has become almost universal for the analysis of linkage data.

The maximum value of the lod score gives a measure of the statistical significance of the result. A value greater than 3 is usually accepted as demonstrating that linkage is present and in most situations it roughly corresponds to the 5% level of significance used in conventional statistical tests. Conversely if lod scores below −2 are obtained, this indicates that linkage has been excluded at the corresponding values of the recombination fraction.

For three-generation phase-known families like family 1 and two-generation phase-unknown families like family 2 the lod scores can be calculated directly or obtained from tables. Computer programs are available to deal with more complex or extensive pedigrees and for the analysis of data involving more than two linked loci (multipoint linkage analysis). The relationship between the recombination fraction and the actual physical distance between loci depends upon several factors. A recombination fraction of 0.1 (10%) corresponds to a map distance of 10

centimorgans (100 centimorgans = 1 morgan), but with increasing distance apart the apparent recombination fraction falls due to the occurrence of double cross-overs (Fig. 9.6). Furthermore, cross-overs for autosomes are more frequent in females than males, and crossing-over frequency also varies in different parts of the chromosome and seems to be greater at the ends than near the centromere.

Thus the physical distance represented by a given recombination fraction needs to incorporate all of these factors. The total length of the haploid genome is estimated to be 3000 centimorgans, and as the DNA therein has 3×10^9 basepairs (bp), on average 1 centimorgan equals 1 megabase (Mb).

In practice it is difficult to detect linkages for loci more than 25 centimorgans apart and thus a linkage search of the genome would require over 120 (3000/25) well-spaced polymorphic markers. Many thousands of DNA polymorphisms have already been identified throughout the genome, thus providing markers for every region of each chromosome.

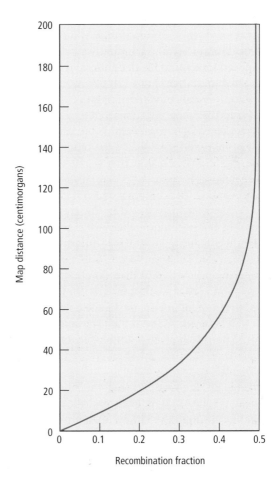

Fig. 9.6 Relationship of physical distance between two loci and the frequency of crossing-over (recombination fraction).

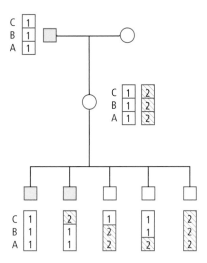

Fig. 9.7 Inheritance of three X chromosomal RFLPs (loci A, B and C with alleles 1 or 2 at each) in a family with colour blindness. Determine which marker is closest to the gene for colour blindness. (Answer p. 215.)

If three loci on the same chromosome are considered then the relative recombination fractions provide evidence for the order of the genes. Figure 9.7 illustrates the inheritance of three X chromosomal RFLPs in a family with colour blindness. The grandfather's X chromosome is transmitted intact into his daughter and the eldest son receives the grandfather's three RFLPs (and colour blindness) without evidence of recombination. The youngest son has received the grandmaternal X chromosome without evidence of recombination. Recombination has occurred at maternal meiosis for the other three sons' X chromosomes. For loci A and B only one recombination out of five meioses is apparent as compared with three out of five for A and C. This suggests that A is closer to B than it is to C. This is also supported by the three-point cross technique. In this technique alternative gene orders are tried for the offspring of a triply informative (phase-known) situation such as this. Double recombination events are much less likely than single recombinations and hence the order which results in the minimum number of recombinations is the likeliest. In this family if locus C was between A and B then the second and third sons would need to have had double recombinations and the order C, B, A is the most likely of the alternative arrangements.

If the three loci are very close together, then recombination between them is very unlikely and alleles at them will pass together through the family. Such a block of closely linked alleles is known as a haplotype and can be clinically useful in predicting the molecular pathology at the associated mutant gene due to linkage disequilibrium. Linkage disequilibrium reflects the background pattern of adjacent DNA markers at the time the original mutation occurred:

due to their proximity and hence lack of recombination they will tend to remain in association as a mutation-specific haplotype. Thus, for example there is a *Hpa*I site next to the beta-globin locus which is polymorphic (RFLP fragment sizes of 7.6 kb or 13 kb). One original mutation for sickle cell disease (p. 71) occurred in a beta-globin gene associated with the 13 kb RFLP and hence the 13 kb RFLP is much commoner amongst patients with sickle cell disease than in the general population. Extended patterns of RFLPs around the beta-globin locus are similarly associated with particular beta-globin mutations which cause beta-thalassaemia (p. 133).

Gene dosage. If a gene's protein product is known, then mapping of the locus may be possible using gene dosage. Autosomal genes are arranged in pairs, and for most loci both alleles are expressed. If two normal alleles are present for an enzyme then the activity of that enzyme will be 100%. Unbalanced autosomal chromosomal aberrations can provide information about genes carried by these chromosomes from dosage studies. If the area of the autosome which contains the enzyme locus is deleted then the residual enzyme activity will be 50%, reflecting the activity of the remaining normal allele. Conversely, if the person is trisomic for that area then the enzyme level will be 150%. By comparing enzyme levels in a variety of aberrations with different break points the location of the gene can be determined. Figure 9.8 shows how this method was used to localize two other red cell enzyme loci to particular regions of chromosome 9.

IN SITU HYBRIDIZATION

When a gene is cloned, a variety of approaches can be used to localize it to a region of a chromosome including *in situ* hybridization, interspecific somatic cell hybridization and flow sorted dot-blot analysis.

The principle of *in situ* hybridization is to use a segment of DNA to identify within the metaphase chromosomes its complementary segment. This DNA segment is labelled and made single-stranded by heating and rapid cooling. It is then applied to a standard air-dried chromosome preparation that has also been denatured. The probe anneals to its complementary sequence on the chromosome, and this is revealed by microscopy. This is now a standard method of mapping cloned DNA sequences especially with the advance of non-isotopic probe labelling which provides an experimental result in 1–2 days as compared with up to 4 weeks using radiolabelling. The non-isotopic labelling is based on the incorporation of biotin (or a similar label) into the DNA probe. The site of hybridization is detected by using an anti-biotin (or streptavidin) molecule coupled

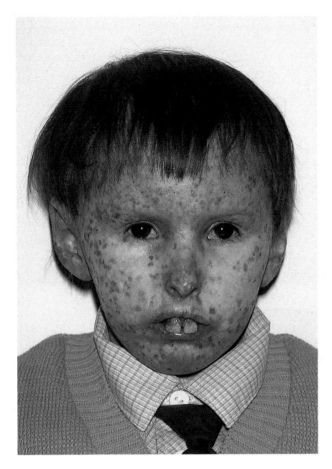

Plate 1 Patient with xeroderma pigmentosum showing multiple ultraviolet-induced skin tumours.

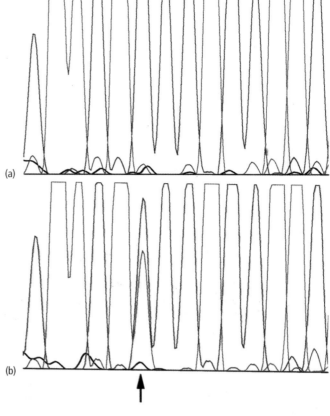

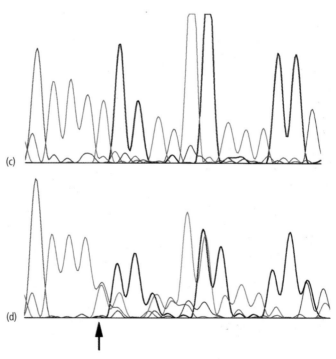

Plate 2 Examples of automated sequencing. Peaks correspond to bases with C in blue, G in black, T in red and A in green. A point substitution (of T to C) is arrowed in (b) with the corresponding normal sequence in (a). A one base (C) insertion causing a frameshift is arrowed in (d) with corresponding normal sequence shown in (c).

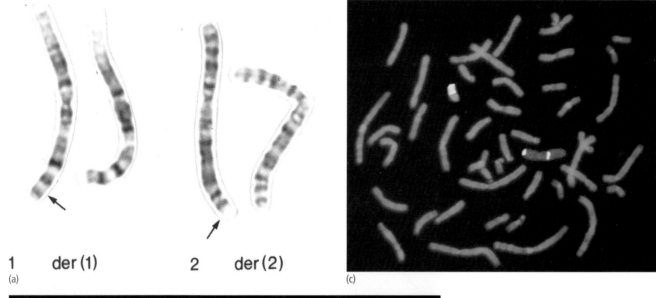

1   der (1)   2   der (2)

(a)

(c)

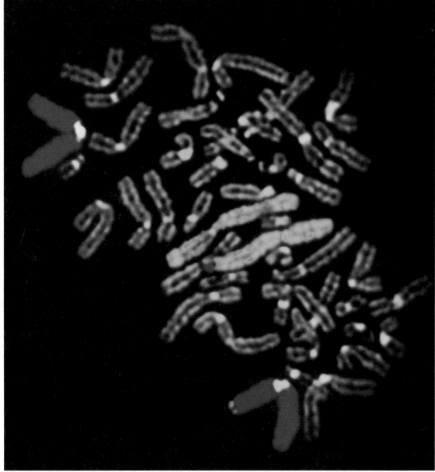

(b)

Plate 3 Examples of chromosome-specific painting. (a) A small reciprocal translocation involving the distal ends of the long arms of chromosome of chromosomes 1 and 2 is difficult to distinguish by G-banding. (b) The same translocation revealed by hybridization with chromosome 1 specific paint (red) and chromosome 2 specific paint (green). (c) The use of X and Y specific chromosome paints to reveal regions of XY homology (yellow) in the sex chromosomes. Specific regions are labelled green and X specific regions are red.

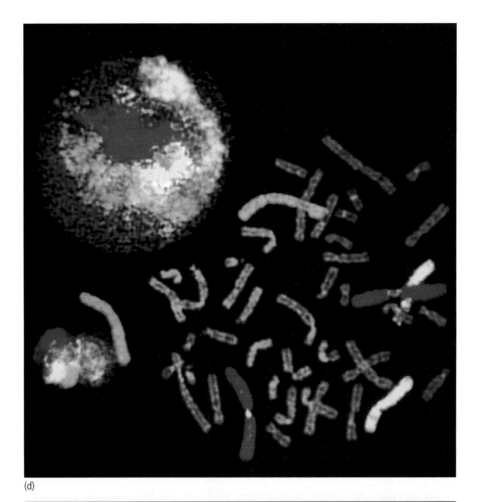

(d)

Plate 3 *Continued.* (d) Example of 3-colour forward chromosome painting. Chromosome 1 (red), chromosome 2 (green) and chromosome 6 (yellow). (e) Karyotype of coloured 'bar code' prepared from Alu-PCR amplification of interspecific somatic cell hybrids containing fragments of normal human chromosomes. Hybrids have been selected to provide adequate coverage and the amplified PCR products separated into two groups for labelling with FITC (green) and Cy-3 (red) respectively. Coincident sequences appear yellow against a blue DAP1 chromosome counterstain. This technique has application in the analysis of intrachromosomal rearrangements (Courtesy of S. Mueller).

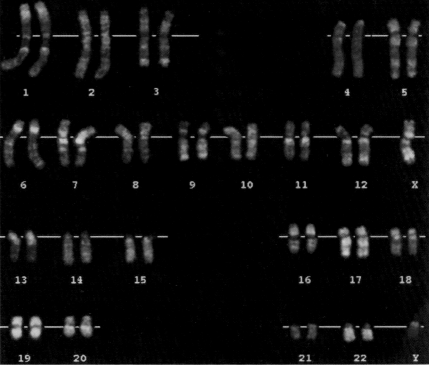

(e)

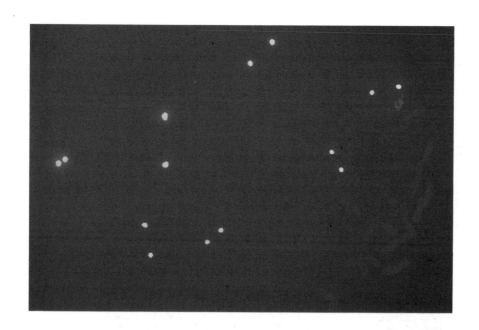

Plate 4 Identification of chromosomes 18 and the X in metaphase and interphase using FISH. Biotinylated alphoid centromeric repeat probes are detected with FITC (chromosome 18) and Texas red (X chromosome), counterstained by propidium iodide. Karyotype 46, XY.

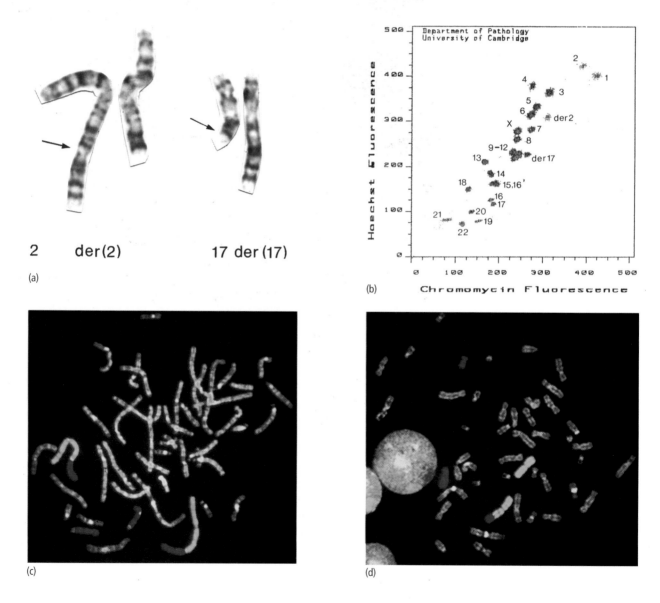

(a)

2   der(2)   17 der(17)

(b)

Department of Pathology
University of Cambridge

500

400

Hoechst Fluorescence

300

200

100

0

0   100   200   300   400   500
Chromomycin Fluorescence

2
1
4
3
5
6
X   der2
7
8
9–12
13   der17
14
18   15.16
16
17
21   20
22   19

(c)

(d)

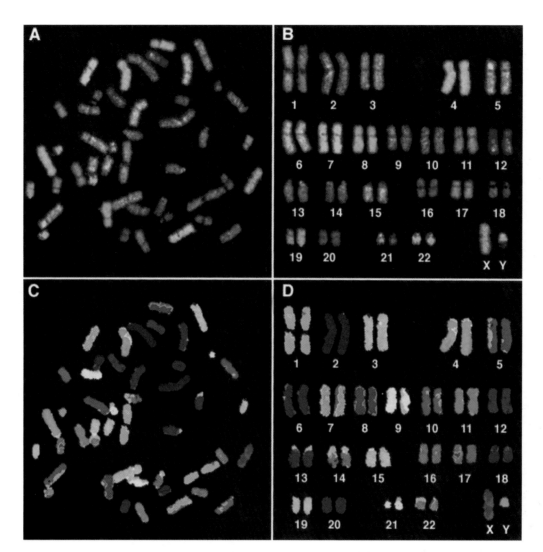

Plate 6 Multicolour FISH using a paint probe composed of a combination of all 24 chromosome-specific probes, each labelled with a different combination of 5 fluorochromes and analysed by spectral imaging (Reprinted with permission from Schröck *et al*, *Science*, 1996; **273**: 494–497. Copyright 1996 American Association for the Advancement of Science.)

Plate 5 *Facing page*. Reverse painting in the analysis of a 46,XX,t(2;17)(q31;q25) translocation. (a) G banded preparation showing chromosomes 2 and 17 and their derivatives from a balanced translocation carrier. (b) Flow karyotype showing the positions of the two derivative chromosomes from which paint probes were prepared following chromosome sorting and amplification. (c) The der 2 probe (green) and the der 17 probe (red) hybridized to a normal male metaphase to confirm the origin and breakpoints of the translocation. (d) The same der 2 and der 17 paints hybridized to a metaphase from the balanced translocation carrier.

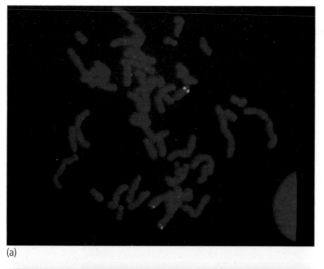

(a)

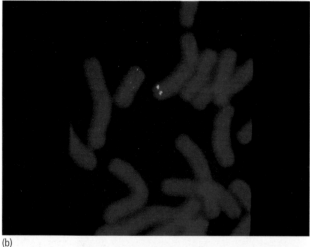

(b)

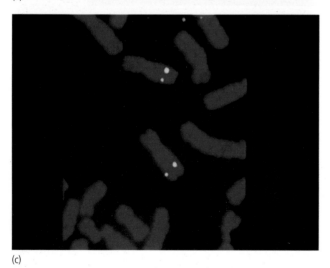

(c)

Plate 7 Metaphase mapping using cosmid or plasmid vectors containing inserts of specific genes which map to 9q. Biotinylated probes detected by FITC, counterstained with propidium iodide. (a) Alphafodrin sequence cloned in a cosmid vector. (b) Adenylate kinase 1 sequence cloned in a plasmid vector. (c) Orosomucoid gene sequence cloned in a cosmid vector. Note ascending order of loci from telomere to centromere.

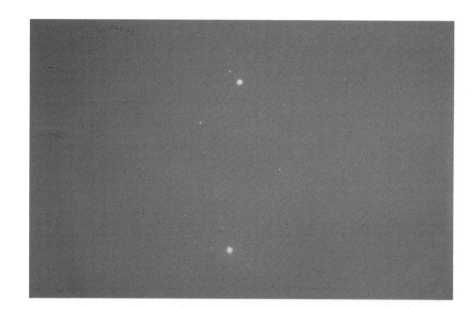

Plate 8 Ordering three sequences on 9q using interphase mapping and cosmid clones. Alphafodrin (green) is distal to adenylate kinase 1 (red) relative to orosomucoid (red) in both chromosomes 9 in an interphase fibroblast nucleus.

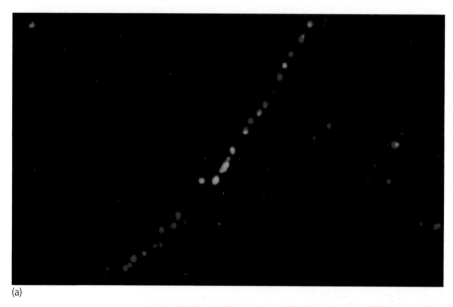

(a)

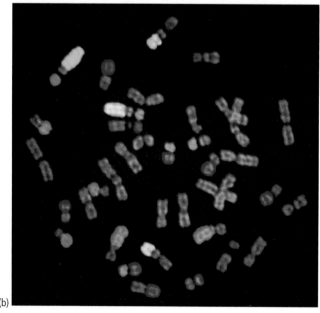

(b)

Plate 9 (a) Extended DNA fibre hybridized with 3 cosmids from the MHC locus. Each cosmid is about 35–40 kilobases (kb). The Texas red-labelled cosmid is separated from the FITC-labelled cosmid by a gap of approximately 10 kb. The third cosmid is labelled with a mixture of Texas red and FITC (Courtesy of M. Leversha). (b) Metaphase from a gibbon (*Hylobates hoolock*) hybridized with human paint probes from chromosomes 1 (red), 2 (green) and 6 (yellow) as shown in Plate 3(d). Note that 5 pairs of gibbon chromosomes contain blocks homologous to human chromosome 1. Similarly, human chromosome 2 is homologous to parts of another 5 pairs of gibbon chromosomes and human chromosome 6 is homologous to parts of 2 pairs of gibbon chromosomes (Courtesy of F. Yang).

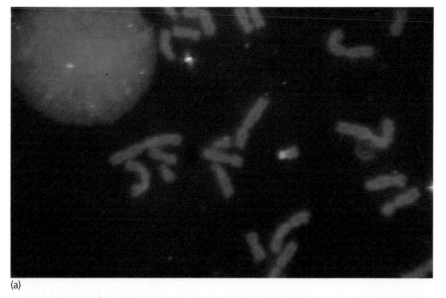

(a)

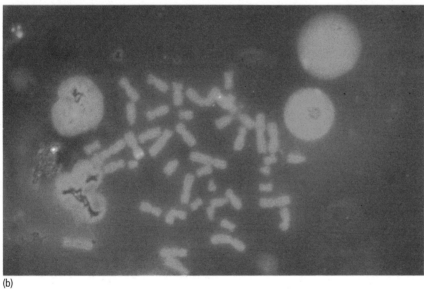

(b)

Plate 10 X–Y interchange demonstrated by *in situ* hybridization. Biotinylated Y probe is labelled with peroxidase-coupled antibody and examined by reflectance contrast microscopy. (a) Normal male control. Y-specific probe (GMG Y10) maps to Y short arm. (b) XX male. Y-specific probe hybridizes to tip of short arm of one of the two X chromosomes, indicating accidental recombination in paternal meiosis between differential part of the Y and the X.

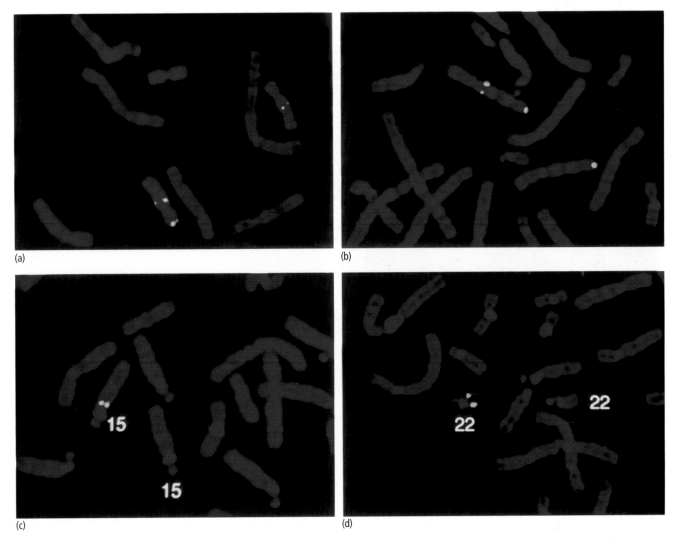

Plate 11 Examples of microdeletion detection using cosmid probes from loci within each microdeletion. In each case, the deletion is identified by the absence of the specific signal which is seen in the normal homologue, and the specific chromosome identified by another chromosome-specific probe (a and b).

(a) Miller–Dieker lissencephaly syndrome, with microdeletion in 17p13. (b) Williams syndrome with deletion at the elastin locus on 7q11. (c) Prader–Willi syndrome with deletion in 15q12. (d) DiGeorge syndrome with deletion in 22q11.

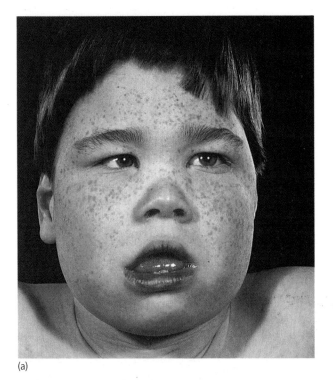

(a)

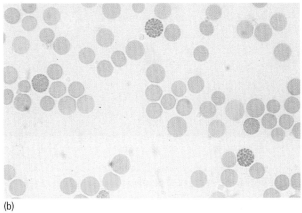

(b)

Plate 12 (a) Facies in the alpha-thalassaemia/mental handicap syndrome. (b) HbH inclusions in an affected boy.

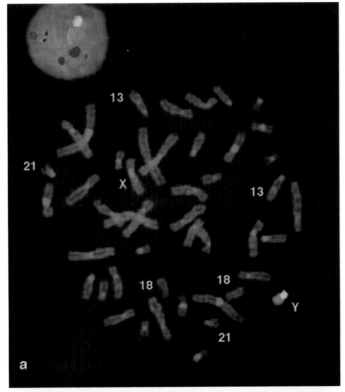

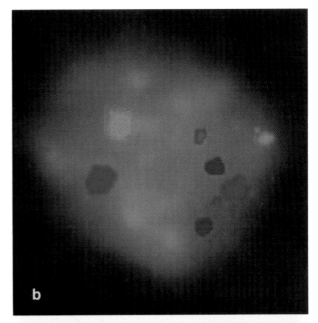

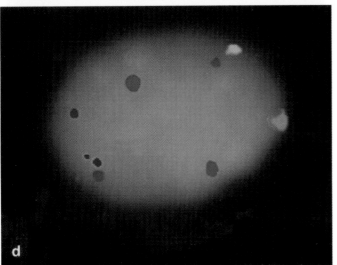

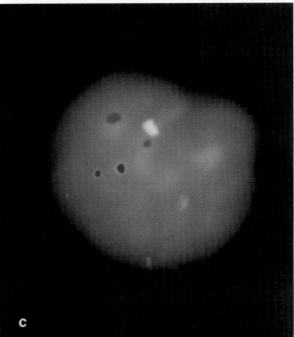

Plate 13 Use of multicolour FISH probes to determine chromosome copy number in interphase nuclei. (a) Lymphocyte metaphase and interphase nuclei showing centromeric probes for X chromosome (lilac), Y chromosome (yellow) and chromosome 18 (dark blue); a YAC clone marks chromosome 13q (green) and a contig of two overlapping cosmid clones marks chromosome 21 (red).

(b) Uncultured amniotic fluid cell nucleus from a female fetus hybridized with the above probes reveals a normal number of each chromosome. (c) As above, from a normal male fetus. (d) As above, from a male fetus with trisomy 21 (Down syndrome) (from Divane *et al*, *Prenatal Diagnosis*, 1994; 14: 1061–1069).

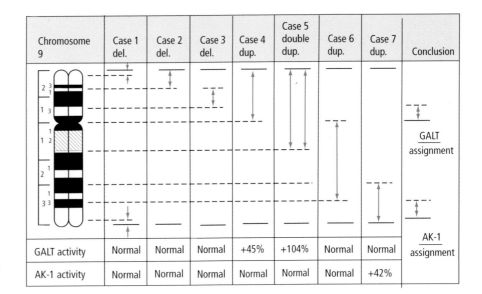

Chromosome 9	Case 1 del.	Case 2 del.	Case 3 del.	Case 4 dup.	Case 5 double dup.	Case 6 dup.	Case 7 dup.	Conclusion
GALT activity	Normal	Normal	Normal	+45%	+104%	Normal	Normal	GALT assignment
AK-1 activity	Normal	Normal	Normal	Normal	Normal	Normal	+42%	AK-1 assignment

Fig. 9.8 Application of gene dosage to localize galactose-1-phosphate uridyltransferase (GALT) and adenylate kinase-1 (AK-1) to particular areas of chromosome 9.

to a fluorescent dye. This can be examined by fluorescence microscopy (Plate 7). Using several different labels, each detected by a different fluorescent dye, it is possible to study several probes simultaneously and so order a series of loci along a metaphase chromosome. Sequences hybridized to chromosomes must be more than 1 Mb apart to be resolved by this method. Greater resolution can be achieved by exploiting the extended chromosomes in interphase nuclei (Plate 8) and it is possible to resolve probes as little as 50–100 kb apart in such preparations.

Even greater resolution can be achieved using techniques which release the chromatin fibre from its protein scaffold. This permits DNA probes to be hybridized directly onto greatly extended fibres fixed on a microscope slide and analysed by FISH. Sequences less than 10 kb apart can be resolved readily (Plate 9a), and distances less than 1 kb have been claimed.

INTERSPECIFIC SOMATIC CELL HYBRIDIZATION

A somatic cell hybrid is produced by fusing two somatic cells which are established in cell culture in the presence or absence of inactivated viruses, such as Sendai, or by some chemical agents. For gene mapping one cell is of human origin and one of a different species, for example a mouse. Initially such a hybrid will have a double chromosome complement, with both human and mouse chromosomes. The human chromosomes are selectively, but randomly, lost, rapidly at first and then more gradually. Mouse and human chromosomes can be distinguished on the basis of their different morphology, and by staining with Giemsa at alkaline pH, when the mouse chromo-

somes are bright purple whereas the remaining human chromosomes are pale blue.

If, for example, the mouse parent line used in the hybrid is homozygous for thymidine kinase deficiency, the presence of this enzyme in a hybrid cell indicates that the human chromosome which produces this enzyme is present in that cell. By studying a selection of hybrids in this way it was possible to correlate the presence of thymidine kinase activity with the presence of human chromosome 17. Thus the locus for thymidine kinase was assigned to chromosome 17.

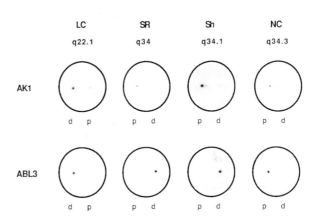

Fig. 9.9 Ordering of adenylate kinase-1 and Abelson oncogene loci using dot-blots of flow sorted translocation chromosomes with break points in 9q as shown: d, derivative 9 translocation in which *distal* long arm is present; p, derivative 9 translocation in which *proximal* long arm is present. Which locus is distal? (Answer p. 215.)

AAC2	8	Arylamine *N*-acetyltransferase 2		*HRAS*	11	Harvey rat sarcoma v-Ha-*ras* oncogene homologue
ABL1	9	Abelson murine leukaemia v-*abl* oncogene homologue 1		*IGH*	14	Immunoglobulin heavy chain gene cluster
ABO	9	ABO blood group		*IGK*	2	Gene (cluster) for kappa light chain
AD1	21	Alzheimer disease, one type		*IGLC*	22	Gene (cluster) for lambda light chain
ALD	X	Adrenoleucodystrophy		*INS*	11	Insulin
ADA	20	Adenosine deaminase		*INT1*	12	Murine mammary tumour virus integration site (v-*int*-1) oncogene homologue
APC	5	Familial adenomatous polyposis				
APOA1	11	Apolipoprotein A-I		*KRAS1*	6	Kirsten rat sarcoma v-Ki-*ras*-1 oncogene homologue
APOB	2	Apolipoprotein B		*KRAS2*	12	Kirsten rat sarcoma v-Ki-*ras*-2 oncogene homologue
APOE	19	Apolipoprotein E		*LDLR*	19	Low density lipoprotein receptor/familial hypercholesterolaemia
APP	21	Amyloid beta (A4) precursor protein		*MEN1*	11	Multiple endocrine neoplasia type 1
APY	11	Atopy		*MEN2*	10	Multiple endocrine neoplasia type 2
ATRX	X	Alpha-thalassaemia/mental retardation syndrome, X-linked		*MET*	7	*MET* proto-oncogene
ATA	11	Ataxia telangiectasia		*MLH1*	3	Hereditary non-polyposis colon cancer
AR	X	Androgen receptor		*MODY*	7	Maturity onset diabetes of the young
BCP	7	Blue cone pigment		*MOS*	8	Moloney murine sarcoma v-*mos* oncogene homologue
BCR	22	Break point cluster region		*MSH2*	2	Hereditary non-polyposis colon cancer
BMD	X	Becker muscular dystrophy		*MYB*	6	Avian myeloblastosis v-*myb* oncogene homologue
BRCA1	17	Breast cancer 1, early-onset		*MYC*	8	Avian myelocytomatosis v-*myc* oncogene homologue
BRCA2	13	Hereditary breast cancer		*NF1*	17	Neurofibromatosis type I
CFTR	7	Cystic fibrosis transmembrane conductance regulator		*NF2*	22	Neurofibromatosis type 2
COL1A1	17	Collagen type I, alpha-1 chain		*NRAS*	1	Neuroblastoma v-*ras* oncogene homologue
COL1A2	7	Collagen type I, alpha-2 chain/osteogenesis imperfecta		*OTC*	X	Ornithine transcarbamylase
COL2A1	12	Collagen type II, alpha-1 chain		*P*	15	Type II oculocutaneous albinism
CYP21	6	Congenital adrenal hyperplasia		*PAH*	12	Phenylalanine hydroxylase/phenylketonuria
CYP2D@	22	Debrisoquine/sparteine polymorphism		*PKD1*	16	Adult polycystic kidney disease
DM	19	Myotonic dystrophy		*PBGD*	11	Porphobilinogen deaminase
DMD	X	Duchenne muscular dystrophy		*PI*	14	Alpha-1-antitrypsin
ERV1	18	Endogenous retroviral sequence 1		*PMP22*	17	Hereditary motor and sensory neuropathy type I
F8C	X	Clotting factor VIII		*PS1*	14	Alzheimer disease, early onset type
F9	X	Clotting factor IX		*RAF1*	3	Murine leukaemia v-*raf*-1 oncogene homologue
FBN1	15	Fibrillin 1/Marfan syndrome		*RB1*	13	Retinoblastoma
FES	15	Feline sarcoma v-*fes* oncogene homologue		*RCP*	X	Red cone pigment (protan colour blindness)
FGFR3	4	Fibroblast growth factor receptor 3		*RH*	1	Rhesus blood group
FGFR2	10	Fibroblast growth factor receptor 2		*RN5S*	1	RNA, 5S
FMS	5	McDonough feline sarcoma v-*fms* oncogene homologue		*RNR*	13–15, 21, 22	Ribosomal RNA
FOS	14	Murine FBJ osteosarcoma v-*fos* oncogene homologue		*RP*	X	X-linked retinitis pigmentosa
FRAXA	X	Fragile X syndrome		*SCA1*	6	Spinocerebellar ataxia, type 1
FRDA	9	Freidreich's ataxia		*SMA*	5	Type 1 Spinal muscular atrophy
FSHD	4	Facioscapulohumeral muscular dystrophy		*SRC*	20	Avian sarcoma v-*src* oncogene homologue
GBA	1	Beta-glucosidase/Gaucher's disease		*TCOF1*	5	Treacher Collins syndrome
GALT	9	Galactosaemia		*TCRA*	14	T-cell receptor alpha polypeptide
G6PD	X	Glucose-6-phosphate dehydrogenase		*TRCB*	7	T-cell receptor beta polypeptide
GCP	X	Green cone pigment (deutan colour blindness)		*TDF*	Y	Testis determining factor
GH1	17	Growth hormone		*TP53*	17	Tumour protein p53
GUSB	7	Beta-glucuronidase		*TSC1*	9	Tuberous sclerosis type 1
HBAC@	16	Haemoglobin alpha globin cluster		*TSC2*	16	Tuberous sclerosis type 2
HBBC@	11	Haemoglobin non-alpha globin cluster		*TYR*	11	Tyrosinase
HD	4	Huntington disease		*VHL*	3	von Hippel–Lindau disease
HEXA	15	Hexosaminidase A		*VWF*	12	Von Willebrand factor/disease
HEXB	5	Hexosaminidase B		*WAGR*	11	Wilm's tumour/aniridia/syndrome
HFE	6	Haemochromatosis		*WND*	13	Wilson disease
HLA	6	Human leucocyte antigens		*WS1*	2	Waardenburg syndrome, one type
HOCM1	14	Hypertrophic obstructive cardiomyopathy		*XG*	X	Xg blood group
HPRT	X	Hypoxanthine-guanine phosphoribosyl transferase				

Fig. 9.10 (*and facing page*). Some of the more important assignments to the human gene map.

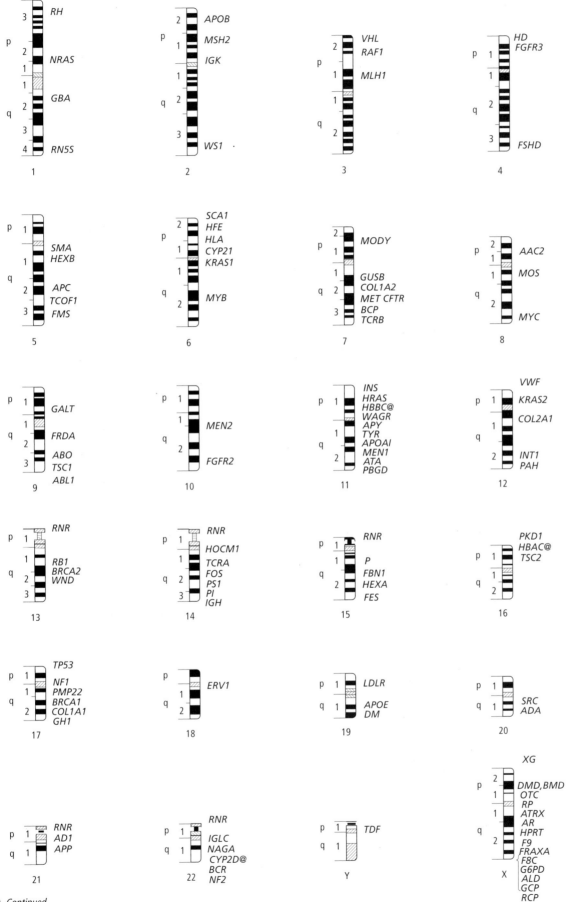

Fig. 9.10 Continued.

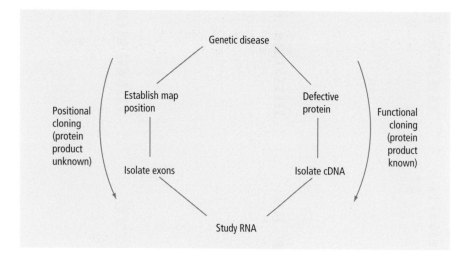

Fig. 9.11 Gene cloning strategies.

FLOW SORTED CHROMOSOME DOT-BLOT ANALYSES

The FACS can not only resolve metaphase chromosomes into a flow karyotype (p. 37) but is also capable of sorting specific chromosomes, or groups of chromosomes, into separate tubes. The sorted chromosomes can then be used for making chromosome-specific genomic DNA libraries, or used for gene mapping. Mapping a DNA sequence by FACS is most readily accomplished by sorting approximately 10 000 chromosomes for each chromosome pair directly onto a nitrocellulose filter. The filters are then denatured and the radiolabelled probe in question is hybridized to the complete filter set. The chromosome location of the probe is determined by autoradiography. Once this is done, the regional location of the probe can be determined by using dot-blots from sorted translocations. Figure 9.9 shows a series of dot-blots in which the two derivative translocation chromosomes from each of four chromosome 9 translocations have been sorted on a separate filter. The four filters have been probed successively with sequences from the adenylate kinase-1 and Abelson oncogene loci. The translocation breakpoints in 9q have been used to determine the regional location and order of the two genes on this chromosome.

STRUCTURE AND ORGANIZATION OF THE GENOME

There are an estimated 60 000–70 000 structural genes encoded in human DNA. Each structural gene usually has only one copy in the haploid genome and these single copy genes and their related regulatory sequences account for 70% of the total DNA (which would predict an average gene size of 30 kb). The remaining 30% of DNA is repeti-tive tandem and interspersed repeats and has no proven function (see Table 2.1, p. 11). The structural genes do not appear to be evenly distributed throughout the genome. CpG islands (p. 14) which are associated with most house-keeping genes and about 40% of tissue-specific genes are more common towards the telomeres, in Giemsa-negative bands and on certain chromosomes (1, 9, 15, 16, 17, 19, 20 and 22). From the genes already mapped, chromosomes 17 and 19 appear to have the highest density and 13 and 18 the lowest.

The clustering of structural genes in part reflects ancestral small duplications with subsequent divergence of function. In this process, some genes become non-functional pseudogenes (e.g. beta-globin cluster), some retain similar functions (e.g. red–green colour vision genes) and some develop novel functions. In contrast, the loci for genes of sequential steps in a metabolic pathway tend to be scattered as are the loci for subunits of complex proteins and the loci for mitochondrial and soluble forms of the same enzyme. Figure 9.10 shows a partial gene map which includes genes of particular relevance to clinical genetics practice.

If a gene's protein product is known, the gene can be cloned by functional cloning (Fig. 9.11). The protein is iso-lated and its partial sequence of amino acids determined. This then allows synthesis of a series of oligonucleotide probes based on the genetic code (Table 2.3) which can be used to identify the complementary gene from a DNA library.

If the gene's protein product is unknown, the gene can be cloned by positional cloning. The first step is to chro-mosomally map the gene and then to identify candidate genes from that region. The correct candidate is then iden-tified by mutational analysis in patients with the disease trait.

C H A P T E R   10

Non-Mendelian Inheritance

CONTENTS

MULTIFACTORIAL DISORDERS 91
TWIN CONCORDANCE STUDIES 91
Determination of concordance 92
Results of twin studies 92
FAMILY CORRELATION STUDIES 93

CONTINUOUS MULTIFACTORIAL TRAITS 93
DISCONTINUOUS MULTIFACTORIAL TRAITS 95
ANALYSIS OF MULTIFACTORIAL TRAITS 96
SOMATIC CELL GENETIC DISORDERS 96
MITOCHONDRIAL DISORDERS 97

In addition to chromosomal disorders (Chapter 6) and single gene (Mendelian) disorders (Chapters 7 & 8), there are three further subgroups of genetic disease, namely multifactorial disorders, somatic cell genetic disorders and mitochondrial disorders.

MULTIFACTORIAL DISORDERS

Multifactorial (or part-genetic) traits may be discontinuous (with distinct phenotypes, e.g. diabetes mellitus) or continuous (with a lack of distinct phenotypes, e.g. height), but in each the trait is determined by the interaction of a number of genes at different loci, each with a small but additive effect, together with environmental factors. For discontinuous multifactorial traits the risk within affected families is raised above the general population risk but the risk within an affected family is low in comparison to Mendelian traits, and rapidly falls towards the general population risk in more distant relatives. Thus, in practice the proband with a discontinuous multifactorial trait is often the only affected person in that family.

Thus, in contrast to Mendelian disorders, pedigree analysis cannot prove multifactorial inheritance and studies of twin concordance and family correlation are necessary.

TWIN CONCORDANCE STUDIES

Twins may be identical (monozygotic) or non-identical (dizygotic). Monozygotic twins are genetically identical as they arise from a single zygote which divides into two embryos during the first 13 days of gestation before the primitive streak forms. Monozygotic twinning has no known predisposing factors and occurs with a frequency of 3–4/1000 births in all populations. Dizygotic twins result from two ova fertilized by two spermatozoa and so have, on average, one-half of their genes in common and are genetically equivalent to brothers and sisters (sibs). The frequency of dizygotic twinning is increased with increasing maternal age, with increased parity, by a positive family history of twins and is associated with tall heavy build in the mother. The frequency of dizygotic twins is low in Japan and Asia at 2–7/1000 births and high in Black Africa at 45–50/1000 births (9–20/1000 in Europe and 7–12/1000 in the USA).

For research purposes, the diagnosis of zygosity cannot be based solely upon a similar appearance and a record of the nature of the placental membranes may be extremely useful. All dizygotic twins have two amniotic sacs and two chorions. The chorions may secondarily fuse, but the circulations of each part of the placenta normally remain separate. The nature of the membranes for monozygotic twins depends upon the timing of separation. In 75% of monozygotic twins there is a single chorion with a common placental circulation—this is diagnostic of monozygosity. In the remaining 25% two chorions are found, and these cannot be distinguished from dizygotic twins by examination of placental membranes (Fig. 10.1) and DNA fingerprinting will be required (p. 26).

Determination of concordance

Twins are concordant if they both show a discontinuous trait, and discordant if only one shows the trait. There is a tendency to report concordant rather than discordant twin pairs in the medical literature, and this bias needs to be considered in the interpretation of twin studies. For continuous traits the extent of the trait, for example height, is directly compared between the twins. As twins usually share a similar family environment it may be difficult to separate the relative extent of environmental (nurture) and genetic (nature) contributions to a multifactorial trait. In this respect the concordance of monozygotic twins who have been adopted and reared apart from infancy is of major importance.

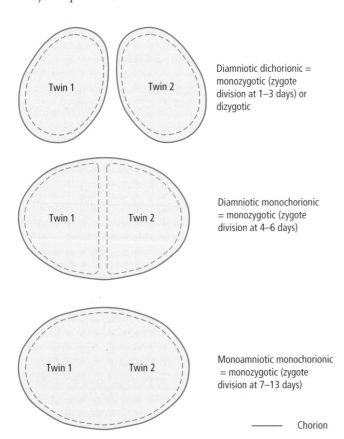

Diamniotic dichorionic = monozygotic (zygote division at 1–3 days) or dizygotic

Diamniotic monochorionic = monozygotic (zygote division at 4–6 days)

Monoamniotic monochorionic = monozygotic (zygote division at 7–13 days)

——— Chorion

– – – – Amnion

Fig. 10.1 Diagnosis of zygosity from the appearance of the placental membranes.

Results of twin studies

Monozygotic twins have identical genotypes whereas dizygotic twins are only as alike as sibs (brothers and sisters). If a condition has no genetic component, for example accidental injury, concordance rates are similar for both types of twins. For a single gene trait or a chromosomal disorder the monozygotic concordance rate will be 100%, whereas the dizygotic rate will be less than this and equal to the rate in siblings. For discontinuous multifactorial traits with both genetic and environmental contributions the rate in monozygotic twins, although less than 100%, will exceed the rate in dizygotic twins (Table 10.1).

Tables 10.2 and 10.3 list the findings in twins for some continuous traits, congenital malformations and common adult disorders. In each multifactorial trait the concordance rate in monozygotic twins exceeds that in the dizygotic twins, although the actual concordance rate in the monozygotic twins ranges from 6% to 100%. This range reflects the heritability of the condition: the higher the monozygotic concordance the more important the genetic contribution and so the higher the heritability.

Table 10.1 Concordance rates in twins.

Disorder	Concordance	
	Monozygotic	Dizygotic
Single-gene	100%	As sibs
Chromosomal	100%	As sibs
Multifactorial	<100% but >sibs	As sibs
Somatic cell genetic	As sibs	As sibs
Mitochondrial	100%	100%
Non-genetic	As sibs	As sibs

Table 10.2 Degree of similarity of twins for continuous traits.

Trait	Degree of similarity	
	Monozygotic (%)	Dizygotic (%)
Height	95	52
IQ	90	60
Finger ridge count	95	49
Diastolic blood pressure	50	27

Table 10.3 Twin concordance for some discontinuous traits.

Trait	Concordance	
	Monozygotic (%)	Dizygotic (%)
Atopic disease	50	4
Cancer	17	11
Cleft lip ± cleft palate	35	5
Cleft palate alone	26	6
Congenital dislocation of the hip	41	3
Diabetes mellitus (insulin-dependent)	30–40	6
Diabetes mellitus (non-insulin-dependent)	100	10
Epilepsy	37	10
Gallstones	27	6
Hypertension	30	10
Hyperthyroidism	47	3
Ischaemic heart disease	19	8
Leprosy	60	20
Manic depression	70	15
Mental handicap, IQ < 50	60	3
Multiple sclerosis	20–30	6
Psoriasis	61	13
Pyloric stenosis	15	2
Rheumatoid arthritis	30	5
Sarcoidosis	50	8
Schizophrenia	45	12
Senile dementia	42	5
Spina bifida	6	3
Talipes equinovarus	32	3
Tuberculosis	87	26

Table 10.4 Proportion of genes shared by relatives.

Degree of relationship	Examples	Proportion of genes in common
First	Parent to child, sib to sib	$1/2$
Second	Grandparent to grandchild, nephew or niece to aunt or uncle	$1/4$
Third	First cousins	$1/8$

FAMILY CORRELATION STUDIES

Relatives share a proportion of their genes (Table 10.4). Thus, if a trait is determined by multifactorial inheritance, relatives should show the trait in proportion to their genetic similarity. This is really only an extension of the twin study technique, and the similarity of different relatives in this respect is known as their correlation. This is measured on a scale of 0–1, where 1 is identical. The more

Table 10.5 Family correlations for some continuous traits.

Trait	Correlation of first-degree relatives	
	Observed	Expected
Height	0.53	0.5
IQ	0.41	0.5
Finger ridge count	0.49	0.5
Diastolic blood pressure	0.18	0.5

closely related the relatives, the higher the correlation should be for a genetically determined trait.

If parents are not blood relatives then they would be expected to be as alike genetically as random members of the population. Thus their correlation for genetically determined traits should be only equal to the general population average. In practice, many slightly exceed this as a result of selective mating for such characteristics as height and intelligence (assortative mating).

Table 10.5 shows the familial correlations for several continuous multifactorial traits. Height, intelligence and total fingertip ridge count provide close family correlations to those predicted from the proportion of genes in common. Table 10.6 shows the frequency of some discontinuous traits in relatives of an affected person. The frequency falls off in proportion to the proportion of genes in common, but is increased in all relatives above the general population frequency.

Hence twin concordance and family correlation studies can provide support for multifactorial inheritance of a trait, whether discontinuous or continuous. Also, the observed frequencies in relatives provide the basis for genetic counselling for multifactorial disorders (empiric risks).

CONTINUOUS MULTIFACTORIAL TRAITS

Many normal human characteristics are determined as continuous multifactorial traits (Table 10.7). These traits by definition have a continuously graded distribution. Thus for height there is a range from the very tall to the markedly short with the mean in English men of 169 cm and a standard deviation of 6.5 cm (Fig. 10.2). As can be seen, the distribution of height in a population is Gaussian, with the majority of individuals centred around the mean. Such a distribution is characteristic (but not diagnostic) of a continuous multifactorial trait.

The interaction of a number of loci to produce such a gradual range can be readily appreciated from the range

Table 10.6 Frequency of discontinuous traits for differing degrees of relationship.

Trait	Frequency (%)			
	First-degree relatives	Second-degree relatives	Third-degree relatives	Population frequency
Cleft lip	4	0.6	0.3	0.1
Spina bifida/anencephaly	4	1.5	0.6	0.3
Pyloric stenosis	2	1	0.4	0.3
Epilepsy	5	2.5	1.5	1
Schizophrenia	10	4	2	1
Manic depression	15	5	3.5	1

Table 10.7 Examples of human continuous multifactorial traits.

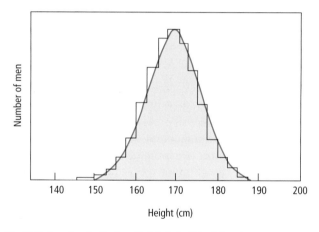

Height	Red cell size
Weight	Blood pressure
Intelligence	Skin colour
Total ridge count	

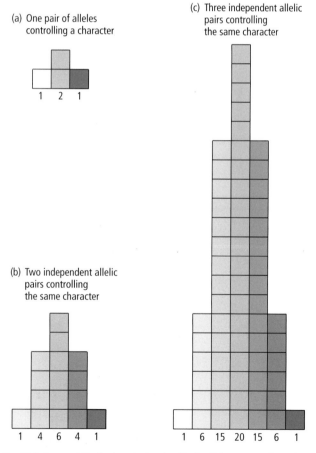

(a) One pair of alleles controlling a character

(b) Two independent allelic pairs controlling the same character

(c) Three independent allelic pairs controlling the same character

Fig. 10.3 Expected distribution of colour in offspring if the trait was due to (a) a single locus with two alleles, (b) two loci each with two alleles and (c) three loci each with two alleles. Note the approach towards a Gaussian distribution.

Fig. 10.2 Gaussian distribution of height in English adult males.

towards the mean. This also operates at the lower end of the normal range of height and tends to be most obvious in families where the degree of parental deviation is extreme.

of shade produced by the interaction of pairs of alleles at one, two and three hypothetical loci for skin colour (Fig. 10.3). Thus relatively small numbers of loci could account for a continuous distribution.

Parents of above average height tend to have children who are taller than average but who are not quite as tall as themselves. As a child only receives half of each parent's genes, the expected correlation to the mid-parents' height would be 0.71 ($\sqrt{0.5}$) if height depended only upon genetic factors. However, environmental factors are also important and as the same combination of environmental and genetic factors which operated for each parent is unlikely to occur in the child, this results in a tendency to regress

DISCONTINUOUS MULTIFACTORIAL TRAITS

More than 20 discontinuous multifactorial traits have been described and Table 10.8 lists some of the commoner discontinuous multifactorial traits which are of medical importance. Broadly, these traits can be divided into congenital malformations and common conditions of adult life.

Cleft lip and palate is a congenital malformation which is inherited as a multifactorial trait (Fig. 10.4). In the mildest form the lip alone is unilaterally cleft, whereas in the most severe form the lip is bilaterally cleft and the palatal cleft is complete. The parents of the child in Fig. 10.4 were unaffected and there was no family history of cleft lip and palate but by virtue of having produced an affected child this indicates that each parent must have

Table 10.8 Discontinuous human multifactorial traits.

Congenital malformations
Cleft lip and palate
Congenital heart disease
Neural tube defect
Pyloric stenosis

Common adult diseases
Rheumatoid arthritis
Epilepsy
Schizophrenia
Manic depression
Multiple sclerosis
Diabetes mellitus
Premature vascular disease
Hyperthyroidism

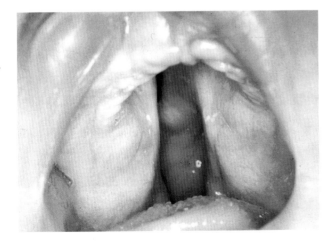

Fig. 10.4 Cleft lip and palate.

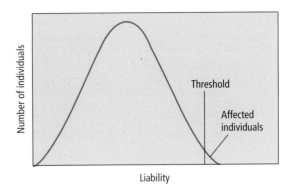

Fig. 10.5 General population liability curve for cleft lip and palate.

some underactive genes for lip and palate formation. However, as they have fully formed lips and palates they must also have, on balance, sufficient normally active genes. For these discontinuous traits it is the critical balance between the number of underactive and the number of normally active genes which is important. Only when the balance exceeds a threshold will the malformation occur, and the further the threshold is exceeded the greater the extent of the malformation. Thus the liability (including both genetic and environmental factors) can be represented as a Gaussian curve (Fig. 10.5). The threshold is indicated, and the proportion of the population to the right of this threshold (0.1%) equals the general population incidence of cleft lip and palate. For parents (first-degree relatives) of an affected child the liability curve is shifted to the right, and so we would expect to find an increased frequency (4%) of this malformation amongst parents and other first-degree relatives (Fig. 10.6). With each further degree of relationship the liability curve moves back a step towards the general population position, with a corresponding reduction in the incidence (Table 10.6).

The more severe the malformation in the affected child the more the parents' liability curve is shifted to the right and the higher the incidence in relatives. Thus 5% of first-degree relatives are affected if the clefting is bilateral and complete, whereas only 2% are affected if unilateral and incomplete.

Some multifactorial traits show an unequal sex ratio (Table 10.9). Thus whilst pyloric stenosis affects 5 in 1000 males, only 1 in 1000 females are affected. The incidence is increased in the relatives of affected males, but is even more increased in the relatives of affected females (the Carter effect; Table 10.10). This indicates that the female threshold is higher than the male threshold for this malformation, and so the parents of an affected female need to have a higher proportion of underactive genes and hence a more displaced liability curve.

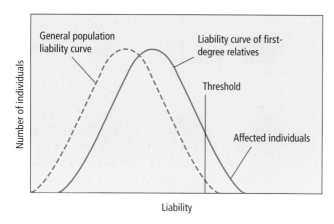

Fig. 10.6 Displaced liability curve in first-degree relatives of a proband with cleft lip and palate.

Table 10.9 Multifactorial conditions with an unequal sex ratio.

Condition	Sex ratio (males to females)
Pyloric stenosis	5 to 1
Hirschsprung disease	3 to 1
Congenital dislocation of the hip	1 to 6
Talipes	2 to 1
Rheumatoid arthritis	1 to 3

Table 10.10 Pyloric stenosis frequency in relatives.

Relationship	Frequency (%)	Increase on general population risk for same sex
Male relatives of a male patient	5	10-fold
Female relatives of a male patient	2	20-fold
Male relatives of a female patient	17	35-fold
Female relatives of a female patient	7	70-fold

ANALYSIS OF MULTIFACTORIAL TRAITS

Currently there is a great deal of interest in the analysis of multifactorial traits to their genetic determinants. Several approaches have been utilized including linkage analysis, sib pair studies, association analysis and mutational analysis of candidate genes.

Linkage analysis is a standard approach for analysis of single gene disorders (Chapter 9) but is more difficult in multifactorial traits especially where these have a continuous distribution. This approach has been more successful when coupled with selective breeding in experimental animals.

Sibs have approximately one-half of their genes in common and thus at a particular locus one-quarter of sibs will share two alleles, one-half will have one allele in common and one-quarter will have different alleles. Affected sib pairs are studied to seek distortion from this expected 1 to 2 to 1 ratio as such distortion with an excess of sharing is a clue that the locus is involved in the causation of the disorder.

Association analysis compares the frequency of particular alleles at a locus between an affected group and an unaffected control group. Differences may be clues to genetic determinants which reflect linkage disequilibrium between causative mutations and the genetic marker under study (p. 86).

The preceding approaches identify chromosomal regions of interest and these can be further analysed by mutational analysis in candidate genes from these regions in affected patients.

SOMATIC CELL GENETIC DISORDERS

When a mutation is present in the fertilized egg then this mutation will be transmitted to all daughter cells. If, however, a mutation arises after the first cell division, then this mutation will only be found in a proportion of cells and the individual is mosaic (two or more different genotypes in one individual). The mutation may be confined to the gonadal cells (gonadal mosaic) or to the somatic cells (somatic mosaic) or occur in a proportion of both. Irrespective of the distribution of the initial mutation within the individual there would be no preceding family history but if the gonad includes the mutation there would be a risk to offspring.

Most, if not all, cancers are now known to be somatic cell genetic disorders. Some familial cancers have germ-

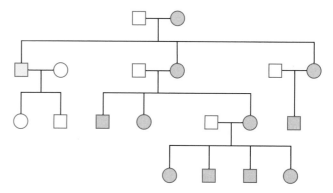

Fig. 10.7 Pedigree from a family with Leber optic neuropathy showing mitochondrial inheritance.

line mutations but in the remainder a succession of mutations occur in the somatic cell(s) which progress to malignancy (Chapter 17).

MITOCHONDRIAL DISORDERS

Each cell has hundreds of mitochondria in the cytoplasm and each mitochondrion has about 10 copies of the circular mitochondrial chromosome (p. 43). The mitochondria (and their chromosomes) are virtually all derived from the mother and hence mitochondrial disorders due to mutations in these chromosomes show characteristic patterns of inheritance with transmission to all children of an affected mother but no risk to the offspring of an affected man (Fig. 10.7). The mitochondrial DNA has a high mutation rate and both point and length mutations occur at a 10-fold higher rate than in nuclear DNA. The phenotypic effect depends on the location and type of mutation and also on the proportion of mitochondrial chromosomes which are involved. Heteroplasmy with some normal and some affected mitochondrial chromosomes in each mitochondrion is common in mitochondrial disorders and, as cells can accumulate variable proportions of mutant and normal mitochondrial DNAs at subsequent cell divisions, this can result in a wide phenotypic range in a single family. The process of replicative segregation of mitochondrial DNA tends to cause cells to drift towards having all mutant or all normal mitochondrial DNA (homoplasmy). The high mutation rate for mitochondrial DNA means that somatic mutations are normal with ageing and this can contribute to disease expression in a patient with inherited heteroplasmy for a mitochondrial mutation.

Mitochondria are important for energy production and different tissues vary in the extent to which they rely on this process. The central nervous system, the heart, skeletal muscle, kidney and endocrine glands are particularly reliant and hence are the main organs and tissues which are involved in mitochondrial diseases. So far, 59 mitochondrial diseases have been identified and all are rare (e.g. Leber hereditary optic atrophy, p. 141).

C H A P T E R 11

Medical Genetics in Populations

CONTENTS

SELECTION FOR SINGLE GENE DISORDERS 98
FOUNDER EFFECT FOR SINGLE
GENE DISORDERS 100

ALTERED MUTATION RATE FOR SINGLE
GENE DISORDERS 100

In contrast to the previous chapters which have focused on the different types of genetic diseases at the level of the affected family, this chapter will consider the factors which can influence the population frequencies of genetic disease. The prevalence of a genetic disorder is the number of patients with the condition per 1000 of a defined population at any point in time (e.g. 10/1000 births affected) whereas the incidence of a genetic disease is the number of new patients with the condition per 1000 of a defined population in a defined time period (e.g. 10 new patients affected/1000 adults per annum).

Most information to date on population genetics has related to single gene disorders which collectively have a birth prevalence of about 20/1000. The population prevalence of individual single gene disorders may be influenced by three main factors: selection, a founder effect and any alteration to the mutation rate.

SELECTION FOR SINGLE GENE DISORDERS

Prior to Darwin, the different species were held to have been fixed since their outright creation. Darwin challenged this view by showing that traits favoured by the environment tended to increase in frequency, as the favoured animals were more successful at reproduction. Conversely, deleterious traits hindered reproduction and thus fell in frequency. This natural selection operates on the phenotype, which in turn is determined by the genotype and evolution is simply a change in gene fre-

quencies as a result of selection and genetic variation is a prerequisite for evolution.

Selection is a powerful means of altering gene frequencies for single gene disorders and it may operate to reduce (negative selection) or increase (positive selection) a particular phenotype and hence its genotype. Selection acts on the individual phenotypes and either favours or hinders reproduction and hence the propagation of that individual's genotype. Many populations tend to increase in size over time but without disturbing factors, such as selection, the relative gene frequencies tend to remain constant. This can be demonstrated mathematically (the Hardy–Weinberg equilibrium, Appendix 4). With negative selection the relative frequency of the condition and its gene frequency will decrease and conversely with positive selection it will increase (Fig. 11.1).

Sickle cell disease (p. 71) is inherited as an autosomal recessive trait and although the carrier parents are asymptomatic, the affected offspring have a severe chronic anaemia and in many parts of the world often die before adulthood (and reproduction). With such an effect on the affected homozygote, the birth frequency would be expected to be low yet in equatorial Africa it is 1 in 40 and 1 in 3 of the population carry the mutant gene. This high gene frequency has arisen due to a selective advantage for the mutant gene carriers in respect of malaria due to *Plasmodium falciparum*. This is a major cause of death in equatorial Africa and sickle cell heterozygotes are at an advantage in that their infected red cells undergo more rapid clearance with a better chance of recovery from the malarial infection. This selective advantage no longer

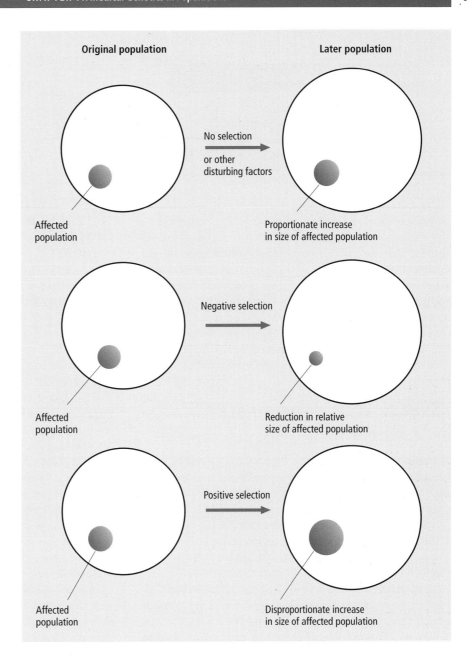

Fig. 11.1 Effect of selection on the frequency of a condition within a population.

operates in regions where malaria has been eradicated and removal of the selective pressure results in a fall in the gene frequency. Thus the sickle cell gene frequency has fallen from about 1 in 3 to 1 in 10 in the descendants of African Blacks who were transported to America some ten generations ago. Selection for a particular allele also influences the allele frequencies at adjacent closely linked loci due to linkage disequilibrium (p. 86) and selection for the sickle cell allele also raised the frequency of the adjacent 13 kb restriction fragment length polymorphism (RFLP).

A selective advantage in respect of malarial infection also operates for heterozygotes for beta-thalassemia

(p. 133) and glucose-6-phosphate dehydrogenase (G6PD) deficiency (p. 138) and in consequence these conditions are also prevalent in regions where malaria is (or was) common. A heterozygote advantage is also evident for carriers of congenital adrenal hyperplasia in respect of *Haemophilus influenzae* type B infection but for the majority of conditions where a natural selective pressure is (or was) operating, its basis is as yet unknown.

Most serious genetic conditions tend to hamper reproduction and so produce negative selection. Advances in treatment can reverse this disadvantage and then the frequency of the condition would rise to a new equilibrium.

Table 11.1 Examples of genetic isolates with high frequencies of certain single gene disorders.

Isolate	Disorder
Cuna Indians of Panama	Albinism
Hopi Indians	Albinism
Finns	Congenital nephrotic syndrome
Afrikaners	Variegate porphyria, familial hypercholesterolaemia

Table 11.2 Equations for prediction of birth frequency of single gene disorders.

> Autosomal dominant disorders
> Birth frequency = $2\mu/(1-f)$
>
> Autosomal recessive disorders
> Birth frequency = $\mu/(1-f)$
>
> X-linked recessive disorders
> Birth frequency = $3\mu/(1-f)$

μ, mutation rate; f, biological fitness.

The rate of change depends upon the mode of inheritance. For an autosomal dominant trait where previously reproduction was impossible, restoration to normality would double the frequency of the disorder in a generation, whereas for an X-linked recessive trait, doubling of the birth frequency would take about four generations and for an autosomal recessive trait it would take about 50 generations. Similarly enforced eugenic programmes which prevented reproduction of affected individuals would result in reduced disease frequencies in similar timescales.

FOUNDER EFFECT FOR SINGLE GENE DISORDERS

For religious, geographical or other reasons, a small group of individuals may become genetically isolated from the rest of the population (a genetic isolate). The founder member of the group will have mutant alleles for some autosomal traits (recessive or late-onset dominant) and so within the population these genes are automatically at a higher frequency than within the general population (Table 11.1).

The Afrikaners who settled in South Africa in the 17th century provide several striking examples of the founder effect. Thus, for example, in variegate porphyria which is inherited as an autosomal dominant trait, many current gene carriers are direct descendants of one couple who emigrated from Holland in the 1680s. In consequence, all will share the same mutation and a similar restricted range of causative mutations is a characteristic of the founder effect.

ALTERED MUTATION RATE FOR SINGLE GENE DISORDERS

The mutation rate (μ) is usually expressed as an incidence with the number of mutations at a locus per million gametes produced per generation and the mutant gene frequency reflects the balance between introduction of new mutant genes to the population and loss of mutant genes from the population when an affected individual fails to reproduce. If there is no impairment of reproductive capacity, the biological fitness (f) is normal (1 or 100%), and if reproduction is impossible, the biological fitness is zero. The impact of changes in the mutation rate on the frequency of a single gene disorder depends upon the mode of inheritance (Table 11.2).

If the condition precludes reproduction ($f = 0$), then the respective birth frequencies for autosomal dominant, autosomal recessive and X-linked recessive conditions will be 2μ, μ and 3μ. Hence, any change in the mutation rate will have most effect for an X-linked recessive trait and least on an autosomal recessive trait. The risk of a new mutation for several autosomal dominant traits and for some X-linked recessive traits has been shown to be increased with increasing paternal age and is increased by exposure to mutagenic chemicals. Mutation rates are difficult to determine and most information relates to autosomal dominant traits and X-linked recessive traits with estimates of 1–100 mutations per million gametes per generation for different loci and an average figure of 10–20 mutations per million gametes per generation.

PART 2

CLINICAL
APPLICATIONS

Genetic Assessment and Counselling

C O N T E N T S

COMMUNICATION OF ADVICE 103
History and pedigree construction 103
Clinical examination 103
Confirmation of diagnosis 105

Counselling 106
Follow-up 107
LEGAL ASPECTS 108
SPECIAL POINTS IN COUNSELLING 108

COMMUNICATION OF ADVICE

Genetic counselling is the communication of information and advice about inherited conditions and a person seeking such advice is called a consultand. This process includes history and pedigree construction, examination, diagnosis, counselling and follow-up.

History and pedigree construction

The affected individual who caused the consultand(s) to seek advice is called the proband. Often the proband is a child, but he or she may also be the consultand or a more distant relative. A standard medical history is required for the proband and for any other affected persons in the family.

Next the pedigree is constructed. A standardized set of symbols is used (Fig. 12.1). The male line is conventionally placed on the left, and all members of the same generation are placed on the same horizontal level. Roman numerals are used for each generation, starting with the earliest, and arabic numerals are used to indicate each individual within a generation (numbering from the left). Thus in Fig. 12.2, III4 is the proband, and his parents who are seeking advice are II5 and II6. When drawing a pedigree it is advisable to start at the bottom of the page with the most recent generation and work upwards. The offspring of each set of parents are given in birth order with the eldest on the left. For each member of the

pedigree, name and age are included. For an extended family study, the full name, age, address and phone number for individuals who need to be contacted should also be included. Miscarriages, neonatal deaths, handicapped or malformed children and parental consanguinity might not be mentioned unless specifically asked about.

Clinical examination

A complete physical examination of the proband is desirable. This examination differs from the routine, however, in that there is often a need to describe dysmorphic features accurately. A dysmorphic feature is by definition some characteristic which is outside the range seen in normal individuals. Table 12.1 and Fig. 12.3 indicate some of the terms used for the description of dysmorphic features.

Clinical impressions can be misleading, and so it is important to make accurate measurements to confirm features such as widely spaced eyes or disproportionate short stature. Table 12.2 lists some commonly used measurements in this context. The normal ranges of each will vary with age and sex and are provided in standard dysmorphology texts. Normally each measurement is close to the same percentile. If not, then the unusual measurements reflect an abnormality. For example, if height and head circumference are on the 10th percentile but interpupillary distance is on the 90th percentile, then relative

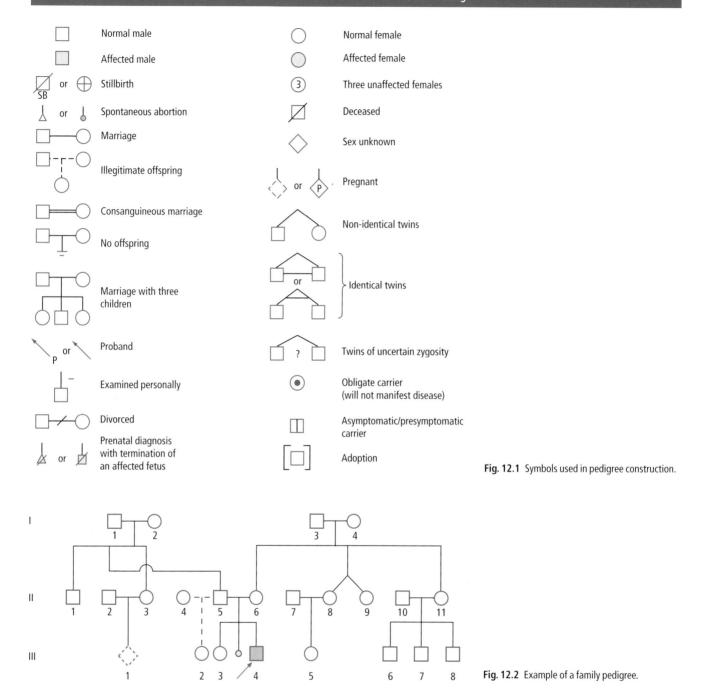

Fig. 12.1 Symbols used in pedigree construction.

Fig. 12.2 Example of a family pedigree.

hypertelorism is present although the actual measurement is within the normal range.

An often neglected aspect of the physical examination is the recording of the fingerprint pattern (dermatoglyphics), which may provide important clues to the diagnosis (Table 12.3). Three common patterns are found: loop, arch and whorl (Fig. 12.4). Loops are further subdivided into ulnar and radial according to the side of the forearm from which they point. In 4% of the population only a single

palmar crease (Simian crease) is present on one hand and in 1% of the normal population single palmar creases are present bilaterally.

In patients with multiple dysmorphic features it is necessary to consider identifiable syndromes. A syndrome (Greek: running together) is the non-random occurrence in the same individual of two or more abnormalities which are aetiologically related. Most syndromes have multiple components, of which few if any are universal or

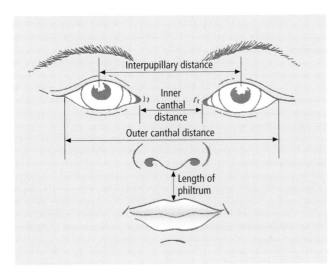

Fig. 12.3 Facial landmarks.

Table 12.1 Descriptive terms used in dysmorphology.

Term	Meaning
Hypertelorism	Interpupillary distance above expected
Hypotelorism	Interpupillary distance below expected
Telecanthus	Inner canthal distance above expected yet interpupillary distance not increased
Low set ears	Upper border of ear attachment below intercanthal line with head upright
Mongoloid slant	Outer canthi above inner canthi
Antimongoloid slant	Inner canthi above outer canthi
Brushfield spots	Speckled iris ring (20% of normal babies)
Simian crease	Single transverse palmar crease
Epicanthic folds	Skin folds over inner canthi
Brachycephaly	Short anteroposterior skull length
Dolichocephaly	Long anteroposterior skull length
Clinodactyly	Incurved fifth fingers

Table 12.2 Standard dysmorphic measurements.

Measurement	Comment
Height	
Arm span	
Weight	
Lower segment	Floor to upper border of pubis
Upper segment	Height minus lower segment
Sitting height	
Interpupillary distance	Fig. 12.3
Inner canthal distance	Fig. 12.3
Head circumference	Maximum occipitofrontal circumference
Testicular volume	Assessed using Prader orchidometer standards
Ear length	Maximum ear length

Table 12.3 Dermatoglyphic abnormalities.

Condition	Dermatoglyphic findings
Trisomy 18	6–10 arches, Simian crease (30%)
Turner syndrome	Predominance of whorls
47, XXY	Excess of arches
5p-	Excess of arches, Simian crease (90%)
Trisomy 13	Excess of arches, Simian crease (60%)
Trisomy 21	Usually all ulnar loops, Simian crease (50%)
Smith–Lemli–Opitz syndrome	Predominance of whorls

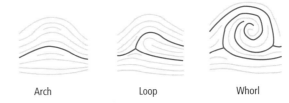

Arch   Loop   Whorl

Fig. 12.4 Fingerprint patterns.

pathognomonic features and thus the average patient will not have every feature listed in the textbook. Furthermore, some abnormalities are non-specific; for example, reduced height and high arched palate may be seen in severe mental handicap of any cause.

The pattern of dysmorphic or other features is generally more important than a single sign, and, as some dysmorphic features are age-related, re-examination at a future date may be helpful. Many syndromes have now been described and differential diagnosis of these is greatly aided by computerized databases in addition to standard reference texts.

Confirmation of diagnosis

Nowhere in clinical medicine is it more essential to obtain an accurate diagnosis, for without it genetic advice can be totally misleading. The history and physical examination may permit a confident diagnosis or may indicate the need for further investigation. A wide variety of investigations may be required, reflecting the wide spectrum of genetic disease (Table 12.4). Indications for chromosomal and DNA analysis are given in Table 12.5. Chromosomal abnormalities may produce diverse dysmorphic features and malformations, and chromosomal analysis should be considered if these are present, especially if accompanied by mental handicap. Conversely there is little point performing chromosomal analysis on patients with single congenital malformations, single gene disorders or with recognizable non-chromosomal syndromes.

Table 12.4 Diagnosis of genetic disease.

Type	Diagnostic test
Chromosomal disorders	Chromosomal analysis
Single-gene disorders	Pedigree analysis Clinical examination Biochemical analysis DNA analysis
Multifactorial disorders	Clinical examination Biochemical analysis DNA analysis Other investigations (imaging, functional studies, etc.)
Mitochondrial disorders	Pedigree analysis Clinical examination DNA analysis
Somatic cell genetic disorders	Histopathology DNA analysis Chromosomal analysis

Table 12.5 Indications for chromosomal or DNA analysis.

Chromosomal analysis
Dysmorphic features suggestive of a chromosomal syndrome
Unexplained mental handicap*
Family study of structural chromosomal abnormality
Multiple congenital abnormalities
Unexplained stillbirth
Female with unexplained short stature
Recurrent miscarriages
Primary infertility
Ambiguous sexual development
Certain types of cancer (Chapter 17)
Suspected contiguous gene disorder

DNA analysis/storage
Known or suspected single-gene disorder (patient)
Known single-gene disorder (family member if linkage study required)
Neonatal death with suspected metabolic disorder
Certain multifactorial disorders (Chapter 16)
Known or suspected mitochondrial disorder

* Also perform DNA analysis to exclude fragile X syndrome.

Occasionally the affected individuals will have died or be otherwise unavailable for assessment, and an attempt should then be made to obtain hospital or other records which might aid definitive diagnosis.

Counselling

Accurate diagnosis is of paramount importance for mean-ingful genetic counselling, and thus counselling should never precede the steps involved in diagnosis as outlined above.

Both parents should be counselled and adequate time allowed in an appropriate setting. Few couples can be counselled in under 30 min, and neither the corner of a hospital ward nor a crowded clinic room is adequate. Further, it is inappropriate to counsel too soon after recent bereavement or after the initial shock of a serious diagnosis.

Counselling needs to include all aspects of the condition, and the depth of explanation should be matched to the educational background of the couple. One might start by outlining the clinical features, complications, natural history, prognosis and treatment/effective management of the condition. Then a simple explanation of the genetic basis of the condition, perhaps with the aid of a diagram, could be given, and a recurrence risk calculated for the consultands. It is often useful to compare this recurrence risk against the general population risk for the condition and for other common birth defects (Table 12.6). Generally medical geneticists consider a risk of more than 1 in 10 as high and of less than 1 in 20 as low, but risks have to be considered in relation to the degree of disability.

Consultands often feel very guilty or stigmatized, and it is important to recognize and allay this. Common misconceptions about heredity may also need to be dispelled (Table 12.7).

The reproductive options open to the couple may now be discussed (Fig. 12.5). In many consultations the couples' fears are unjustified and they can undertake a pregnancy with the reassurance that their risk of genetic disease is no different from other couples in the general population. Where there is an increased risk, and especially where the disease burden is significant, then other options need to be considered. In this context disease burden is the consultand's perception of the cost (physical, emotional and financial) of the disorder. The possibility of prenatal diagnosis for the condition needs to be considered, as, if available, this often encourages a couple

Table 12.6 General population risks.

Condition	Risk
Spontaneous miscarriage	1 in 6
Perinatal death	1 in 30–100
Neonatal death	1 in 150
Cot death	1 in 500
Major congenital malformation	1 in 33
Serious mental or physical handicap	1 in 50
Adult cancer	1 in 4

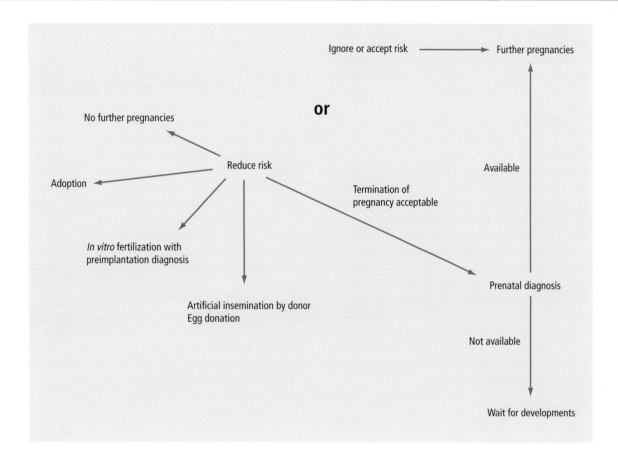

Fig. 12.5 Reproductive options.

Table 12.7 Common misconceptions about heredity.

- Absence of other affected family members means that a disorder is not genetic and vice versa
- Any condition present at birth must be inherited
- Upsets, mental and physical, of the mother in pregnancy cause malformations
- Genetic diseases are untreatable
- If only males or females are affected in the family this indicates sex linkage
- A 1 in 4 risk means that the next three children will be unaffected
- All genetic disorders and their carrier state can be detected by chromosomal analysis
- Confusion of odds, fractions and percentage risks

to undertake a further pregnancy which otherwise they would be reluctant to contemplate. Where the couple decide not to undertake a further pregnancy it is necessary for the counsellor to ensure that contraception is adequate and to mention other means of family extension. About 1% of all artificial insemination by donor (AID) is per-

formed for genetic indications, such as a husband with an autosomal dominant trait or when both parents are carriers for a serious autosomal recessive disease for which prenatal diagnosis is unavailable. Although this substantially reduces the risk of an autosomal recessive trait, some risk will remain in proportion to the population carrier frequency.

Counselling must be non-judgemental and non-directive. The aim is to deliver a balanced version of the facts which will permit the consultands to reach their own decision with regard to their reproductive future.

For certain conditions, such as balanced chromosomal rearrangements, autosomal dominant traits and X-linked recessive traits, an extended family study will be required and it is useful to enlist the aid of the consultands in approaching other family members at risk.

Follow-up

Many consultands can be fully counselled at one sitting, but some will require follow-up sessions. Our policy is to follow the counselling with a letter to the consultands which summarizes the information given and invites them to return if new questions arise. Also, if new opportunities arise (e.g. an improved carrier or prenatal diagnostic test) consultands can be contacted and offered a return appointment through the regional genetic register.

LEGAL ASPECTS

Genetic counselling

In the UK under the Congenital Disabilities (Civil Liability) Act of 1976 legal action can be brought against a person whose breach of duty to parents results in a child being born disabled, abnormal or unhealthy. In both the UK and the USA there has been an escalation of litigation concerning genetic disease. Most cases concern physician errors of omission, and it behoves all doctors who provide genetic advice to ensure the validity and up-to-dateness of that information. Thus failure (whether from ignorance or religious objections) to take a family history and to follow up with appropriate tests or referrals and failure to give correct genetic advice may constitute medical negligence. The claim would fail if at any time both parents knew and accepted that the child might be abnormal.

Prenatal diagnosis

Prenatal diagnosis with selective termination of pregnancy became a reality in the UK with the Abortion Act of 1967. Under this Act one ground for termination of pregnancy is '. . . a substantial risk that if the child were born it would suffer from such physical or mental abnormality as to be seriously handicapped'. The legal position in other countries varies from total prohibition of abortion for fetal abnormality to relative liberality. Prenatal diagnostic tests need informed consent, and parents should be reminded that no single test excludes all known fetal abnormalities, and that occasionally the test fails to give a result. The indications for, and limitations of, prenatal diagnosis are discussed further in Chapter 19.

Consanguinity

All human societies in existence prohibit the mating of first-degree relatives (incest). Marriage between relatives less close than sibs or parents and offspring is not necessarily outlawed, but the dividing line between legal and illegal varies somewhat between countries. Thus, in about one-half of the USA uncle–niece, aunt–nephew and first-cousin matings are forbidden by law, and in most African societies consanguineous marriage is not allowed. In contrast, in parts of the Middle East, Pakistan and India marriage between relatives is common, and up to 20% of marriages are consanguineous. The marriage of double first cousins (both sets of grandparents in common) is the closest legal union in the UK and overall, about 1 in 200 marriages in the UK are consanguineous (usually the parents are first cousins).

SPECIAL POINTS IN COUNSELLING

There are several pitfalls for the unwary who practise genetic counselling (Table 12.8). Precision of diagnosis is fundamental to meaningful genetic counselling, and most mistakes arise from an inaccurate or incomplete diagnosis. Incomplete knowledge of the literature is especially important for syndromic assessment and in relation to genetic heterogeneity.

In the following sections some general points are made, and the counselling details for individual conditions are covered in other chapters.

Chromosomal disorders

The exact recurrence risk varies with the abnormality, but for couples at high risk prenatal diagnosis is always an option. Parental karyotypes need not be performed if the child has regular aneuploidy but must be examined if the child has a partial duplication or deficiency. Extended family studies will be required if a parent has a balanced structural rearrangement.

Autosomal dominant traits

The risk to each child of an affected person is, on average, 1 in 2, whereas the risk to the offspring of an unaffected person is negligible provided the disorder has high penetrance. This information needs to be modified accordingly as the penetrance falls. Further, most dominant traits show variable expression. Where dominant traits have an age-dependent onset, such as Huntington disease, the conditional information that a person is unaffected at a given age can be combined with the pedigree risk using Bayes' theorem (Appendix 2).

Increasingly, DNA analysis is becoming available for families with dominant traits to provide presymptomatic and prenatal diagnosis. General principles of indirect

Table 12.8 Pitfalls and problems in genetic counselling.

No diagnosis in the proband
Incorrect or incomplete diagnosis
Genetic heterogeneity
Non-penetrance
Variable expression
Inadequate knowledge of the literature
Previously undescribed disease
Gonadal mosaicism
Unstable mutations

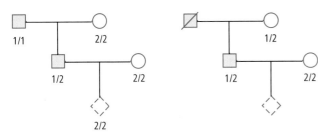

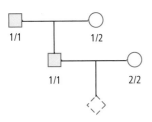

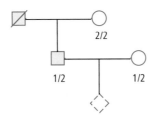

Fully informative situation. If marker is intragenic, fetus is unaffected. If extragenic, the error rate equals the recombination fraction

Although heterozygous for the marker the phase is unknown and the risk to the fetus remains at 50%

Non-informative situation. Risk to fetus remains at 50%

Marker informative in only one-half of pregnancies. If the fetus is 1/1 then it is affected, if 2/2 it is unaffected. But if 1/2 risk remains at 50%

Fig. 12.6 General principles of indirect DNA analysis, using marker with polymorphic fragments of sizes 1 and 2 in four different families with an autosomal dominant trait who are seeking prenatal diagnosis.

DNA analysis are outlined in Fig. 12.6 and the combination of this and other information is covered in Appendix 2.

For autosomal dominant traits extended family studies will often be required to counsel all at risk.

Autosomal recessive traits

Figure 12.7 shows a family with an autosomal recessive condition. For the carrier parents the risk of recurrence is on average 1 in 4. For each normal sib there will be a 2 in 3 chance of being a carrier (not 3 in 4, as one possibility, namely homozygous affected, is excluded); see Fig. 7.8 (p. 73). The carrier risk is indicated for other family members. The carrier frequency in the general population needs to be known in order to provide a recurrence risk for relatives other than the parents. For example, the chance that the unaffected sib of the proband and his spouse are both carriers is the carrier frequency in the population multiplied by two-thirds. The risk that their present pregnancy will produce an affected child is one-quarter of this, or $2/3 \times f \times 1/4$ (where f is the general population carrier frequency, Appendix 4).

Figure 12.8 illustrates general principles of application of indirect DNA analysis in families with an autosomal recessive trait.

X-linked recessive traits

Figure 12.9 indicates an X-linked recessive pedigree and, as indicated, certain of the females are obligate carriers. For each obligate carrier, on average one-half of her sons will be affected and one-half of her daughters will be carriers. If affected males reproduce then their sons will be normal but their daughters will be obligate carriers. The difficulty arises in the counselling of the non-obligate carrier females. Biochemical tests may be available for carrier detection, but, because of X inactivation few of these are absolute, and this information needs to be combined with the pedigree risk using Bayes' theorem (Appendix 2).

Figure 12.10 illustrates general principles of application of indirect DNA analysis in families with an X-linked recessive trait.

For X-linked recessive traits, extended family studies will often be required to counsel all females at risk.

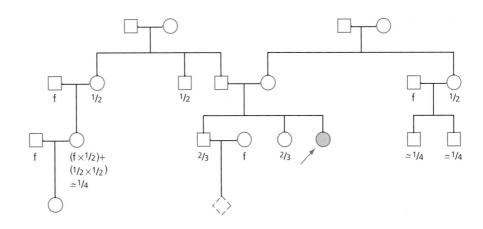

Fig. 12.7 Autosomal recessive trait in a family; carrier risks indicated for each individual; f, general population carrier frequency.

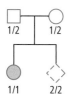

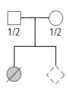

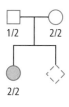

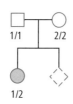

Fully informative situation. If marker is intragenic, the fetus is unaffected. If extragenic, there will be an error rate

Both parents heterozygous for each marker but no living affected child, hence phase unknown and DNA prenatal diagnosis not possible

Marker informative in only one-half of pregnancies. If the fetus is 1/2 then it is unaffected. If the fetus is 2/2, the risk is 50%

Non-informative situation. Risk to fetus remains at 25% and would not be influenced by the marker result

Fig. 12.8 General principles of indirect DNA analysis using a marker with polymorphic fragments of sizes 1 and 2 in four different families with an autosomal recessive trait who are seeking prenatal diagnosis.

Multifactorial disorders

For discontinuous multifactorial traits empiric recurrence risks are used. These are the observed (rather than the calculated) recurrence risks for different relatives of an affected individual. Strictly, empiric recurrence risks apply only to the population from which they were collected.

Infertility

One in 10 of all couples are involuntarily infertile. As part of the investigation of such a couple chromosomal analysis of both partners is indicated to exclude a balanced structural rearrangement and Klinefelter syndrome.

Recurrent miscarriages

One in six of all recognized pregnancies ends as a spontaneous miscarriage. If a couple has had three or more first-trimester spontaneous miscarriages then, in addition to gynaecological examination and exclusion of hormonal dysfunction and anti-phospholipid antibodies in the wife, chromosomal analysis is indicated for each, as in 3–5% of cases one partner will have a balanced structural rearrangement.

Stillbirth

Five in 1000 babies are stillborn and in about 50% no cause can be identified. In that event the empiric recurrence risk is 7%.

Perinatal death with multiple malformations

Seven in 1000 total births have multiple congenital malformations. The aetiology is diverse (Chapter 18) but genetic counselling is facilitated by chromosome analysis, autopsy, whole body radiography and clinical photographs (hence the mnemonic CARP). Chromosomal analysis may still be possible even 2–3 days after death by culturing and karyotyping fibroblasts from a post-mortem sample of fascia lata. Recurrence risks depend upon aetiology, but if these investigations are all normal, no syndrome is identified in the literature and the parents are non-consanguineous, the specific recurrence risk is 2–5% (in addition to the general population risk), and reassurance by means of detailed ultrasound might be offered during subsequent pregnancies.

Disorders of sexual differentiation

Many factors can interfere with the process of normal sexual differentiation and clinically these may be considered under three headings: ambiguous genitalia, female pubertal failure and male pubertal failure (Table 12.9). Differential diagnosis within each group will generally require cytogenetic analysis in addition to hormonal studies. There is an added urgency in infants with ambiguous genitalia in view of the need to assign gender for rearing and to diagnose and treat salt-losing variants of congenital adrenal hyperplasia.

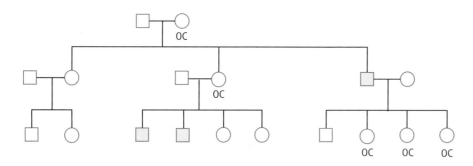

Fig. 12.9 X-linked recessive trait in a family with obligate carriers indicated (OC).

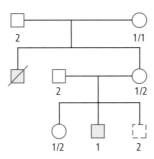

Full informative situation. If marker intragenic, the male fetus is unaffected and the daughter is a carrier. If extragenic, the error rate equals the recombination fraction

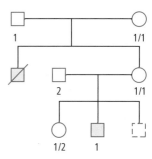

Non-informative situation. Risk to male fetus is 50% and would not be influenced by the marker result

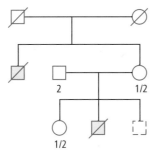

Mother heterozygous for marker but phase unknown. Risk to male fetus is 50%

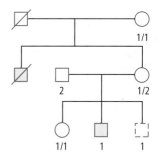

Informative mother with affected male fetus if the marker is intragenic. Non-paternity evident for daughter, but as she is homozygous for the marker she is a carrier if the marker is intragenic

Fig. 12.10 General principles of indirect DNA analysis using a marker with polymorphic fragments of sizes 1 and 2 in four different families with an X-linked recessive trait who are seeking prenatal diagnosis.

Sudden infant death syndrome

Two in 1000 babies die unexpectedly during infancy. Typically these deaths occur at 2–6 months of age in a previously healthy child, and, by definition, no cause can be identified at post-mortem. Some cases have undiagnosed inborn errors of metabolism and so samples of serum, red cells, white cells, urine, skin fibroblasts, muscle and liver should be stored at –70°C pending analysis in the absence of a defined cause. There is clearly an increased risk to sibs (between 4- and 7-fold) which merits the use of an apnoea monitor during infancy.

Mental handicap

Moderate and severe mental handicap (IQ < 50) affects 1% of newborns but this falls to 0.3–0.4% in children of school age due to deaths in infancy from associated abnormalities or rapidly progressive disorders. The cause can be identified in about 75% (Table 12.10).

Trisomy 21 is the single commonest cause of mental handicap in this age group and a variety of other chromosomal abnormalities comprise the additional 2%. Over 240 single gene disorders have been described for which mental handicap is a consistent or common feature. Numerically the most frequent amongst the autosomal dominant traits is tuberous sclerosis. Amongst autosomal recessive disorders phenylketonuria, cerebral degenerative disorders and recessive microcephaly predominate whereas amongst the X-linked disorders the fragile X syndrome is the single commonest cause.

Genetic assessment will thus be directed towards establishing the cause of the handicap in the family and counselling will be as outlined elsewhere for each condition. When the cause is obscure and no other relatives are affected to suggest a pattern of inheritance then observed (empiric) risks need to be used and prenatal reassurance

Table 12.9 Disorders of sexual differentiation.

Ambiguous genitalia
Female pseudohermaphroditism (46,XX and ovaries but virilized external genitalia)
　*Congenital adrenal hyperplasia (especially 21- or 11-hydroxylase deficiency)
　Maternal androgens or progesterone
　Localized malformation

Male pseudohermaphroditism (46,XY and testes but underdeveloped external genitalia)
　*Turner syndrome mosaic (45,X/46,XY)
　*Localized malformation (isolated or a syndrome component, e.g. Smith–Lemli–Opitz syndrome or autosomal chromosomal imbalance)
　Enzyme defect (e.g. 17α-hydroxylase, 17-ketosteroid reductase, 5α-reductase)
　Incomplete androgen insensitivity (Reifenstein syndrome, incomplete testicular feminization)

True hermaphrodite (46,XX or 46,XY or mosaic with ovarian and testicular tissue)

Female pubertal failure (female hypogonadism)
Hypogonadotrophic hypogonadism (reduced gonadotrophins)
　*Gonadotrophin deficiency (isolated or secondary, e.g. Kallman syndrome)
　Hypopituitarism

Hypergonadotrophic hypogonadism (increased gonadotrophins)
　*Turner syndrome
　*46,XX gonadal dysgenesis
　46,XY gonadal dysgenesis
　Agonadia
　Germinal cell aplasia

Other
　*Complete androgen insensitivity (testicular feminization—normal FSH but elevated LH)
　*Malformations of uterus or vagina (isolated or syndrome components)
　Enzyme defects (17α-hydroxylase, 17-ketosteroid reductase, 5α-reductase)
　True hermaphrodite

Male pubertal failure (male hypogonadism)
Hypogonadotrophic hypogonadism (reduced gonadotrophins)
　*Constitutional delay
　Gonadotrophin deficiency (isolated or secondary, e.g. Kallman syndrome)
　Hypopituitarism
　Multiple malformation syndromes

Hypergonadotrophic hypogonadism (increased gonadotrophins)
　*Klinefelter syndrome
　45,X/46,XY mosaic
　Reifenstein syndrome
　46,X–Y interchange males
　Bilateral anorchia
　Germinal cell aplasia
　Acquired disease (e.g. mumps, irradiation)
　Multiple malformation syndromes

Other
　Multiple malformation syndromes
　True hermaphrodite

*　Commoner causes.

Table 12.10 Causes of moderate and severe mental handicap in children of school age.

Chromosomal disorders	
Trisomy 21	25%
Other	2%
Single-gene disorders	
Autosomal dominant	1%
Autosomal recessive	10%
X-linked	
Fragile X syndrome	4%
Other	4%
* Brain malformations * Idiopathic dysmorphic syndromes	14%
Environmental factors	15%
Unexplained	25%

* Excluding recognized chromosomal and single gene disorders.

during a subsequent pregnancy cannot be offered (Fig. 12.11).

Mild mental handicap (IQ 50–70) affects at least 0.4% of children of school age and in about one-half a cause can be identified (perinatal asphyxia, fetal alcohol syndrome, fragile X syndrome, neurofibromatosis type I, 47,XXY). Again genetic counselling depends upon the cause and empiric risks need to be used if the cause cannot be established.

Congenital deafness

Congenital deafness affects 1 in 1000 children and in one-half the cause is genetic (Table 12.11). Genetic heterogeneity is apparent with different modes of inheritance in different families and multiple loci for each type of inheritance.

For normal parents of a congenitally deaf child with no identifiable enviromental cause, such as fetal infection with rubella or cytomegalovirus and no recognized single-gene disorder, the risk of recurrence is 1 in 6. This composite figure reflects the clinical inability to distinguish autosomal dominant families with a negligible new recurrence risk from autosomal recessive families with a 1 in 4 risk. If a subsequent child is affected then autosomal recessive inheritance is accepted and the recurrence risk is modified to 1 in 4.

The empiric risk for the first child of a congenitally deaf parent with no family history and a normal spouse is 1 in 20. If the child is deaf then autosomal dominant

Table 12.11 Causes of congenital deafness.

Single gene disorders	50%
Autosomal dominant	6%
Autosomal recessive	43.5%
X-linked	0.5%
Environmental	30%
Idiopathic	20%

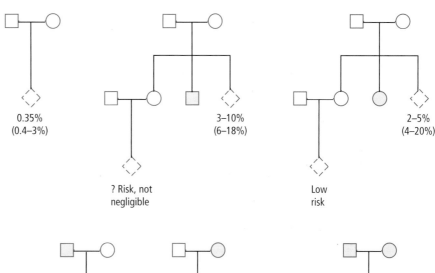

Fig. 12.11 Empiric recurrence risks for severe (IQ < 50) mental handicap and any degree (IQ < 70) of mental handicap (with the latter in parentheses) for various pregnancies when a proband has idiopathic severe mental handicap.

Table 12.12 Causes of congenital cataract.

Chromosomal disorders	22%
Single gene disorders (mostly autosomal dominant with several loci involved some autosomal recessive)	10%
Environmental	
Prenatal infection	25%
Metabolic	9%
Unexplained	34%

inheritance is accepted and the recurrence risk is modified to 1 in 2.

When both parents are deaf a variety of outcomes are observed. In 80% of such families all children will have normal hearing, 10% will have some deaf children (autosomal dominant inheritance) and 10% will have only deaf children (both parents homozygous for the same autosomal recessive condition).

Congenital cataract

One in every 250 babies is affected with a genetic basis in 32% (Table 12.12). For the normal parents of an affected child the composite recurrence risk is 1 in 10.

Consanguinity

A consanguineous couple are at increased risk for autosomal recessive and multifactorial traits, including several congenital malformations. If there is no previous consanguinity in the family the risk of serious disease or major malformations in the offspring of a first-cousin marriage is 1 in 20 (i.e. double the population risk). For the offspring of a first-cousin marriage in an inbred family the risk is 1 in 11 and the risk rises to 1 in 2 for offspring of incestuous unions. No special screening is indicated before a pregnancy unless indicated by other factors such as ethnic origin, but during a pregnancy detailed ultrasound scanning for malformations might be considered. For a consanguineous mating with an autosomal recessive condition in a relative the recurrence risk can be calculated from the proportion of genes in common (Appendix 3).

Short stature

Multiple factors can interfere with normal growth and clinically these can be subdivided according to the mode of presentation and the presence or absence of disproportion (Tables 12.2 and 12.13).

Amongst patients with proportionate short stature the commonest diagnoses are non-genetic causes and polygenic short stature. The latter is characterized by a normal birth weight, a slow pace of linear growth (but normal bone age), puberty at the normal age and parents who are in the lower percentiles for height but who are otherwise normal.

Over 100 different conditions may result in disproportionate short stature. A skeletal survey is invaluable for differential diagnosis and it is particularly important that this is not overlooked for a baby dying in the neonatal period with skeletal disproportion as otherwise meaningful genetic counselling will be impossible.

Exposure to irradiation or mutagens

In the UK the average annual irradiation dose from all sources is under 2 mSv (10 mSv = 1 rem). In the male diagnostic X-rays are of little genetic significance. Therapeutic irradiation with 2–4 Gy (10 mGy = 1 rad) kills most spermatogonia but more mature germ cells survive. Hence there is little reduction in fertility in the first 6 weeks but thereafter sterility may ensue depending upon the dose. In the long term there is a small increase in autosomal dominant point mutations after gonadal irradiation, but the overall risk is probably only 1 in 500.

The female oocyte is especially radiosensitive around the time of fertilization. Outside this period the risks are similar to, or less than, those for the male. An accidental diagnostic X-ray (of 0.01 Gy or less) during the early stages of pregnancy results in a total added risk of 1 in 1000 to the fetus for congenital malformation, mental handicap or cancer in children. Neither termination of pregnancy nor amniocentesis is indicated. The fetal risks increase in relation to the dose of X-rays, and termination is generally advised if a fetus less than 8 weeks is exposed

Table 12.13 Causes of short stature.

Proportionate short stature
Non-genetic (multiple causes—chronic infection, nutritional deficiency, etc.)
Familial short stature (polygenic)
Turner syndrome
Autosomal imbalance (usually associated with mental handicap)
Dysmorphic syndromes (de Lange, Noonan, Rubinstein–Taybi, Russell–Silver, Smith–Lemli–Opitz, Williams, others)
Disproportionate short stature
Lethal (neonatal presentation)
Thanatophoric dysplasia, osteogenesis imperfecta (congenital variant),   achondrogenesis, others
Non-lethal (neonatal or later presentation)
Short trunk
Spondyloepiphyseal dysplasia (various types), mucopolysaccharidosis   type IV, others
Short limbs
Achondroplasia, hypochondroplasia, others

to more than 0.25 Gy (25 rads). Exposure to 2–4 Gy usually results in female sterility.

Exposure of either sex to therapeutic doses of irradiation results initially in structural chromosomal abnormalities (rings, dicentrics, translocations; Fig. 6.12, p. 63) in 25–35% of lymphocytes. These tend to disappear with time and most have resolved by two years although the translocations tend to persist.

Paternity testing

Historically, disputed paternity was tested using a series of polymorphic blood groups and enzymes. With a combination of these markers paternity could be excluded in at least 95% of cases but could never be proven, only excluded. This area has been transformed by the use of variation at the DNA level and in particular by DNA fingerprinting. The probes used identify multiple (about 60) dispersed sequences of variable size (essentially multiple VNTRs) and the pattern produced is characteristic for an individual (see Fig. 3.7, p. 28). The hypervariability of size of each fragment is such that the chance of two unrelated individuals having an identical pattern is less than 3×10^{-11} with one probe and less than 5×10^{-19} if two probes are employed. A child's fragment pattern is a combination of some of the fragments from each parent, and a putative father can be either excluded or positively identified. The DNA fingerprints are identical in monozygotic twins and this approach is also employed to resolve family relationships in immigration disputes and for forensic testing of DNA from semen or dried blood spots.

C H A P T E R 13

Chromosomal Disorders

C O N T E N T S

TRANSLOCATIONS 116
PERICENTRIC INVERSIONS 117
TRISOMY 21 (MONGOLISM, DOWN SYNDROME) . . . 118
47,XYY 120
47,XXY (KLINEFELTER SYNDROME) 120
47,XXX 121
46,XX MALES 121
45,X (TURNER SYNDROME) 121
TRISOMY 18 (EDWARDS SYNDROME) 122

TRISOMY 13 (PATAU SYNDROME) 123
TRIPLOIDY 123
DELETIONS AND DUPLICATIONS 124
MARKER CHROMOSOMES 125
PRADER–WILLI SYNDROME 126
ANGELMAN SYNDROME (HAPPY PUPPET
   SYNDROME) 126
OTHER MICRODELETION DISORDERS 129

Chromosomal disorders include all conditions associated with visible changes of the chromosomes. Approximately 20% of all conceptions have a chromosomal disorder, but most of these fail to implant or are spontaneously aborted so the birth frequency is 0.6% (Fig. 13.1). Amongst early spontaneous abortions, the frequency of chromosomal disorders is 60%, whereas in late spontaneous abortions and stillbirths the frequency is 5%. The types of chromosomal abnormality differ within these different groups. Table 13.1 shows the types of chromosomal abnormality seen in early spontaneous abortions. With the exception of chromosome 1, each type of autosomal trisomy has been seen, and trisomy 16 is especially frequent. In contrast, trisomy 16 is never seen in the newborn because no recognizable embryo is formed. Triploid fetuses may survive to term, but the majority abort. Thus, in general, the chromosomal abnormalities which cause early spontaneous abortion tend to be those with the most severe effects on the fetus. Sex chromosome abnormalities are rare amongst early abortuses, with the notable exception of 45,X.

Table 13.2 indicates the commonest chromosomal disorders seen in newborns. Not all of these chromosomal changes are associated with disease, but in general autosomal abnormalities tend to be more severe than sex chromosomal abnormalities, and deletions tend to be more severe than duplications. In the autosomal abnormalities mental handicap, multiple congenital malformations, dysmorphic features and growth retardation (pre- and postnatal) are usual. Although the pattern of features may suggest the chromosomal disorder, no individual clinical feature is pathognomonic for a given chromosomal abnormality.

TRANSLOCATIONS

A translocation is the transfer of chromosomal material between chromosomes. Three main types are identified: reciprocal, centric fusion and insertional (p. 58). Centric fusion translocations only involve the acrocentric chromosomes 13–15, 21 and 22, whereas reciprocal translocations may involve any of the chromosomes, including the sex chromosomes. If the transfer results in no overall loss or gain of chromosomal material then the person will be healthy and is said to have a balanced translocation. The birth frequency for balanced translocations is 1 in 500, with approximately equal numbers of the centric fusion (mostly inherited, 10% de novo) and reciprocal (half inherited half de novo) types but relatively few insertional translocations.

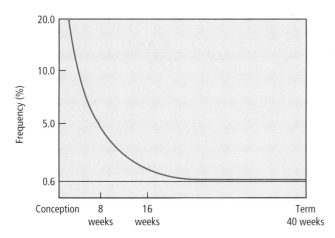

Fig. 13.1 Frequency of chromosomal abnormalities.

Table 13.1 Chromosomal findings in early spontaneous abortions.

40% apparently normal	
60% abnormal	
Trisomy	30%
45,X	10%
Triploid	10%
Tetraploid	5%
Other	5%

Table 13.2 Chromosomal disorders in newborns.

Disorder	Birth frequency
Balanced translocation	1 in 500
Unbalanced translocation	1 in 2000
Pericentric inversion	1 in 100
Trisomy 21	1 in 700
Trisomy 18	1 in 3000
Trisomy 13	1 in 5000
47,XXY	1 in 1000 males
47,XYY	1 in 1000 males
47,XXX	1 in 1000 females
45,X	1 in 5000 females

The carrier of a balanced translocation can be reassured that health and lifespan will be unaffected. Problems may arise, however during meiosis with production of chromosomally unbalanced offspring. Some of these fetuses will spontaneously abort, but if liveborn they show multiple dysmorphic features and mental handicap. On theoretical grounds the majority of offspring should be unbalanced, but the actual risk is much lower because of embryonic inviability and gametic selection (p. 58). The risk for unbalanced offspring depends upon the type of

Table 13.3 Risks of chromosomally unbalanced offspring for carriers of balanced structural rearrangements.

Rearrangement	Carrier	Risk of unbalanced offspring at amniocentesis (%)
Centric fusion 13;14	Either parent	1
Centric fusion 14;21	Father	1
Centric fusion 14;21	Mother	15
Centric fusion 21;22	Father	5
Centric fusion 21;22	Mother	10
Centric fusion 21;21	Either parent	100
Reciprocal (any)	Either parent	12
Insertional (any)	Either parent	50
Pericentric inversion*	Father	4
Pericentric inversion*	Mother	8

* Excluding the common pericentric inversion of chromosome 9.

translocation and which parent is the carrier (Table 13.3). The risks for reciprocal translocations vary somewhat in different families, reflecting the wide variety of possible break points and rearrangements. Exchanges of whole arms of non-acrocentrics rarely produce viable offspring, and in general if ascertainment is via recurrent miscarriages the risk of chromosomally abnormal viable offspring is 5% or less. However, if ascertainment is via a handicapped child, if the likely imbalance is only 1–2 bands or if chromosome 9 is involved, the risk is 20% or greater. Reassurance may be given in a pregnancy at risk by fetal karyotyping after amniocentesis or chorionic villus sampling. At the time of chorionic villus sampling the overall risk of unbalanced offspring for a reciprocal translocation carrier is 23%, of which about one-half would have spontaneously aborted before amniocentesis.

A family study should always be undertaken to determine other outwardly healthy carriers who will be at similar reproductive risk. A *de novo* translocation where both parents have normal chromosomes is usually not associated with clinical abnormality. Occasionally (<10%) in reciprocal but not in centric fusion translocations, genes may be damaged at the break points and produce chromosomal imbalance and an abnormal phenotype, and this is a cause for concern when a *de novo* reciprocal translocation is an incidental finding at amniocentesis.

PERICENTRIC INVERSIONS

Paracentric (i.e. excluding the centromere) inversions do not produce a clinical abnormality in the carrier, nor do they usually constitute an indication for prenatal diagnosis, because if a cross-over occurs within the inversion loop the degree of imbalance generated is such that it would be incompatible with viability in all but the most exceptional cases (p. 64).

Pericentric inversion carriers are not clinically abnormal, but there is a risk of producing chromosomally unbalanced offspring, particularly when the inversion involves a large part of the chromosome. This risk is 8% for a carrier mother and 4% for a carrier father. Small pericentric inversions of chromosome 9, which are found in 1% of the population, are an exception to this, and no chromosomally abnormal offspring resulting from cross-over within the inversion have ever been described.

TRISOMY 21 (MONGOLISM, DOWN SYNDROME)

Incidence

The overall birth incidence of trisomy 21 is 1 in 700 livebirths. The incidence at conception is, however, much greater, but more than 60% are spontaneously aborted, and at least 20% are stillborn. The incidence increases with increasing maternal age (Table 13.4). Thus the incidence at the 16th week of pregnancy (a common time for amniocentesis) is 1 in 300 for a 35-year-old mother, rising to 1 in 22 at 45 years.

Clinical features

The facial appearance often permits a clinical diagnosis. The palpebral fissures are upslanting, with specking of the iris (Brushfield spots), the nose is small, and the facial profile flat (Fig. 13.2). In the neonate, hypotonia may be

marked and redundant folds of skin about the neck are a feature of this and several other chromosomal disorders. The skull is brachycephalic with misshapen, low set ears. A single palmar crease (Simian crease) may be present (50%) and the little fingers are short and incurved (clinodactyly, 50%). A wide gap between the first and second toes may be present.

Mental handicap is the most serious complication. The IQ is usually less than 50, and if not mosaicism should be suspected. Congenital heart malformations, especially endocardial cushion defects, are present in 40%, and duodenal atresia may occur. Other complications include cataracts (2%), epilepsy (10%), hypothyroidism (3%), acute leukaemia (1%) and atlantoaxial instability (symptomatic in 2–3% but radiologically evident in 18%).

When serious cardiac malformations are present, death during infancy is common, but otherwise life expectancy is little reduced. Trisomy 21 accounts for about one-quarter of all moderate and severe mental handicap in children of school age. Most will walk and develop simple language. Puberty is often delayed and incomplete, with adult heights about 150 cm. Presenile dementia commonly supervenes after 40 years of age.

Aetiology

Most cases (95%) are regular trisomy 21 (Fig. 13.3). This arises from non-disjunction usually at the first (80%) but sometimes at the second meiotic division. Overall, the mother contributes the extra chromosome in 85% of cases, and the father in 15%. At least 1% of patients have mosaicism with normal and trisomy 21 cell lines. This may arise from mitotic non-disjunction in a trisomy 21 zygote (80%) or in a normal zygote (20%). The clinical features in these individuals tend to be milder than in the full syndrome. In 4% of cases the child received the extra copy of chromosome 21 from a parent who is a carrier of a balanced translocation involving chromosome 21 (see previous section and Fig. 6.8) or has a *de novo* translocation.

Recurrence risk

For young parents who have produced a child with trisomy 21 (or mosaic trisomy 21) the risk of recurrence of trisomy 21 or other major chromosomal abnormality at amniocentesis is 1.5% (risk at birth 1%). This is a low risk, but many couples still seek reassurance by fetal karyotyping in future pregnancies. When the mother is over 35 years of age the age-specific risk should be added (Table 13.4). The recurrence risks of carriers of a balanced translocation are given in Table 13.3.

Affected persons rarely reproduce. There is no evidence of a patient fathering a child, but offspring of female patients with trisomy 21 are recorded, and rather less than one-half are affected.

Table 13.4 Frequency of trisomy 21 at birth and at prenatal diagnosis in relation to maternal age.

| Maternal age | Frequency of trisomy 21 | | |
	At birth	At amniocentesis	At chorionic villus sampling
20	1 in 1500	1 in 1200 (E)	1 in 750 (E)
25	1 in 1350	1 in 1000 (E)	1 in 675 (E)
30	1 in 900	1 in 700 (E)	1 in 450 (E)
35	1 in 380	1 in 300	1 in 240
37	1 in 240	1 in 190	1 in 130
39	1 in 150	1 in 120	1 in 75
41	1 in 85	1 in 70	1 in 40
43	1 in 50	1 in 40	1 in 25
45	1 in 28	1 in 22	1 in 13

(E), estimated frequency.

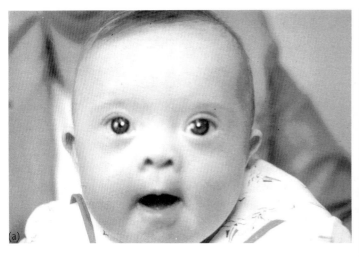

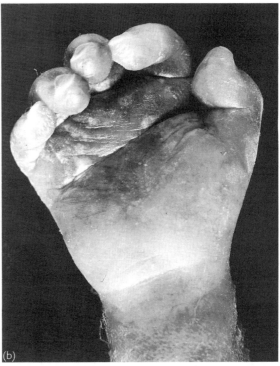

Fig. 13.2 Trisomy 21 phenotype. (a) Facies. (b) Single palmar crease in affected fetus.

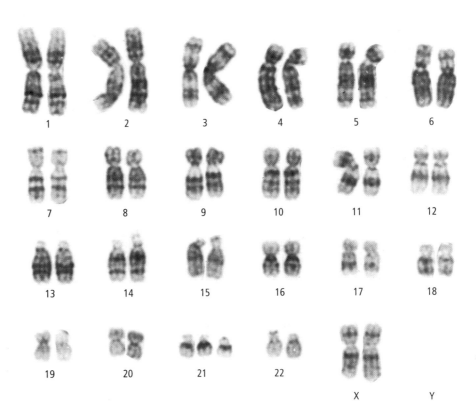

Fig. 13.3 Trisomy 21 karyotype.

47,XYY

Incidence

The incidence of 47,XYY is 1 in 1000 male births with no apparent parental age effect. The frequency is increased in males in penal institutions for the mentally subnormal (20 in 1000) and in mentally handicapped adult males (3 in 1000).

Clinical features

This chromosome disorder is often asymptomatic, although intelligence tends to be 10–15 points less than the normal sibs, and behaviour problems with easy frustration and aggression may occur. Patients tend to be tall, but have normal body proportions and no other clinical signs.

Aetiology

47,XYY arises from the production of a YY sperm at the second paternal meiotic division, or post-fertilization non-disjunction of the Y.

Recurrence risk

The recurrence risk is probably not increased for the parents of an affected child. For a person with 47,XYY the expected offspring would be 2XXY to 2XY to 1XX to 1XYY. In practice, fertility appears unimpaired in most cases, yet only XX and XY offspring have been observed.

47,XXY (KLINEFELTER SYNDROME)

Incidence

Overall the birth incidence of 47,XXY is 1 in 1000 males with an increased risk at increased maternal age. The frequency is increased amongst azoospermic infertile males (100 in 1000) and in males in institutions for the mentally handicapped (10 in 1000).

Clinical features

The diagnosis is generally made during adult life at the investigation of infertility, since this is the single commonest cause of hypogonadism and infertility in men. The testes are small (less than 2 cm long in the adult) and fail to produce adult levels of testosterone. This leads to poorly developed secondary sexual characteristics and gynaecomastia (40%). The limbs are elongated from early childhood and the upper to lower segment ratio is abnormally low with a mean adult height close to the 75th centile (Fig. 13.4). Scoliosis, emphysema, diabetes mellitus (8%) and osteoporosis may occur and the frequency of carcinoma of the breast (7%) is similar to that for normal females.

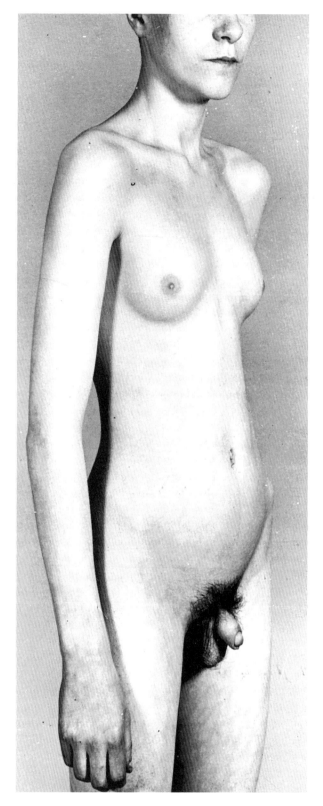

Fig. 13.4 Klinefelter syndrome.

Testosterone replacement therapy from early adolescence will improve secondary sexual characteristics, but infertility is the rule, except in mosaics. There is a 10–20 point reduction in verbal skills but performance scores are usually normal and severe mental handicap is uncommon.

Aetiology

The extra X chromosome is of maternal origin in 56% and paternal in 44%. It usually arises by non-disjunction at either the first (36%) or second (10%) maternal meiotic division, occasionally at the second maternal meiotic division and rarely as a mitotic error after fertilization. In the male it arises when the first meiotic division produces an XY sperm and this is favoured if the normal single XY cross-over is lost or fails to occur during male meiosis. About 15% are mosaic 46,XY/47,XXY.

Recurrence risk

The recurrence risk does not appear to be increased above the general population risk.

47,XXX

Incidence

The birth frequency is 1 in 1000 females with a maternal age effect.

Clinical features

Individuals appear clinically normal, but 15–25% are mildly mentally handicapped.

Aetiology

47,XXX may arise from non-disjunction at either the first (65%) or second (24%) maternal meiotic divisions, as a post-zygotic mitotic error (3%) or from non-disjunction at the male second meiotic division (8%).

Recurrence risk

The recurrence risk does not appear to be increased above the general population incidence. About three-quarters of affected females are fertile. One-half of their offspring would be expected to be affected, but in practice they are usually normal.

46,XX MALES

Incidence

One in 20 000 males have an apparently normal female karyotype, but in 80% careful banding studies reveal transfer of Yp11.2 to Xp, and in most of the others Y-specific sequences can be identified by DNA analysis or by *in situ* hybridization (Plate 10).

Clinical features

Patients are sterile and have the endocrine features of Klinefelter syndrome, including small testes. However, intelligence is usually normal and there is no skeletal disproportion. Stature tends to be within the normal female range. The diagnosis is usually made during the investigation of infertility, and occasionally following prenatal diagnosis when the predicted female infant proves to be an apparently normally developed male.

Aetiology

The condition is due to accidental recombination between the short arm of the Y chromosome and the short arm of the X in paternal meiosis. This X–Y interchange results in transfer of Y sequences, including the testis-determining factors, from the Y to the X.

Recurrence risk

The recurrence risk appears to be no greater than the population risk.

45,X (TURNER SYNDROME)

Incidence

The overall incidence of Turner syndrome is 1 in 5000 female births. The frequency at conception is much higher but over 99% spontaneously abort.

Clinical features

The diagnosis may be suggested in the newborn by redundant neck skin and peripheral lymphoedema (Fig. 13.5). However, not infrequently the diagnosis is only made later, during the investigation of short stature or primary amenorrhoea.

Proportionate short stature is apparent from early childhood, no adolescent growth spurt occurs, and the mean adult height, if untreated, is 145 cm with a corrrelation to mid-parental height. The chest tends to be broad, with the impression of widely spaced nipples, the hair line is low, and the neck may be webbed (Fig. 13.6). The carrying angle may be increased and the fourth metacarpals short. Hypoplasia of the nails and multiple pigmented naevi are common. Peripheral lymphoedema occurs at some stage in 40%. The ovaries develop normally until the 15th week of gestation, but then ova begin to degenerate and disappear, so that at birth the ovaries are represented by streaks, and this results in failure of secondary sexual development. Occasionally, ovarian degeneration is incomplete,

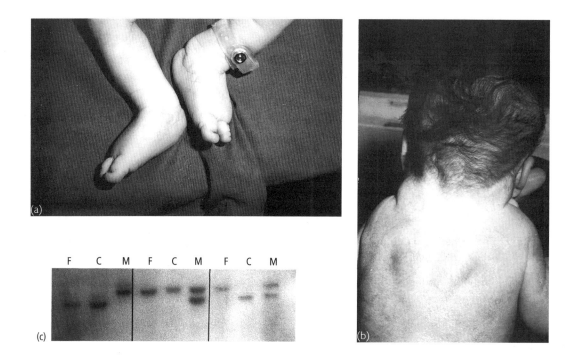

Fig. 13.5 (a) Neonatal lymphoedema in Turner syndrome. (b) Redundant neck skin in Turner syndrome. (c) Application of an X chromosomal RFLP to determine the origin of the abnormality in three children (C) with 45,X. M, mother; F, father. (Answers p. 215).

menses may occur (10–15%) and, rarely, a pregnancy may be possible.

Congenital heart disease, notably coarctation of the aorta and atrial septal defect, is present in 20%, and there is also an increased risk of unexplained systemic hypertension (27%), renal malformations, Hashimoto thyroiditis, Crohn's disease and gastrointestinal bleeding. Intelligence and lifespan are normal. Sex hormone replacement will allow the development of secondary sexual characteristics and treatment with growth hormone in childhood has been shown to increase the final height by 3–5 cm. Normal childbirth has been achieved by IVF using donor oocytes.

Aetiology

Monosomy X may arise from non-disjunction in either parent. In 80% with monosomy X only the maternal X chromosome is present, and thus the error occurred in spermatogenesis or post-fertilization. Overall 50% of patients have 45,X, 17% have an isochromosome of the long arm of X, 24% are mosaics, 7% have a ring X and 2% have a short arm deletion of one X. In general, deletion of the short arm of the X is associated with the Turner pheno-

type, whilst long arm deletions alone produce streak ovaries without the associated dysmorphic features. In 4% of patients, mosaicism with a second cell line containing a Y chromosome is found. In these patients, there is a risk of up to 20% that the streak gonad will develop a gonadoblastoma (which can progress to a dysgerminoma) and gonadal removal is generally recommended.

Recurrence risk

The recurrence risk does not appear to be increased above the general population risk.

TRISOMY 18 (EDWARDS SYNDROME)

Incidence

The incidence of trisomy 18 is 1 in 3000 livebirths with a maternal age effect. The incidence at conception is much higher, but 95% of affected fetuses abort spontaneously. At birth there is a preponderance of females, which may reflect an excess of spontaneous abortion in the affected males.

Clinical features

The birth weight is low, and multiple dysmorphic features are apparent in the newborn. These include: a characteristic skull shape with a small chin and prominent occiput, low set malformed ears, clenched hands with overlapping index and fifth fingers, single palmar creases, rockerbot-

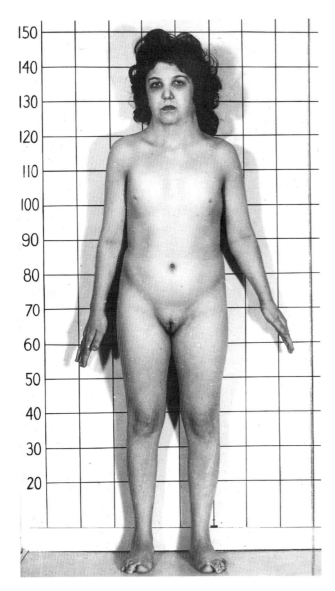

Fig. 13.6 Adult female with untreated Turner syndrome.

tom feet and a short sternum (Fig. 13.7). The dermato-glyphics show a predominance of arches, and in males cryptorchidism is usual.

Malformations of the heart, kidneys and other organs are frequent, and 30% die within a month. Only 10% survive beyond the first year, and these children show profound developmental delay.

Aetiology

Trisomy 18 usually results from maternal non-disjunction (95%, especially at the first meiotic division). Paternal non-disjunction is less common (5%) and rarely a parental translocation is responsible. Occasionally, mosaicism is seen with a milder phenotype.

Recurrence risk

For parents of a child with regular trisomy 18 the risk of recurrence or of other major chromosomal abnormality is 1.5% at amniocentesis.

TRISOMY 13 (PATAU SYNDROME)

Incidence

The incidence of trisomy 13 is 1 in 5000 livebirths, with a maternal age effect.

Clinical features

Multiple dysmorphic features are apparent at birth. These include: hypotelorism reflecting underlying holoprosen-cephaly, microphthalmia, cleft lip and palate, abnormal ears, scalp defects, redundant skin about the nape, clenched fists, single palmar creases (60%), post-axial (little finger side) polydactyly, prominent heels and cryp-torchidism in the male (Fig. 13.8).

Congenital heart disease is usual, and 50% die within a month. Only 10% survive beyond the first year and these children show profound developmental delay.

Aetiology

Trisomy 13 usually results from maternal non-disjunction (65%, especially the first meiotic division). Paternal non-disjunction is less common (10%). In about 20% of cases one parent is a translocation carrier and in about 5% of patients mosaicism is present.

Recurrence risk

The recurrence risk is less than 1% provided a parent is not a carrier of a balanced translocation.

TRIPLOIDY

Incidence

Triploidy occurs in 2% of all conceptions, but early sponta-neous abortion is usual and survival to term exceptional.

Clinical features

The neonate with triploidy has marked low birth weight, disproportionately small trunk to head size, syndactyly, multiple congenital abnormalities and a large placenta with hydatidiform-like changes in many cases (Fig. 13.9).

Aetiology

In most cases the extra set of chromosomes is paternally derived, with 66% due to double fertilization, 24% due to fertilization with a diploid sperm and 10% due to fertiliza-tion of a diploid egg. Sixty per cent are 69,XXY and most of

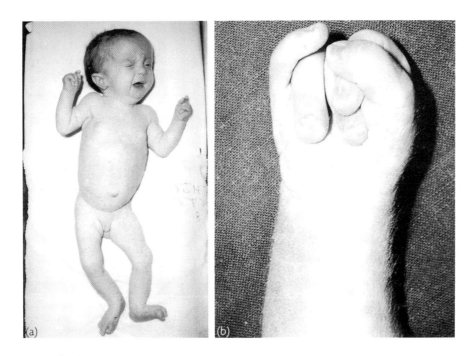

Fig. 13.7 Trisomy 18 phenotype. (a) General view. (b) Close-up of hand showing characteristic posture.

the remainder are 69,XXX. Hydatidiform change is found only when there is a double paternal contribution (p. 54).

Recurrence risk

The recurrence risk is not known but is probably not increased above the general population risk.

DELETIONS AND DUPLICATIONS

A large number of chromosomally unbalanced children have been described with visible deletions or duplications, or combinations of the two. Overall the birth incidence is 1 in 2000.

These may arise from meiosis where a parent has a balanced structural rearrangement (10–15%), or as new mutations. Any visible chromosomal imbalance of the autosomes almost invariably produces an abnormal phenotype with multiple dysmorphic features and mental handicap. The clinical features tend to be fairly non-specific, although similar in sibs with the same aberration. The presence of duplicated or deleted genes in the involved areas of the chromosomes may be confirmed by gene dosage studies. These not only prove the chromosomal imbalance but also aid gene localization. (The children with chromosome 9 imbalance in Fig. 13.12 helped to localize galactose-1-phosphate uridyltransferase and adenylate kinase-1; see Fig. 9.8 p. 87.) For any of these chromosomal duplication–deletions, parental chromosomes must be examined to exclude balanced structural rearrangements. If parental chromosomes are normal then

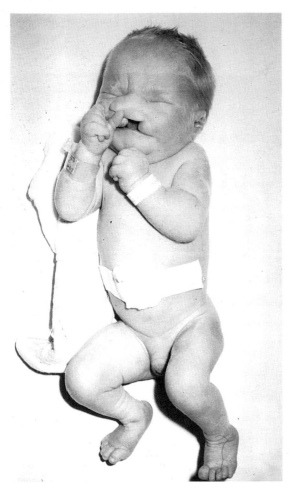

Fig. 13.8 Trisomy 13 phenotype.

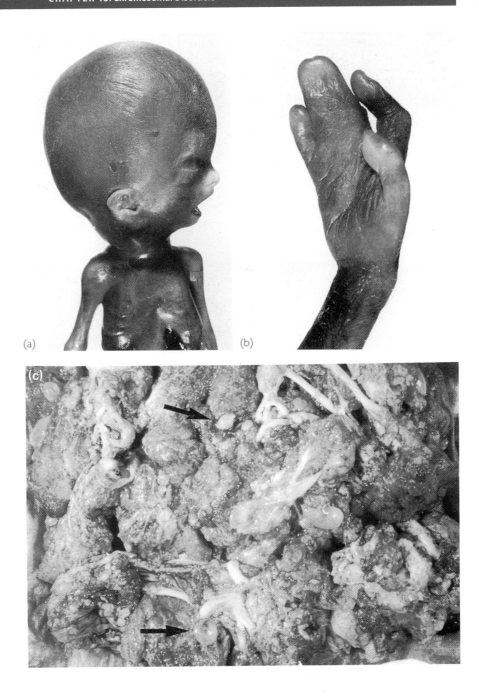

Fig. 13.9 Triploidy showing (a) trunk to head disproportion and (b) syndactyly. (c) Partial hydatidiform changes in the placenta.

the recurrence risk is not increased above the general population incidence unless gonadal mosaicism is present. If a parent is a balanced carrier then recurrence risks are as given in Table 13.3.

The child shown in Fig. 13.10 has mental handicap, an iris coloboma and a dysmorphic facial appearance due to a partial deletion of the short arm of chromosome 4. In this case the parents' chromosomes were normal and the recurrence risk was thus low (Fig. 13.11). In contrast, in the family shown in Fig. 13.12 the two children have partial duplication of 9p and partial deficiency of 15p, which results in a dysmorphic facial appearance and mental handicap. Their mother is clinically normal but carries the balanced translocation, as does their brother, whose wife has had prenatal diagnosis in each pregnancy with termination of one chromosomally unbalanced fetus.

MARKER CHROMOSOMES

A small additional chromosome of unknown origin (termed a marker chromosome) is found in one per 2500

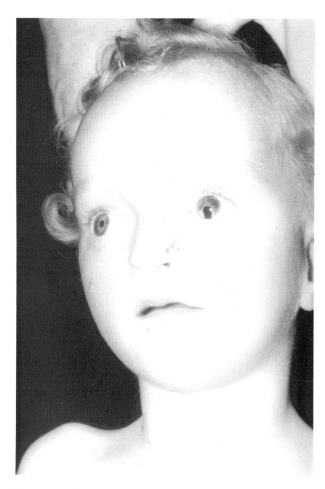

Fig. 13.10 Facial appearance in partial deletion of the short arm of chromosome 4 (4p–, Wolf syndrome).

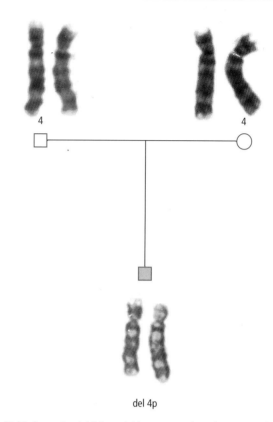

del 4p

Fig. 13.11 Parental and child's partial karyotype to show *de novo* partial deletion of the short arm of chromosome 4.

pregnancies. About 90% are thought to be derived from the short arms and pericentromeric regions of acrocentric chromosomes (with about one-half from chromosome 15; hence the value of DAPI + distamycin A staining, p. 34). Parental karyotypes should be examined and an attempt might be made to identify the nature of the additional chromosomal material using chromosome painting (p. 65).

PRADER–WILLI SYNDROME

Clinical features
In the newborn with Prader–Willi syndrome, hypotonia and poor swallowing may be marked. The face is flat with a tented upper lip, and the external genitalia are hypoplastic. In later childhood the hypotonia improves and overeating with obesity occurs. The forehead tends to be prominent with bitemporal narrowing. The palpebral fissures are almond-shaped and the hands and feet are small (Fig. 13.13). Mental handicap is usual with an IQ range of 20–80 and a mean of 50.

Genetic aspects
The frequency is 1 in 10 000 and in 50% a cytogenetic microdeletion is apparent at 15q11–13. In a further 25%, a deletion of chromosome 15q of variable size can be detected by fluorescence *in situ* hybridization (FISH) or DNA analysis with probes from the deleted region (Plate 11). In contrast to Angelman syndrome the deleted chromosome in Prader–Willi syndrome is invariably paternal in origin. Recurrence has not been documented where the child has a *de novo* deletion but 2% arise from a parental structural rearrangement and here prenatal diagnosis needs to be considered. In the remaining 25% of Prader–Willi patients, there is no 15q deletion but DNA analysis reveals maternal uniparental disomy (p. 68) and the consequent lack of paternally expressed genes from the critical region results in the phenotype.

ANGELMAN SYNDROME (HAPPY PUPPET SYNDROME)

Clinical features
Developmental delay, very poor speech, jerky movements, paroxysms of inappropriate laughter and a dysmorphic facies are characteristic (Fig. 13.14). The EEG

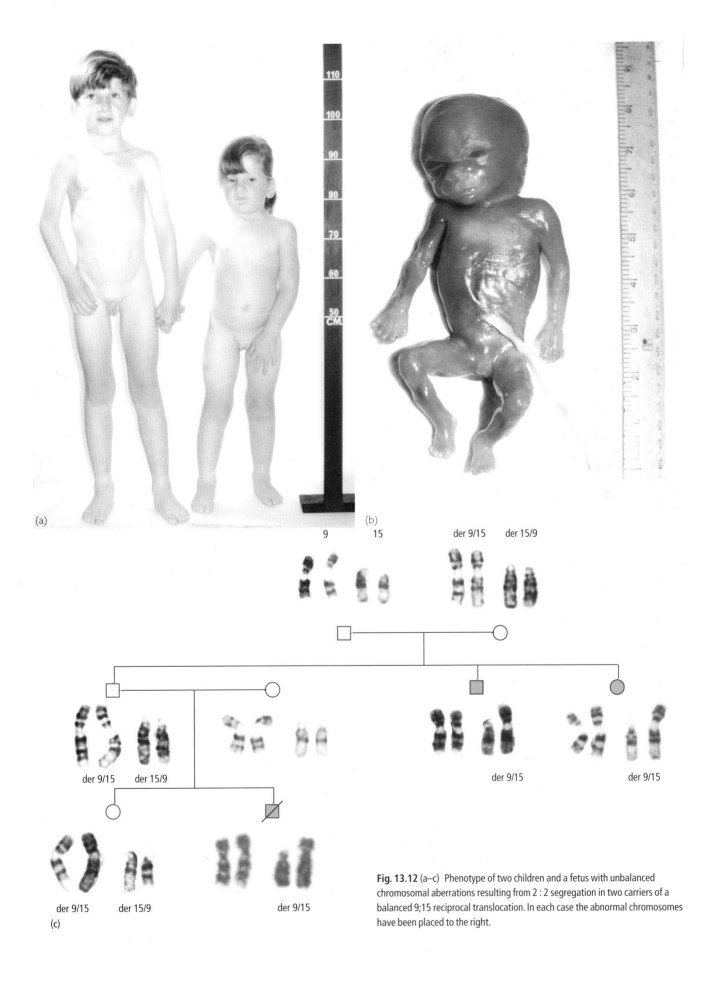

Fig. 13.12 (a–c) Phenotype of two children and a fetus with unbalanced chromosomal aberrations resulting from 2 : 2 segregation in two carriers of a balanced 9;15 reciprocal translocation. In each case the abnormal chromosomes have been placed to the right.

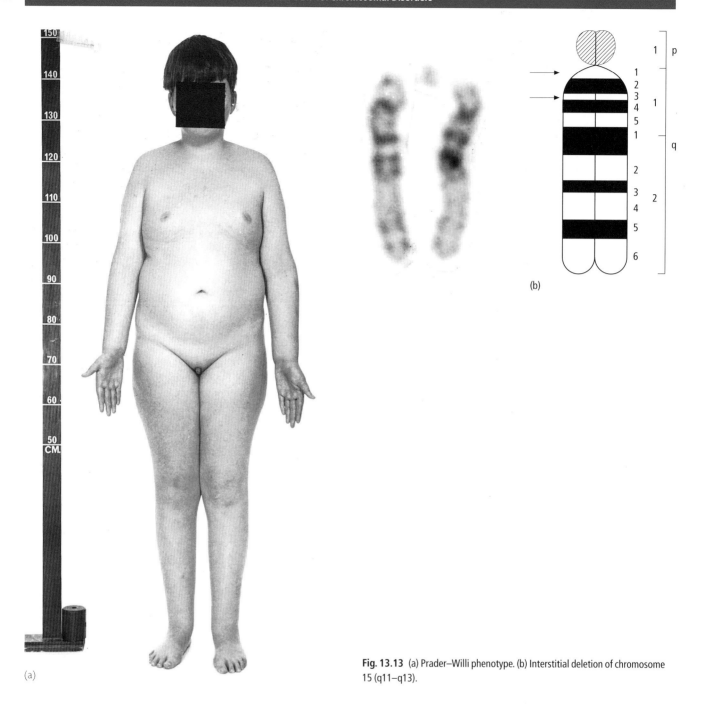

(a)

(b)

Fig. 13.13 (a) Prader–Willi phenotype. (b) Interstitial deletion of chromosome 15 (q11–q13).

is always abnormal with posterior high voltage sharp waves and posterior spike and wave on eye closure.

Genetic aspects

The frequency is 1 in 20 000 and about 50% of patients show a visible cytogenetic microdeletion at 15q12 and a deletion can be identified in a further 25% using FISH or DNA analysis with probes from the deleted region. In contrast to the Prader–Willi syndrome, which shows a similar cytogenetic microdeletion, the deleted 15 is invariably maternal in origin in Angelman syndrome (Fig. 13.15). The recurrence risk in families with a *de novo* deletion is low but familial recurrences have been described and in these affected children no deletion is apparent on DNA analysis. In a further 5% of patients, DNA analysis reveals paternal uniparental disomy but the molecular pathology in the remaining 20% is unknown.

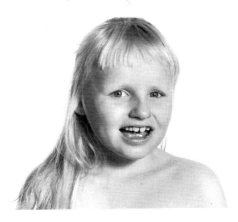

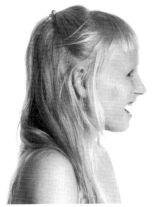

Fig. 13.14 Facies in Angelman syndrome.

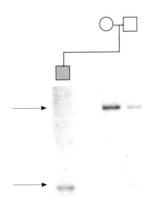

Fig. 13.15 DNA analysis in a family with Angelman syndrome using a polymorphic probe from chromosome 15q12. The polymorphic fragments are arrowed and the child has failed to inherit a maternal fragment.

OTHER MICRODELETION DISORDERS

In addition to Prader–Willi and Angelman syndromes several other conditions have been shown to be due on occasion to a visible microdeletion (Table 13.5).

The smallest visible deletion involves 4000 kb, and thus large numbers of genes can be lost or gained without producing visible changes. The clinical effects of such abnormalities would be mental handicap, multiple congenital abnormalities and/or dysmorphic features. In some cases a deletion can result in the occurrence of more than one single gene disorder in the same patient because they happen to map close to one another. The best-known example of such a deletion syndrome (contiguous gene disorder or segmental aneusomy) is the association of Duchenne muscular dystrophy, adrenal hypoplasia and glycerol kinase deficiency (and sometimes chronic granulomatous disease) due to a 6000–8000 kb deletion in Xp21.2.

Table 13.5 Conditions which may be caused by visible chromosomal microdeletions.

Condition	Site of microdeletion
Alagille syndrome	20p
Alpha-thalassaemia with mental handicap (p. 132)	16p
Angelman syndrome (p. 126)	15q11–12
DiGeorge syndrome (p. 192)	22q11
Langer–Giedion syndrome	8q24
Miller–Dieker lissencephaly	17p13
Prader–Willi syndrome (p. 126)	15q11–12
Retinoblastoma (p. 175)	13q14
Rubinstein–Taybi (p. 193)	16p
Williams syndrome (p. 194)	7q
Wilms tumour–aniridia syndrome (WAGR) (p. 176)	11p13

CHAPTER 14

Single Gene Disorders

CONTENTS

Single gene disorders discussed in this chapter
are arranged in alphabetical order

To date, more than 6600 human single gene disorders have been described, which collectively affect about 2% of the population. Their identification is vital in order to provide meaningful genetic counselling and, when appropriate, prenatal diagnosis. This is hampered by the similar phenotypes exhibited by different single gene defects and by some commoner multifactorial disorders (genetic heterogeneity).

The commoner and clinically most important single gene disorders are outlined here in alphabetical order, together with some rarer conditions which illustrate important genetic principles. These outlines should serve to allow the reader to select appropriate reference texts for further information.

Acetylator status

Diagnosis. Quantitative studies of metabolic rate of drugs (e.g. isoniazid, hydralazine, nitrazepam) which are metabolized by acetylation. DNA analysis for specific point mutations.

Prognosis. Rapid metabolizers need increased doses of drugs to produce therapeutic effects and slow metabolizers have abnormally high circulating levels on standard doses and are thus prone to side effects.

Genetics. Autosomal recessive trait due to defects in hepatic arylamine *N*-acetyltransferase 2 (*AAC2*). In Caucasians, mutant alleles (especially R197Q — 36%, I114T — 34%) are commoner than the normal allele (26%) and as slow acetylators are homozygotes or compound heterozygotes for these mutant alleles, 50–65% of Caucasians are

slow acetylators. Only 10–20% of Orientals are slow acetylators as 69% of their alleles are normal (with R197Q in 24% and G286E in the remaining 7%).

Achondroplasia

Diagnosis. Short limbs especially proximally (rhizomelia); normal length trunk with lumbar lordosis; prominent forehead with depressed nasal bridge; trident hand; X-ray caudal narrowing of lumbar interpedicular distance (Fig. 14.1).

Prognosis. Mean adult height 132 cm in male, 123 cm in female; normal IQ and lifespan; backache common with a 5–10% lifetime risk for spinal cord compression.

Genetics. Autosomal dominant trait due to a specific point mutation (G380R) in fibroblast growth factor receptor 3 (*FGFR3*). The trait shows full penetrance and little variation in expressivity (the latter presumably reflects the consistency of the molecular pathology). Frequency 1 in 15 000–77 000 live births in different surveys with 80–90% of patients due to new mutations.

Acute intermittent porphyria (AIP)

Diagnosis. Episodes of abdominal pain, vomiting and red urine. Assay of red cell porphobilinogen deaminase and leucocyte ALA synthase.

Prognosis. Most patients (80%) are asymptomatic until exposed to an environmental trigger (drugs — barbiturates, sulphonamides, griseofulvin, diphenylhydantoin, oestrogens; infections; starvation; or alcohol). The

Behaviour disturbance, dementia, spastic paraparesis. Increased plasma long chain fatty acids (C26 : C22 ratio).

Genetics. X-linked recessive trait due to mutations in adrenoleucodystrophy protein gene (*ALD*). Variety of molecular pathology observed (including an exon 5 deletion of AG in 16%) with no genotype–phenotype correlation. Female carriers can be identified by combined indirect or direct DNA analysis and measurement of fatty acid ratios in plasma and cultured skin fibroblasts. Prenatal diagnosis is possible by either DNA or biochemical analysis of chorionic villus samples. Frequency 1 in 20 000 males.

Agammaglobulinaemia (Bruton type)

Diagnosis. Recurrent bacterial infections from 6 months onwards. Reduced serum immunoglobulins, failure to respond to injected antigens.

Prognosis. Excellent outlook with adequate immunoglobulin replacement therapy.

Genetics. Bruton agammaglobulinaemia is inherited as an X-linked recessive trait and is caused by mutations in the Bruton agammaglobulinaemia tyrosine kinase gene (*BTK*). Female carriers can be detected by indirect or direct DNA analysis and prenatal diagnosis is possible by either DNA analysis or immunological studies on fetal blood samples.

Other less common genetic causes of agammaglobulinaemia (X-linked and autosomal recessive) occur and overall the combined frequency of genetic agammaglobulinaemia is 1 in 10 000.

Albinism (oculocutaneous)

Diagnosis. Pink–red skin which fails to tan, white hair, blue or pink irides and a prominent red reflex. Abnormal visual evoked response due to misrouting of optic fibres. Absent hair root tyrosinase in most (90–95%) patients with type I.

Prognosis. Variable phenotype depending upon the level of residual protein activity. Non-progressive reduction in visual acuity. Increased risk of basal cell carcinoma and melanoma.

Genetics. Type I oculocutaneous albinism is inherited as an autosomal recessive trait and is caused by a variety of mutations in tyrosinase (*TYR*). Carrier detection within an affected family may be possible by DNA analysis and prenatal diagnosis has been reported by electron microscopy of fetal skin biopsies (and would also be possible by DNA analysis). Type I oculocutaneous

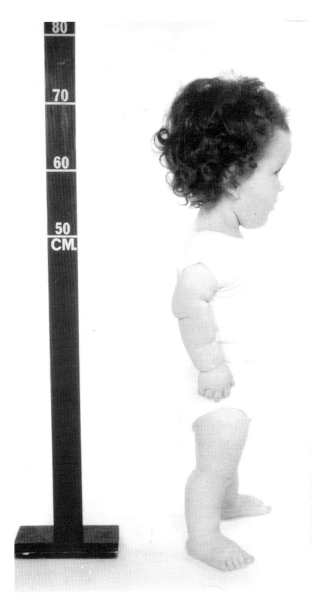

Fig. 14.1 Achondroplasia.

porphyric crisis may cause a neuropathy which can result in respiratory paralysis. Porphyric crises severe enough to cause hospitalization occur in 1 in 75 000 of the population and carry a mortality rate of 5%.

Genetics. Autosomal dominant trait due to mutations in porphobilinogen deaminase (*PBGD*). Family members at risk can be screened biochemically (see 'Diagnosis') or by direct or indirect DNA analysis.

Adrenoleucodystrophy

Diagnosis. Variable clinical picture with symptoms due to neurological involvement and/or adrenal insufficiency.

albinism has a similar frequency in many populations of 1 in 40 000.

Type II oculocutaneous albinism is also inherited as an autosomal recessive trait and is caused by a variety of mutations in the *P* gene. The frequency of type II oculocutaneous albinism is 1 in 40 000 in Caucasians but much higher in equatorial Africa (e.g. 1 in 1400 in Tanzania with 75–80% due to a 2.7 kb deletion) and in Hopi Indians (1 in 227).

Alpha₁-antitrypsin deficiency

Diagnosis. Assay of protease inhibitor activity and typing by isoelectric focusing. DNA analysis for specific mutations.

Prognosis. Only ZZ homozygotes affected; juvenile cirrhosis (5–10%) but if a ZZ sib has juvenile liver disease this rises to 40–78%; pulmonary emphysema in third or fourth decade, especially in those who smoke cigarettes (60–70%). These patients account for about 2% of patients with emphysema.

Genetics. Autosomal recessive trait due to a variety of mutations in antitrypsin (*PI*). The Z allele is a point mutation (E342K) which interferes with its release from its site of production in hepatocytes. The carrier frequency of the Z allele in Europe and the USA is 3% and this results in a ZZ homozygote frequency of 1 in 4400. Carrier detection is possible by biochemical or DNA analysis and prenatal diagnosis by DNA analysis of a chorionic villus sample can be offered.

Alpha-thalassaemia

Diagnosis. Homozygotes for alpha-thalassaemia 1 show 80% haemoglobin Bart's with four gamma chains and a persistence of embryonic haemoglobins. Patients with HbH show reduced MCHC and reduced MCV with HbH (four beta chains) 5–30% and some haemoglobin Bart's. Alpha-globin synthesis is reduced or absent.

Prognosis. Normally there are two functional alpha-globin genes on each copy of chromosome 16 (αα/αα). If no functional alpha-globin genes are present (−−/−−, alpha-thalassaemia type 1 homozygote) then profound anaemia occurs *in utero* with hydrops fetalis and intrauterine or early neonatal death. Presence of a single functional alpha-globin gene (−−/−α) results in a chronic haemolytic anaemia (Haemoglobin H disease). Individuals with two (−α/−α, alpha-thalassaemia type 2 homozygote; or −−/αα, alpha-thalassaemia type 1 heterozygote) or three (−α/αα, alpha-thalassaemia type 2 heterozygote) functional alpha-globin loci are asymptomatic.

Genetics. Autosomal recessive trait due to a variety of mutations in the alpha-globin gene cluster (*HBAC@*). Detection of the severe (alpha-thalassaemia 1) carrier is possible by routine haematological analysis but the mild (alpha-thalassaemia 2) carrier may not be readily detected. Prenatal diagnosis by DNA analysis is possible for couples at risk of alpha-thalassaemia type 1 homozygotes (−−/−−). Five to eight per cent of Thais are alpha-thalassaemia 2 heterozygotes and 6% are alpha-thalassaemia 1 heterozygotes. In contrast in US Blacks, 25% are alpha-thalassaemia 2 heterozygotes but heterozygotes for alpha-thalassaemia 1 are rare.

Alpha-thalassaemia/mental handicap syndrome

Diagnosis. Haemoglobin H inclusions (in 1–40% of red cells) in a mentally handicapped microcephalic male with a characteristic facies (small triangular nose with anteverted nares, hypertelorism and carp-like lips, Plate 12) and genital abnormalities in most cases.

Prognosis. Mental handicap is severe with absent or very limited speech.

Genetics. X-linked recessive trait with transacting downregulation of alpha-globin (chromosome 16) synthesis due to *ATRX* mutations. Obligate female carriers have occasional HbH inclusions. Carrier detection and prenatal diagnosis are possible by direct or indirect DNA analysis.

Several children (males and females) have also been described with variable degrees of mental handicap, variable dysmorphic features and alpha-thalassaemia associated with microdeletions of 16p which include the alpha-globin locus.

Alport syndrome

Diagnosis. Nephritis with proteinuria and haematuria, progressive sensorineural deafness, electron microscopy of a renal biopsy shows extensive thickening of the glomerular basement membrane and splitting of the lamina densa.

Prognosis. Chronic renal failure is usual in adulthood in affected males. One-third of female carriers become hypertensive in middle age and 5–10% develop chronic renal failure.

Genetics. X-linked recessive trait due to a variety of mutations in the gene for the type of collagen (*COL4A5*) which is a specific component of the glomerular basement membrane. Female carriers are usually asymptomatic although most have microscopic haematuria. DNA analysis (mutation or mutant gene tracking) can be used for carrier detection and early prenatal diagnosis. Frequency 1 in 5000 males.

Androgen insensitivity syndrome (testicular feminization syndrome)

Diagnosis. Female phenotype with normal breast development but primary amenorrhoea and paucity of pubic and other body hair; blind vaginal pouch, intra-abdominal testes; 46,XY karyotype.

Prognosis. Inguinal herniae (50%); gonadal neoplasms if not removed (5–20%); infertility (100%); normal IQ and lifespan.

Genetics. X-linked recessive trait due to a variety of mutations in the androgen receptor (*AR*) which interfere with binding and hence effects of testosterone and dihydrotestosterone. Carrier detection possible by direct or indirect DNA analysis. Frequency 1 in 62 000 males.

Apert syndrome

Diagnosis. Craniosynostosis of several sutures; bony syndactyly of digits 2–5 (Fig. 14.2).

Prognosis. Mental handicap (mild in 31%, severe in 7%); cleft palate (25%).

Genetics. Autosomal dominant trait due to mutations in the fibroblast growth factor receptor 2 gene (*FGFR2*). Most patients represent new mutations and the birth frequency is 1 in 10 000.

Craniosynostosis is a feature of a large number of rare single gene disorders.

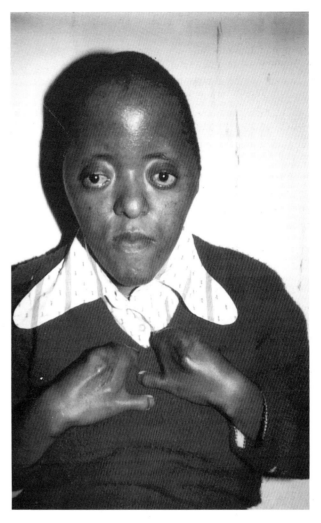

Fig. 14.2 Apert syndrome.

Ataxia telangiectasia

See p. 171.

Beta-thalassaemia

Diagnosis. Blood film in homozygotes shows severe hypochromia, microcytosis with target cells and increased haemoglobin F. Haemoglobin A_2 is usually increased. Beta-globin synthesis is reduced or absent.

Prognosis. Homozygotes (or compound heterozygotes) have a severe chronic anaemia due to ineffective erythropoesis and haemolysis and need repeated blood transfusions. Lifespan is often reduced despite such supportive measures. There is a range of clinical severity depending upon the molecular lesions and the coexistence of other haemoglobinopathies.

Genetics. Autosomal recessive trait due to a variety (over 120) of mutations in the beta-globin gene cluster (*HBBC@*).

Selection has resulted in a high carrier frequency for beta-thalassaemia in Mediterranean (e.g. 1 in 6 Cypriots and 1 in 14 Greeks), Asiatic Indian (1 in 6 to 1 in 50) and Chinese (1 in 50) populations and in each population particular mutations tend to be prevalent (e.g. a beta-globin splice site mutation G → C at nucleotide 5 of intron 1 in Indians and Q39X in Sardinians). Carriers can be detected by haematological analysis (microcytosis with MCV < 80 fl and/or low MCH, <27 pg and increased haemoglobin A_2, >3.5%). Prenatal diagnosis can be offered by direct or indirect DNA analysis on chorionic villus samples or by fetal blood sampling and haematological analysis.

Branchio–oto–renal syndrome

See p. 187.

Colour blindness

Diagnosis. Detected by colour vision charts or anomaloscopy.

Prognosis. Normal visual acuity.

Genetics. Normal colour vision depends upon the products of three loci — blue (*BCP*) on chromosome 7 and red (*RCP*) and green (*GCP*) in Xq28. Unequal crossing-over is common for the red and green genes (see p. 17) to produce loss or altered absorption spectra for the red or green gene products. X-linked recessive defects of red–green colour vision affect 8% of male Caucasians (rarer in Blacks and Orientals) with absent red or green genes in one-quarter and altered genes in the remainder.

Congenital adrenal hyperplasia (21-hydroxylase deficiency)

Diagnosis. Neonatal vomiting, shock and death in the salt-losing form; virilization of the female with ambiguous genitalia; precocity in the male; elevated urinary ketosteroids and pregnanetriol; markedly elevated serum 17α-hydroxyprogesterone and ACTH; biochemical abnormalities restored to normal with therapy.

Prognosis. Normal lifespan, health and fertility if promptly diagnosed and replacement therapy with hydrocortisone and fludrocortisone instituted.

Genetics. Autosomal recessive trait due to gene conversion (70%) or unequal crossing-over (30%) involving the active cytochrome P450 genes involved in steroid 21-hydroxylation, which are linked to the MHC on chromosome 6 (see Fig. 15.6, p. 154). In the UK the commonest mutation is a gene conversion of the active *CYP21B* to the form of the neighbouring pseudogene *CYP21A* and this mutation shows linkage disequilibrium with the HLA A11, B55, DR4 haplotype. Non-salt-losing and salt-losing (50%) forms are allelic and reflect the residual level of enzyme activity. Carrier detection is possible by direct or indirect DNA analysis. Prenatal diagnosis is available by assay of 17α-hydroxyprogesterone in amniotic fluid or by DNA analysis of a chorionic villus sample in order to administer maternal dexamethasone 1.5 mg day^{-1} in divided doses for prevention of virilization in an affected female fetus. Incidence 1 in 8000–26 000 births in USA, 1 in 17 000 in UK and 1 in 500 in Yupik Eskimos. Deficiency of 21-hydroxylase is the commonest cause (95%) of congenital adrenal hyperplasia, but rarer enzyme deficiencies are known, which have different clinical features and biochemical abnormalities.

Congenital spherocytosis

Diagnosis. Chronic haemolytic anaemia with splenomegaly and unconjugated hyperbilirubinaemia; spherocytes with increased MCHC; reduced red cell survival and increased osmotic fragility.

Prognosis. Splenectomy abolishes the need for repeated blood transfusion; normal lifespan.

Genetics. Genetically heterogeneous due to mutations in ankyrin, β-spectrin, α-spectrin or protein 4.2. Most families show autosomal dominant inheritance but can be autosomal recessive. Frequency 1 in 5000.

Cystic fibrosis

Diagnosis. Sodium exceeds 60 mmol l^{-1} and chloride exceeds 70 mmol l^{-1} in a sample ($\geqslant$100 mg) of sweat induced by pilocarpine iontophoresis; absent trypsin in pancreatic juice; elevated serum immunoreactive trypsin levels in newborn permit neonatal screening.

Prognosis. Pancreatic insufficiency (85–90%); chronic lung disease secondary to recurrent infection; rectal prolapse (5–10%); male infertility (98%) meconium ileus (5–10%); cirrhosis of the liver (1–5%); median survival 25 years but variable clinical severity.

Genetics. Cystic fibrosis is inherited as an autosomal recessive trait and is caused by a variety (over 500) of mutations in the cystic fibrosis transmembrane conductance regulator gene (*CFTR*). A 3 bp deletion at position 508 (ΔF508) is the single commonest mutation. This mutation accounts for 70–80% of mutant alleles in northern Europe and the USA but is less common in southern Europe (45–55%), US Blacks (37%) and Ashkenazi Jews (30%). The protein in patients with ΔF508 is abnormally processed after translation and is degraded before it reaches its site of function. Of the remaining mutations, most are missense (40%), frameshift (30%), nonsense (20%) or splicing mutations (10%) — large length mutations are rare. Most of these other mutations are individually uncommon with occasional exceptions in association with particular ethnic groups (e.g. W1282X accounts for 48% of mutant alleles in Ashkenazi Jews).

Homozygosity of ΔF508 (about half of northern European and US patients) or other mutations with no residual function are associated with pancreatic insufficiency but the genotype (even within a family) is not predictive of the severity of pulmonary involvement which is the main prognostic factor. Homozygotes and compound heterozygotes for certain mutations where there is residual function retain pancreatic function, and in some, the only symptoms are chronic sinusitis or male infertility due to congenital absence of the vas deferens (where it accounts for 6% of all male infertility).

Carrier detection and prenatal diagnosis are possible by direct or indirect DNA analysis.

The frequency of affected homozygotes is 1 in 2500 in northern Europe with a carrier frequency of 1 in 25 but it is less common in Blacks (1 in 17 000 in US Blacks) and Orientals.

Cystinuria

Diagnosis. Increased urinary excretion and reduced intestinal absorption of cystine, lysine, arginine and ornithine.

Prognosis. Recurrent urinary calculi but lifespan normal with therapy.

Genetics. Autosomal recessive trait due to a variety of mutations in the gene for solute carrier family 3 member 1 (*SLC3A1*). Carrier detection and prenatal diagnosis possible by biochemical or direct or indirect DNA analysis. Frequency 1 in 10 000.

Debrisoquine/sparteine polymorphism

Diagnosis. Quantitative studies of metabolic rate of drugs (e.g. debrisoquine, sparteine, beta-blockers) which are metabolized by 4-hydroxylation or by DNA analysis to demonstrate specific point mutation.

Prognosis. Extensive metabolizers need increased doses of drugs to produce therapeutic effects and poor metabolizers have abnormally high circulating levels on standard doses and are thus prone to side effects.

Genetics. Autosomal recessive trait due to mutations in the hepatic cytochrome P450 for 4-hydroxylation (*CYP2D@*). Two common mutations in *CYP2D6*, a nucleotide deletion (2637A) and a splice site defect (1934 G → A), account for 70% of the total. Homozygotes or compound heterozygotes for the mutant alleles are poor metabolizers whereas mutant/normal heterozygotes and normal homozygotes are extensive metabolizers. Poor metabolizers have a frequency of 8% in Caucasians, 16% in Nigerians and 1% in Japanese.

Ehlers–Danlos syndrome

Diagnosis. Numerous variants are known with variable combinations of lax joints, hyperelastic skin, vascular fragility and poor wound healing (Fig. 14.3).

Prognosis. Lifespan is normal except in the variant with marked vascular fragility.

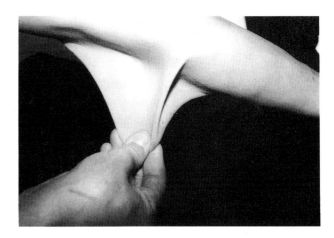

Fig. 14.3 Hyperelastic skin in Ehlers–Danlos syndrome.

Genetics. The three commonest types are inherited as autosomal dominant traits but X-linked and autosomal recessive forms are known; overall frequency 1 in 150 000.

Epidermolysis bullosa

Diagnosis. Multiple subtypes exist with a wide phenotypic range of severity of skin blistering in response to trauma. Skin histology, including electron microscopy, is usually required for classification.

Prognosis. Variable depending upon the subtype (ranges from neonatal death to normal lifespan).

Genetics. The commonest type is epidermolysis bullosa simplex where the split occurs in the epidermal basal cells. Several subtypes each inherited as an autosomal dominant trait due to mutations in keratin genes (e.g. keratin 14) or their control genes (e.g. keratin 14 or keratin 5) are known.

The dystrophic form also shows autosomal dominant inheritance and is linked to the Type VII collagen gene (*COLVIIA1*).

The lethal forms show autosomal recessive inheritance and prenatal diagnosis can be offered by fetal skin biopsy for electron microscopy.

Fabry disease (angiokeratoma corporis diffusum, Anderson–Fabry disease)

Diagnosis. Deficient alpha-galactosidase A activity in plasma, leucocytes and skin fibroblasts.

Prognosis. Childhood onset in affected males of episodic limb pains, skin lesions (angiokeratomas, especially on the lower trunk or upper legs), corneal streaks (on slit-lamp examination) and lens opacities. Chronic renal failure usually ensues in adulthood. Carrier females may be asymptomatic or show attenuated features of affected males.

Genetics. X-linked recessive trait due to a variety of mutations in alpha-galactosidase (*GLA*). Carrier detection by clinical examination (including slit lamp examination), assay of alpha-galactosidase A and direct or indirect DNA analysis. First-trimester prenatal diagnosis is possible by a combination of fetal sexing and biochemical or DNA analysis in a chorionic villus sample.

Familial spastic paraplegia

Diagnosis. Several subtypes with variable neurological features but including progressive spastic paraplegia.

Prognosis. Variable depending upon the subtype.

Genetics. Genetically heterogeneous with autosomal dominant, autosomal recessive and X-linked modes of inheritance evident in different families.

Fanconi syndrome

See p. 172.

Fragile X syndrome

Diagnosis. Under specialized culture conditions (thymidine or deoxycytidine starvation), cytogenetic analysis in mentally handicapped males and females with the full fragile X mutation usually shows a fragile site at Xq27.3 in 10–40% of cells (Fig. 14.4). One-half of unaffected female carriers of the full mutation also show the fragile site but the remainder and carriers (male or female) of the premutation have a normal cytogenetic analysis.

   DNA analysis usually shows an unstable length mutation in the CGG trinucleotide repeat (normally 6–52 repeats, median 30 repeats) in the 5′ UTR of the *FMR1* gene. In males with the premutation the size of the DNA fragment with the CGG repeat is usually increased by 150–500 bp (corresponding to 60–200 repeats). A similar increase in size is seen in females with the premutation and their second band represents the normal X chromosome (Fig. 14.5). In affected males the normal band is replaced by a single (1–4 kb corresponding to 230 to over 1000 repeats) larger band, multiple discrete larger bands or a smear of fragments (representing somatic instability of the mutation). Female carriers of the full mutation (whether normal or mentally handicapped) have a normal sized band in addition to the mutant band or bands as seen in the affected males (Fig. 14.5). In the full mutation, *FMR1* becomes hypermethylated and transcription is suppressed.

Prognosis. Male and female carriers of the premutation (small length mutations) are clinically normal. Females with the full mutation may be normal, or show mild (20–30%) or moderate (1%) mental handicap. Males with the full mutation are mentally handicapped and 50% have enlarged testes after puberty. Less consistent features include large ears, a long face and prognathism (Fig. 14.6).

Genetics. The instability of the length mutation results in atypical X-linked inheritance for the fragile X syndrome. All daughters of clinically normal males with the premutation (normal transmitting males) inherit the premutation which may be passed on either intact or with expansion to the full mutation. Further expansion of the full mutation can occur in somatic tissues or at female meiosis. Thus affected relatives usually have different length mutations and show phenotypic variability. In practice all mothers of affected males have either the premutation or the full mutation. For mothers with the full mutation one-half of their sons will be handicapped and one-half of their daughters will receive the full mutation (and about one-half of these daughters will have mental handicap to some extent). Prenatal diagnosis by DNA

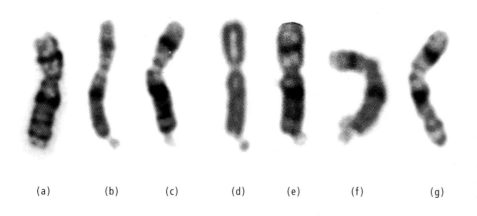

(a)   (b)   (c)   (d)   (e)   (f)   (g)

Fig. 14.4 Fragile site at Xq27.3. (a) Normal X chromosome (G-banding). (b) Site shown as a gap. (c–e) Site shown as chromatid break at gap (d; aceto-orcein). (f) Triradial produced by chromatid break at previous division followed by non-disjunction of distal fragment. (g) Loss of Xq28 following double chromatid break.

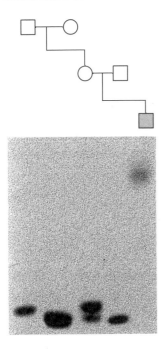

Fig. 14.5 DNA analysis of a family with the fragile X syndrome. (Note instability of the larger mutant allele.)

analysis is possible in the first trimester but prediction of which females with the full mutation will be handicapped is not yet possible. For mothers with the premutation the risk of expansion to the full mutation at meiosis depends upon the size of the mother's premutation and ranges from 16% (61–70 CGG repeats) to 70% (71–80 CGG repeats) to 100% (for over 80 CGG repeats).

The fragile X syndrome is the commonest inherited cause of mental handicap with a frequency of 1 in 1250 males. The frequency of the premutation is even higher (1 in 500–1500 males, 1 in 255–510 females).

Friedreich's ataxia

Diagnosis. Progressive ataxia from 6 to 8 years; pes cavus; loss of deep tendon reflexes in legs; extensor plantar response.

Prognosis. Progressive disability, 95% chairbound by 45 years.

Genetics. Autosomal recessive trait usually due to length mutations in *FRDA*. The GAA triplet in intron 1 normally has 7–22 repeats and patients commonly have expansion to 700–800 repeats. Prenatal diagnosis and carrier detection possible by direct (or indirect) DNA analysis.

This is the commonest (50% of the total) inherited cause of cerebellar ataxia but other rarer types are known (genetic heterogeneity). Frequency 1 in 50 000.

Galactosaemia

Diagnosis. Neonatal weight loss, vomiting, hepatomegaly, jaundice, cataracts and susceptibility to infection; reducing substance in the urine (galactose); absent red cell galactose-1-phosphate uridyl transferase (GALT).

Prognosis. Exclusion of milk and milk products from the diet is necessary for life; with such a diet lifespan is normal

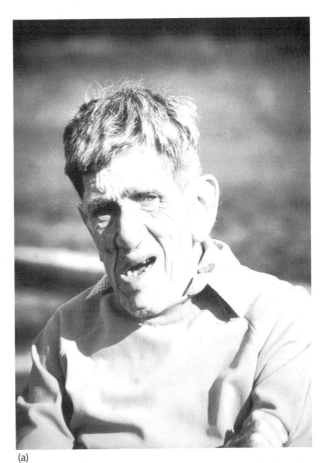

(a)

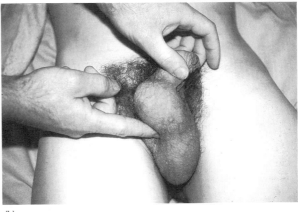

(b)

Fig. 14.6 Fragile X syndrome. (a) Typical facies. (b) Macro-orchidism.

but developmental delay, specific speech abnormalities and ovarian dysfunction are frequent. Mental handicap is invariable if therapy is delayed until after 1 month—hence the value of neonatal screening.

Genetics. Autosomal recessive trait due to a variety of mutations in *GALT*. Carrier detection possible (assay red cell GALT or DNA analysis). Prenatal diagnosis possible (assay of GALT in amniocytes or chorionic villi or assay of galactitol in amniotic fluid or DNA analysis). Allelic Duarte variant with higher residual GALT activity has no symptoms even in the homozygote but may be symptomatic in the Duarte–galactosaemia genetic compound. Incidence of galactosaemia 1 in 50 000 in Europe.

Gaucher disease

Diagnosis. Chronic adult type (Type I) results in bone pain and splenomegaly; acute infantile form (Type II) is a progressive neurological illness with hepatosplenomegaly; intermediate variants known (Type III); reduced leucocyte beta-glucosidase in all types.

Prognosis. One to two years' survival in infantile form; death in the second to fourth decade in Type III; normal lifespan in adult form and beneficial results from modified enzyme replacement.

Genetics. Autosomal recessive trait due to mutations in beta-glucosidase (*GBA*). Two common (N370S and L444P) and many rarer mutations. N370S accounts for 67–73% of mutant alleles amongst Ashkenazi Jews. N370S homozygotes and compound heterozygotes (N370S/ other) have Type I disease. L444P homozygotes have Type III Gaucher disease and compound heterozygotes (L444P/other inactivating mutation) have Type II disease.

Type I disease is particularly frequent in Ashkenazi Jews as 1 in 400 are affected and 1 in 10 are carriers (1 in 12–13 have N370S). Type III is frequent in Sweden.

For each type, carrier detection and prenatal diagnosis are possible by beta-glucosidase assay or by DNA analysis.

Gilles de la Tourette syndrome

Diagnosis. Onset in childhood of motor and vocal tics, obsessive–compulsive behaviour, attention deficit and learning difficulties.

Prognosis. Tics often (two-thirds) improve with age.

Genetics. Autosomal dominant trait with incomplete penetrance. Frequency 1 in 2000.

Glucose-6-phosphate dehydrogenase deficiency (G6PD deficiency)

Diagnosis. Deficiency of erythrocyte G6PD (may be false negative soon after a haemolytic crisis).

Prognosis. Clinical findings are variable. Affected males may be asymptomatic or present with prolonged neonatal jaundice, episodic haemolysis or a chronic haemolytic anaemia. Episodes of haemolysis may be triggered by drugs (e.g. primaquin or sulphonamides), chemicals (e.g. naphthalene in mothballs), ingestion of fava beans (favism) or by infections.

Carrier females are usually asymptomatic but may manifest with prolonged neonatal jaundice or haemolytic episodes with environmental triggers.

Genetics. X-linked recessive trait due to a variety of mutations in *G6PD*. Over 300 variants have been described but most have normal levels of enzyme activity and are asymptomatic. Almost all Caucasians and most Blacks have the normal electrophoretic B type of G6PD. The A type has an altered electrophoretic mobility but has near normal enzyme activity. This is present in 20% of Blacks and is due to a point mutation N126D. The A– variant, which is found in 10–25% of Blacks, has only 15% G6PD activity and is due to a second point mutation (V68M) on the A background (i.e. two point mutations in A– as compared with normal). The clinical features for families with this A– variant tend to be milder than for mutations which are commoner in Chinese (e.g. G163S) and Mediterraneans (e.g. S188F). G6PD deficiency occurs in 0–5% of Chinese, 0–20% of Italians, 0–32% of Greeks and 5–65% of Saudis.

Female carrier detection is possible by quantitation of erythrocyte G6PD or by direct or indirect DNA analysis.

Haemochromatosis

Diagnosis. Homozygotes have increased serum iron, transferrin saturation, serum ferritin and increased iron in a liver biopsy. The heterozygotes are normal except for a 3- to 10-fold increase in serum ferritin.

Prognosis. Untreated the complications include diabetes mellitus, hepatic cirrhosis, cardiomyopathy and arthropathy. Repeated venesection to reduce the iron overload improves the prognosis.

Genetics. Autosomal recessive trait with a gene locus (*HFE*) in 6p21. Frequency 1 in 400 Caucasians with 1 in 10 carriers. Carrier detection within an affected family may be possible using a combination of biochemical analysis and indirect or direct DNA analysis.

Haemophilia A

Diagnosis. Recurrent haemorrhage postoperatively and spontaneously into soft tissues and joints; factor VIII levels less than 30% of normal (<1% severe, 1–5% moderate, 5–30% mild).

Prognosis. With factor VIII intravenous replacement therapy lifespan near normal.

Genetics. X-linked recessive trait due to a variety of mutations in the gene for factor VIII (*F8C*). One mutation (an inversion rearrangement) is particularly common and accounts for one-half of all severe patients (and 20% of all haemophilia A mutations). Other loss of function mutations are associated with severe disease and missense mutations with mild-to-moderate disease. Carrier detection is possible by a combination of haematological analysis (Fig. 14.7) and indirect or direct DNA analysis. Prenatal diagnosis can be offered by DNA analysis of a chorionic villus sample (or by haematological analysis of a fetal blood sample). Haemophilia A affects 1 in 5000 males and accounts for 85% of all patients with haemophilia.

Haemophilia B (Christmas disease)

Diagnosis. Clinically indistinguishable from haemophilia A; factor IX level less than 30% of normal.

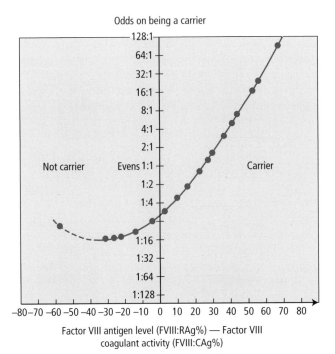

Odds on being a carrier

Fig. 14.7 Application of coagulation analysis to determine carrier risks in females at risk of haemophilia A.

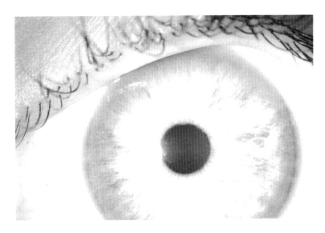

Fig. 14.8 Kayser–Fleischer ring in hepatolenticular degeneration.

Prognosis. With factor IX intravenous replacement therapy lifespan near normal.

Genetics. X-linked recessive trait due to a variety of mutations in the gene for factor IX (*F9*). Loss of function mutations are associated with severe disease and missense mutations with mild-to-moderate disease. Carrier detection is possible by a combination of haematological analysis and indirect or direct DNA analysis. Prenatal diagnosis can be offered by DNA analysis of a chorionic villus sample (or by haematological analysis of a fetal blood sample). Haemophilia B affects 1 in 30 000 males.

Hand–heart syndrome

See p. 189.

Hepatolenticular degeneration (Wilson disease)

Diagnosis. Juvenile or later (rare beyond 30 years) onset of progressive liver disease, basal ganglial disturbance and psychiatric and behavioural changes; Kayser–Fleischer rings of greenish brown pigmentation at periphery of iris (after 7 years of age, Fig. 14.8). Defective copper metabolism with reduced serum caeruloplasmin, increased hepatic copper and increased urinary copper on treatment with D-penicillamine.

Prognosis. Untreated results in chronic active hepatitis and neurological sequelae; normal lifespan with therapy.

Genetics. Autosomal recessive trait with locus a variety of mutations in a copper transporting beta polypeptide (*WND*). Carrier detection within a family and prenatal diagnosis are possible by direct or indirect DNA analysis. Homozygote frequency 1 in 33 000 (carrier frequency 1 in 90).

Hereditary angio-oedema (hereditary C1-inhibitor deficiency)

Diagnosis. Recurrent self-limiting episodes of oedema of the subcutaneous tissues or intestinal walls due to a functional deficiency of the complement C1 esterase inhibitor. Reduced C4 titres, especially when symptomatic.

Prognosis. Episodes tend to settle in later adult life, but death may occur during an attack if laryngeal oedema occurs, and prophylaxis with medications such as danazol or stanazolol should be considered. Attacks may be spontaneous (50%) or precipitated by trauma (e.g. dental extraction).

Genetics. Autosomal dominant trait due to a variety of mutations in the C1 inhibitor gene (*CINH*). DNA analysis (direct or indirect) for presymptomatic carrier detection.

Hereditary haemorrhagic telangiectasia (Osler–Weber–Rendu disease)

Diagnosis. Recurrent epistaxes (94%) or gastrointestinal bleeding (16%) with mucocutaneous telangiectases (Fig. 14.9).

Prognosis. Pulmonary arteriovenous malformations occur in 13%.

Genetics. Inherited as an autosomal dominant trait with age-related penetrance (50% by 12 years, 80% by 25 years and 100% by 45 years). Genetically heterogeneous with one locus on 9q (mutations in endoglin gene) and further loci on 3p and 12q. Frequency 1 in 100 000.

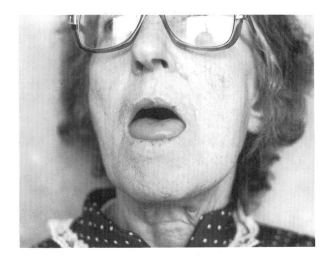

Fig. 14.9 Hereditary haemorrhagic telangiectasia.

Hereditary motor and sensory neuropathy Type I (peroneal muscular atrophy, Charcot–Marie–Tooth disease)

Diagnosis. Onset in the teens with bilateral foot drop; enlarged peripheral nerves; inverted champagne bottle legs; pes cavus; reduced ankle jerks; some sensory loss, especially for vibration; reduced nerve conduction velocity; nerve biopsy shows demyelination.

Prognosis. Normal lifespan with mild to moderate disability.

Genetics. Inherited as an autosomal dominant trait and in most families is associated with a localized duplication of 17p11.2 which includes the gene for peripheral myelin protein 22 (*PMP22*). This can be demonstrated by DNA analysis (routine cytogenetic analysis is normal) and this and nerve conduction studies can be helpful for counselling presymptomatic relatives at risk.

The frequency of HMSN1 is 1 in 2600 but rare variants occur with autosomal dominant, autosomal recessive and X-linked dominant inheritance.

Hereditary thrombophilia

Diagnosis. Recurrent superficial and deep vein thrombosis with either reduced plasma protein C, reduced protein S, reduced antithrombin III or factor V resistance.

Prognosis. Variable depending upon the site and extent of lesions.

Genetics. Each condition is inherited as an autosomal dominant trait. Presymptomatic screening of relatives by haematological analysis and indirect or direct DNA analysis (90% of factor V-resistant patients have the same mutation R506Q). Factor V resistance is present in 2–4% of the Dutch population but not all are symptomatic.

Huntington disease (HD, Huntington's chorea)

Diagnosis. Onset usually between 30 and 50 years; psychiatric symptoms; progressive chorea and dementia. Computed tomography (CT) scan may show caudate atrophy. Neuropathological changes tend to lag behind the clinical manifestations, but are specific with atrophy of the small neurones in the caudate and putamen and of the large neurones in the globus pallidus.

Prognosis. Progressive disability; death occurs on average 17 years from onset. Three per cent have onset under 15 years of age with intellectual decline, seizures, rigidity, myoclonus or dystonia. Occasional onset only after 60 years of age with chorea and slow progression.

Genetics. Huntington disease is inherited as an autosomal dominant trait and is caused by an unstable length mutation in huntingtin (*HD*). Normally 10–29 copies (median 18) of a CAG repeat are found at the 5′ end of the coding DNA whereas in patients the repeat is amplified to 36–120 copies (commonly 40–55). The patients with the juvenile form tend to show the largest expansions but a wide range of age of onset is observed for any specific repeat number. The repeat size is generally stable at maternal transmission but tends to increase at male transmission. Presymptomatic carrier detection and prenatal diagnosis can be offered by direct DNA analysis.

Hypercholesterolaemia (familial hypercholesterolaemia, FH, hyperlipidaemia II)

Diagnosis. Onset in third or fourth decade with xanthomata, xanthelasma, corneal arcus and evidence of ischaemic heart disease. Markedly increased fasting low density lipoproteins (including cholesterol) due to reduced clearance by defective low density lipoprotein receptors. In the absence of a family history routine laboratory distinction from polygenic hypercholesterolaemia (5% of the population) may be difficult.

Prognosis. Premature death from ischaemic heart disease with 50% of affected males dead by 60 years of age unless treated. This condition accounts for 3–8% of males with premature ischaemic heart disease.

Genetics. Autosomal dominant trait due to a variety of mutations in the low density lipoprotein receptor (*LDLR*). Prenatal and presymptomatic diagnosis possible by direct or indirect DNA analysis. Identification of heterozygotes by measurement of total cholesterol or LDL cholesterol is not fully reliable, especially in children. General population frequency of familial hypercholesterolaemia is 1 in 500.

Hyperthermia of anaesthesia (malignant hyperpyrexia)

Diagnosis. Asymptomatic until exposed to succinylcholine or halothane during a general anaesthetic. This causes muscle rigidity and a progressive rise in body temperature with very high levels of serum creatine kinase.

Prognosis. Mortality rate of 60% for an episode.

Genetics. Autosomal dominant trait with genetic heterogeneity. Some families have mutations in the ryanodine receptor (*RYR1*). Family members at risk can be screened by rectus abdominis muscle biopsy and *in vitro* exposure of the muscle to trigger agents such as halothane or caffeine or by increased cytoplasmic ionized calcium in peripheral blood mononuclears with exposure to halothane (or by DNA analysis if molecular pathology known). One in 15 000–150 000 affected.

Hypertrophic cardiomyopathy (HOCM)

Diagnosis. Asymmetric septal hypertrophy on cardiac ultrasound scan (two-dimensional echocardiography); wide clinical spectrum (asymptomatic mid-systolic ejection murmur, fatigue, dyspnoea, syncope, sudden death).

Prognosis. Annual mortality of 2–4% for sudden death due to arrhythmias.

Genetics. Autosomal dominant trait with genetic heterogeneity. Mutations in cardiac myosin in some families. Overall frequency 1 in 1000.

Ichthyosis vulgaris

Diagnosis. Onset after 3 months with ichthyosis, especially of extensor surfaces.

Prognosis. Normal lifespan.

Genetics. Autosomal dominant trait with variable expression. Affects 1% of the population and accounts for 95% of ichthyosiform dermatoses.

Incontinentia pigmenti

Diagnosis. Onset in infancy of vesicular skin rash followed by irregular whorled pigmentation; partial alopecia, hypodontia.

Prognosis. Mental handicap (30%); ocular problems (30%).

Genetics. X-linked dominant trait with *in utero* lethality for hemizygous males and thus a marked excess of affected females.

Intestinal polyposis

See p. 171.

Leber hereditary optic neuropathy (LHON)

Diagnosis. Acute or subacute visual loss at any age but most commonly in the second or third decade. Demonstration of specific mutations in mitochondrial DNA.

Prognosis. Loss of central vision is usually progressive and bilateral. May be cardiac conduction defects.

Genetics. LHON shows mitochondrial inheritance and is due to mutations in mitochondrial gene components of complex I. In 50% of patients at point mutation G to A at position 11 778 is present in *ND4* (the Wallace mutation) and in about 20% of patients a G to A point mutation is found at position 3460 in *ND2*. Patients are usually homoplasmic for these mutations and not all with the mutations develop symptoms, which suggests a role for as yet unidentified environmental factors.

Lesch–Nyhan syndrome

Diagnosis. Onset in infancy with progressive spasticity and choreoathetosis; later mental handicap is evident and self-mutilation; renal calculi and gouty arthritis. Increased serum uric acid (not invariable), high ratio of uric acid to creatinine in morning urine and reduced red cell hypoxanthine-guanine phosphoribosyl transferase (HPRT).

Prognosis. Allopurinol will lower the uric acid and prevent gouty arthritis and renal calculi, but does not prevent or ameliorate the neurological features.

Genetics. X-linked recessive trait due to a variety of mutations in *HPRT*. Carrier detection is possible using direct or indirect DNA analysis. Prenatal diagnosis can be offered by DNA analysis of chorionic villus samples. Frequency 1 in 10 000 males.

Marfan syndrome

Diagnosis. Wide clinical spectrum including arachnodactyly, long limbs with reduced upper to lower segment ratio, lax joints and evidence of complications (Fig. 14.10). Cultures of skin fibroblasts may show reduced, absent or structurally abnormal fibrillin.

Prognosis. Lens subluxation; scoliosis; aortic fusiform or dissecting aneurysm; average lifespan 40–50 years. Treatment with beta-blockers may retard progressive aortic dilatation and regular screening for cardiac and ocular complications should be offered.

Genetics. Autosomal dominant trait due to a variety of mutations in fibrillin 1 (*FBN1*). Tracking of the mutation or the mutant gene can be used for presymptomatic detection. Population frequency 1 in 10 000 with 25% representing new mutations.

Meckel syndrome

See p. 188.

Medium chain acyl-CoA dehydrogenase deficiency (MCAD deficiency)

Diagnosis. Deficiency of MCAD in liver, fibroblasts or leucocytes.

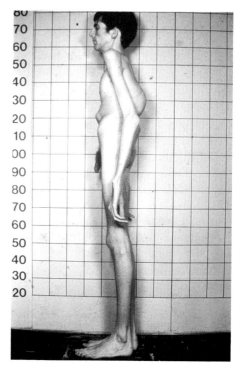

Fig. 14.10 Marfan syndrome.

Prognosis. Variable from no symptoms to episodic hypoglycaemia and sudden death.

Genetics. Autosomal recessive trait due to *MCAD* gene mutations. Commonest mutation (90%) is K329E. Population frequency 1 in 6000.

Mucopolysaccharidoses

Diagnosis. Four main types (although seven types known):

1 Type I (Hurler syndrome): mucopolysacchariduria; deficiency of alpha-1-iduronidase;
2 Type II (Hunter syndrome): mucopolysacchariduria; deficiency of iduronate-2-sulphatase;
3 Type III (Sanfilippo syndrome): mucopolysacchariduria; deficiency of heparan sulphate sulphatase or *N*-acetyl-alpha-D-glucosaminidase;
4 Type IV (Morquio disease): mucopolysacchariduria; deficiency of fibroblast 6-sulpho-*N*-acetylhexosaminidosulphatase.

Prognosis

1 Type I: consistent features include coarse facies in infancy, corneal clouding, umbilical hernia, short stature, progressive mental handicap and death in second decade (Fig. 14.11).

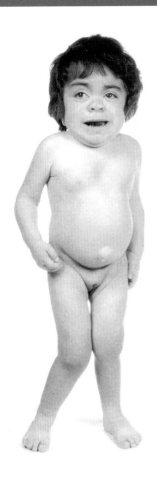

Fig. 14.11 Mucopolysaccharidosis type I (Hurler syndrome).

2 Type II: as type I but later onset and clear corneae; death in third decade.
3 Type III: progressive mental handicap in early childhood; normal facies, stature and corneae; death in second decade.
4 Type IV: short stature with scoliosis; normal intelligence, facies and corneae; atlantoaxial subluxation; death in third decade.

Genetics. All are inherited as autosomal recessive traits with exception of type II which is an X-linked recessive trait. Combined frequency 1 in 20 000 with type III most common. Prenatal diagnosis possible by analysis of glycosaminoglycans in amniotic fluid by two-dimensional electrophoresis and by enzyme assay in cultured amniocytes or chorionic villi; carrier detection is possible in females at risk for type II by biochemical analysis of white cells and hair roots and by the use of mutation or mutant gene tracking.

Multiple endocrine neoplasia

See p. 173.

Multiple exostoses

See p. 173.

Multiple self-healing squamous epithelioma

See p. 173.

Muscular dystrophy—facioscapulohumeral

Diagnosis. Onset is usually in the teens with proximal limb, perioral and periorbital muscle weakness; serum creatine kinase may be normal or increased; abnormal electromyogram and muscle biopsy.

Prognosis. Variable progression but the majority of patients will have moderate to severe disability by middle age (15–19% chairbound by 40 years).

Genetics. Autosomal dominant trait with complete but age-related penetrance (95% symptomatic by 20 years); gene tracking using extragenic RFLPs or localized duplications on 4q can be used for presymptomatic carrier detection; frequency 1 in 20 000.

Muscular dystrophy—X-linked

Diagnosis. Two main types:
1 Duchenne muscular dystrophy (DMD): onset in early childhood (90% < 5 years) of progressive proximal muscle weakness; walking often delayed, rarely able to run properly; calf pseudohypertrophy; marked elevation of serum creatine kinase; abnormal electromyogram and muscle biopsy which shows characteristic histology and absence of dystrophin;
2 Becker muscular dystrophy (BMD): onset of progressive muscular weakness in late childhood; calf pseudohypertrophy; marked elevation of serum creatine kinase; abnormal electromyogram and muscle biopsy which shows characteristic histology and reduced (3–10%) levels of dystrophin.

Prognosis. Duchenne: mild mental handicap (25%), chairbound in mid-childhood (95% by 12 years); death about 20 years. Becker: often chairbound about 25 years from onset; lifespan may be normal.

Genetics. Duchenne and Becker muscular dystrophy are inherited as X-linked recessive traits and are both caused by mutations in dystrophin (*DMD*). Partial deletions of variable size are commonest (65%) followed by a variety of point mutations. DMD is associated with null mutations resulting from frameshifts (due to out of frame deletions) or nonsense point mutations which prevent dystrophin production whereas in BMD dystrophin is produced albeit in reduced amounts or with aberrant function.

Carrier detection is possible by combined biochemical and DNA analysis. Assay of serum creatinine kinase (median of three separate assays; Fig. 8.3, p. 78) may be combined with pedigree risk information and information from direct or indirect DNA analysis (Appendix 2). Prenatal diagnosis can be offered by DNA analysis of chorionic villus samples.

If there is no family history, two-thirds of mothers of affected boys will be carriers with a high risk of recurrence for themselves and other female relatives. Frequencies are 1 in 3000 male births for DMD and 1 in 20 000 male births for BMD.

Myotonic dystrophy

Diagnosis. Progressive muscle weakness in early adult life, especially of the face, sternomastoids and distal limb muscles; difficulty relaxing clenched hands due to myotonia which will be evident on clinical examination or electromyography.

Prognosis. Cataracts, especially in the posterior part of the lens (85%); frontal baldness and gonadal atrophy in males; pigmentary retinopathy; cardiac conduction defects; severe disability usual 15–20 years from onset. General anaesthesia may be hazardous and the anaesthetist should be warned of the patient's diagnosis.

Genetics. Autosomal dominant trait due to an unstable length mutation of a CTG repeat at the 3′ UTR of *DM*. Normal individuals show stable minor length variations of this region (with 5–37 repeats) whereas in myotonic dystrophy expansion from 50 to over 2000 repeats is seen and these larger repeats are unstable. There is a general (but incomplete) correlation between the size of the repeat sequence and the clinical severity (mild 50–99, classic 100–1000 and congenital (1000–2000). Carriers of small amplifications may have no symptoms and normal electromyograms and normal slit-lamp examinations but can show further amplification with more severely affected offspring. Conversely, the length mutation may decrease at transmission and this is more common for paternal (10%) than maternal (3%) transmission. For an affected female: 50% of children unaffected, 29% affected in later life, 12% neonatal deaths, 9% severe neonatal hypotonia and mental handicap (Fig. 14.12). For an affected male: half offspring affected, half unaffected, with no neonatal cases. Presymptomatic carrier detection is possible by DNA analysis. Prenatal diagnosis is possible by direct DNA analysis. Frequency 1 in 7500.

Nephrolithiasis (X-linked)

Diagnosis. Urinary calculi, increased urinary calcium, reduced serum phosphate.

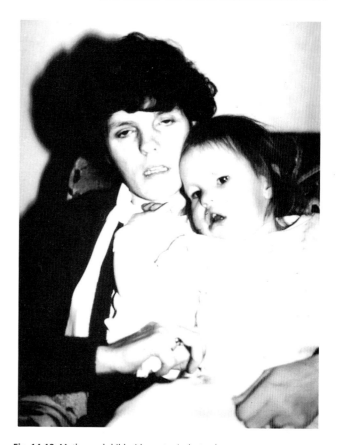

Fig. 14.12 Mother and child with myotonic dystrophy.

Prognosis. Variable.

Genetics. Inherited as an X-linked recessive trait and caused by a variety of mutations in a renal chloride channel (*CLCN5*).

Neurofibromatosis type I

See p. 174.

Neurofibromatosis type II

See p. 174.

Noonan syndrome

See p. 193.

Opsonic defect

Diagnosis. Low serum mannose binding protein.

Prognosis. Frequent unexplained infections in childhood, chronic diarrhoea.

Genetics. Autosomal dominant trait due to a variety of

mutations in the mannose binding protein (*MBL*) which binds glycoproteins prior to leucocyte phagocytosis. Frequency 5–7% of the population.

Osteogenesis imperfecta

Diagnosis

1 Type I: brittle bones with recurrent fractures, blue sclerae, conductive deafness due to otosclerosis, discoloured teeth due to dentinogenesis imperfecta.
2 Type II: perinatal lethal with multiple fractures at birth (Fig. 14.13).
3 Other: several other types with brittle bones and fractures of severity intermediate between types I and II, sclerae usually white.

Prognosis

1 Type I: variable number of fractures, lifespan normal.

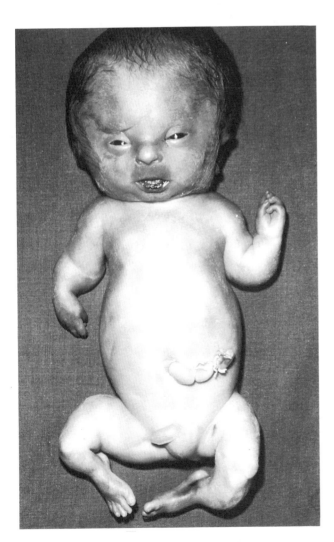

Fig. 14.13 Perinatal lethal variant of osteogenesis imperfecta.

2 Type II: perinatal lethal.
3 Other: variable degrees of physical disability.

Genetics

1 Type I is inherited as an autosomal dominant trait.
2 Type II is genetically heterogeneous with a composite recurrence risk of 3%. Prenatal reassurance is possible with ultrasound.
3 The other group is also genetically heterogeneous with a composite recurrence risk of 7%.

Combined birth frequency 1 in 20 000. A diversity of molecular lesions has now been identified in the structural genes for various collagen components and in the type I variant cosegregation consistently occurs with the collagen genes on chromosomes 7 or 17 (*COL1A2* and *COL1A1*, respectively).

Otosclerosis

Diagnosis. Progressive conductive hearing loss in middle age with normal tympanic membranes.

Prognosis. Hearing is restored by surgery.

Genetics. Autosomal dominant trait with 25–40% penetrance; frequency 1 in 330 in Caucasians, 1 in 3300 in Blacks, 1 in 333 000 in Orientals.

Phenylketonuria

Diagnosis. Elevated blood and urine phenylalanine.

Prognosis. Normal development and lifespan with a diet low in phenylalanine and supplemented with tyrosine; mental handicap if untreated; risk of mentally handicapped and malformed offspring for treated female unless diet is reintroduced *prior* to pregnancy to keep the maternal blood phenylalanine at 120–480 µmol l^{-1}.

Genetics. Autosomal recessive trait due to a variety of mutations in phenylalanine hydroxylase (*PAH*). Pattern of predominant mutations shows ethnic variation (e.g. R408W accounts for two-thirds of mutations in eastern Europe compared with 24% in Scotland and a splicing mutation in intron 10 accounts for 40% of Turkish mutations). Within affected families carrier detection and prenatal diagnosis are possible by DNA analysis. Frequency 1 in 10 000 in Europe (except for Ireland, 1 in 4000 and Turkey, 1 in 3000), rare in Afro-Caribbeans, Ashkenazi Jews and Indians.

Polycystic kidney disease

See p. 188.

Pseudoxanthoma elasticum

Diagnosis. Characteristic flexural skin changes (Fig. 14.14), retinal angiod streaks and diagnostic skin histology.

Prognosis. Systemic hypertension, occlusion of small to medium sized arteries and gastrointestinal haemorrhages result in a reduced lifespan.

Genetics. Genetic heterogeneity is apparent with most families showing autosomal recessive inheritance (remainder autosomal dominant).

Retinitis pigmentosa

Diagnosis. Progressive visual loss with clumps of retinal pigment resembling bone corpuscles.

Prognosis. Early loss of night vision and tunnel vision, later loss of central visual acuity. Progression varies within and between families.

Genetics. Genetically heterogeneous with autosomal dominant (15%, due to mutations in rhodopsin in some families and peripherin in others), autosomal recessive (70%) and X-linked recessive variants (15%) with a combined frequency of 1 in 3000–5000. These types are clinically difficult to distinguish and, in the absence of other affected family members to indicate a mode of inheritance, empiric risks need to be used. Thus the risk to a child of an affected parent with no family history is 1 in 8.

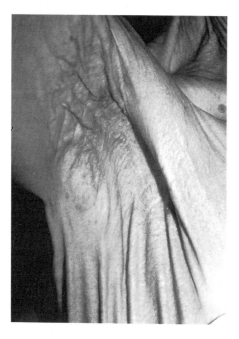

Fig. 14.14 Pseudoxanthoma elasticum.

In families with X-linked recessive inheritance carrier females can be identified using a combination of ophthalmic examination and indirect or direct DNA analysis.

Retinoblastoma

See p. 175.

Rett syndrome

Diagnosis. Onset at 6–18 months with developmental arrest then regression, 'hand-washing' automatisms and later seizures.

Prognosis. Anticonvulsants are helpful for seizure control but do not influence the disease course, and severe handicap is usual (chairbound at about 10 years).

Genetics. ? X-linked dominant trait with lethality in males to account for only females being affected and the low recurrence risk for normal parents. Frequency 1 in 10 000 females.

Severe combined immunodeficiency (SCID)

Diagnosis. Onset in the first few months of life with failure to thrive and recurrent infections (viral, fungal and bacterial). Reduced lymphocyte count, marked reduction in immunoglobulins, no ABO isoagglutinins.

Prognosis. Death in infancy unless a marrow transplant is successful.

Genetics. Genetically heterogeneous. Overall sex ratio 4 males to 1 female. At least two X-linked types and at least four autosomal recessive types. Carriers for the X-linked types cannot be detected immunologically but can be detected by molecular analysis which shows non-random X inactivation in T-lymphocytes. Two of the autosomal recessive types have defined enzyme deficiencies—adenosine deaminase (*ADA*) and purine nucleoside phosphorylase (*NP*)—and in these types prenatal diagnosis is possible by biochemical analysis of chorionic villus samples. In the remainder immunological studies of fetal blood samples will be required (in addition to fetal sexing in the X-linked types).

Sickle cell disease

Diagnosis. Blood film shows anaemia with distorted red cells and haemoglobin electrophoresis shows mainly HbS with some HbA_2 and some persistence of HbF (5–15%).

Prognosis. Severe chronic haemolytic anaemia in homozygotes. Recurrent episodes of infarction especially of the lungs, spleen and bones. Prone to pneumococcal infections and salmonella osteomyelitis. Lifespan is shortened despite supportive care. The outlook is greatly improved for patients who have concurrently inherited hereditary persistence of haemoglobin F.

Genetics. Autosomal recessive trait due to a point mutation in amino acid position 6 of beta-globin (E6V) which results in substitution of valine for glutamic acid. Carrier detection possible by haematological analysis (Sickledex test and Hb electrophoresis). Prenatal diagnosis possible in the first trimester by DNA analysis (direct detection of mutation, Fig. 3.11) or in the second trimester by haematological analysis.

Spinal muscular atrophy type I (Werdnig–Hoffmann disease)

Diagnosis. Progressive weakness due to anterior horn cell loss; reduced or absent deep tendon reflexes; fasciculation; normal creative kinase; EMG shows denervation, and muscle biopsy shows atrophy.

Prognosis. Death usual by 3 years.

Genetics. Type I spinal muscular atrophy is inherited as an autosomal recessive trait and is caused by a variety of mutations (especially deletions) in *SMA*. Carrier detection and prenatal diagnosis within a family may be offered by indirect or direct DNA analysis. Frequency 1 in 10 000 births (carrier frequency 1 in 50).

This is the commonest type of spinal muscular atrophy but there are several later onset variants.

Spinocerebellar ataxia type I (olivopontocerebellar ataxia)

Diagnosis. Onset usually in third or fourth decade with progressive cerebellar ataxia and spastic paraparesis. DNA analysis for specific length mutations.

Prognosis. Variable rate of progression.

Genetics. Inherited as an autosomal dominant trait due to unstable length mutations in a CAG polyglutamine repeat in ataxin-1 (*SCA1*). Normal individuals show stable inheritance of 19–36 repeats whereas in affected patients the repeat length is expanded to 42–81 and is unstable with a strong tendency for further expansion at paternal transmission. The size of the repeat is inversely correlated with age of onset (i.e. earlier in larger repeats). Presymptomatic and prenatal diagnosis can be offered by direct DNA analysis.

Type I is the commonest (50%) type of spinocerebellar ataxia but other variants with autosomal dominant and autosomal recessive inheritance are known.

Steroid sulphatase deficiency

Diagnosis. Commonest cause of ichthyosis presenting in the first 3 months; in adults, abdomen, legs and popliteal fossae most often affected; absent steroid sulphatase in hair roots.

Prognosis. May have corneal opacities (asymptomatic).

Genetics. Inherited as an X-linked recessive trait and caused by mutations (usually deletions) in steroid sulphatase (*STS*). Carrier detection possible by steroid sulphatase assay in hair roots and DNA analysis. Frequency 1 in 6000 males.

Succinylcholine sensitivity

Diagnosis. Asymptomatic until exposed to succinylcholine (suxamethonium) during induction of general anaesthesia when prolonged muscle paralysis with apnoea occurs. Quantitative assay of serum cholinesterase and its percentage inhibition by dibucaine.

Prognosis. Artificial ventilation is required until spontaneous recovery ensues.

Genetics. Autosomal recessive trait due to mutations in cholinesterase 1 (*CHE1*). Homozygote frequency 1 in 3500, carrier frequency 1 in 30, carriers can be detected by quantitative assay of cholinesterase.

Tay–Sachs disease

Diagnosis. Progressive neurological abnormalities from late infancy; cherry-red macular spot (90%); reduced serum beta-*N*-acetylhexosaminidase A activity.

Prognosis. Death usual by 3–4 years.

Genetics. Autosomal recessive trait due to mutations in the alpha chain of beta-*N*-acetylhexosaminidase A (*HEXA*). In Ashkenazi Jews the two commonest mutations are a 4 bp insertion in exon 11 and a splice site mutation in intron 12. Carrier detection is possible by assay of serum beta-*N*-acetylhexosaminidase A and DNA analysis. Prenatal diagnosis possible by assay of beta-*N*-acetylhexosaminidase A in chorionic villi (or amniocytes) and by DNA analysis. Highest frequency in Ashkenazi Jews (1 in 3600 births), carrier frequency 1 in 30. Carrier frequency in non-Jews 1 in 300.

Thrombocytopenia—absent radius (TAR syndrome)
See p. 189.

Treacher Collins syndrome (mandibulofacial dysostosis)

Diagnosis. Small mandible, malar hypoplasia and malformed ears (Fig. 14.15).

Prognosis. Conductive deafness (28%); cleft palate (32%); mental handicap (5%).

Genetics. Autosomal dominant trait with full penetrance but very variable expression; 60% of cases are new mutations. Indirect or direct DNA analysis can be considered for counselling at-risk relatives. Frequency 1 in 50 000.

Tuberous sclerosis

See p. 175.

van der Woude syndrome

See p. 186.

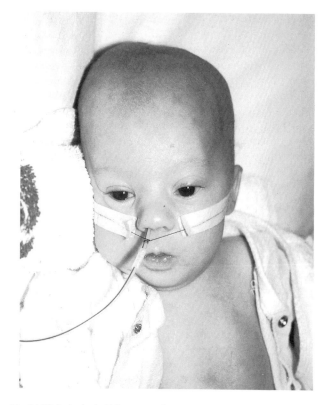

Fig. 14.16 Facies in the Zellweger syndrome.

Vitamin D resistant rickets (familial hypophosphataemic rickets)

Diagnosis. Growth retardation and childhood rickets, reduced serum phosphate.

Prognosis. Treatable with large doses of vitamin D (or its active metabolite calcitrol) and oral phosphate.

Genetics. Inherited as an X-linked dominant trait. Presymptomatic carrier detection possible using indirect DNA analysis. Frequency 1 in 20 000.

von Hippel–Lindau disease

See p. 176.

von Willebrand disease

Diagnosis. Quantitative or qualitative (e.g. reduced platelet aggregation with ristocetin or multimer pattern) defects in von Willebrand factor (vWF).

Prognosis. Patients may be asymptomatic or have excessive bleeding after trauma.

Genetics. Most families show autosomal dominant inheritance and a variety of mutations in *VWF* have been found.

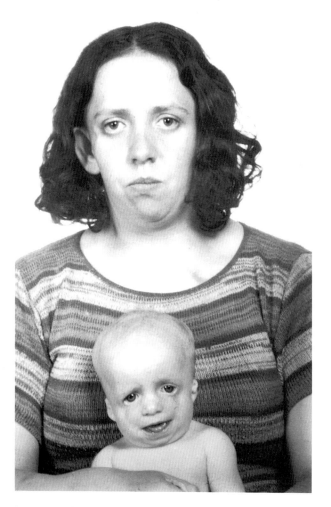

Fig. 14.15 Mother and child with Treacher Collins syndrome. Note variable expression.

In families with apparent autosomal recessive inheritance parents can often be shown to have mild *VWF* mutations which produce severe symptoms in the compound heterozygote (or homozygous) children. Population frequency for vWF heterozygotes may be higher than 1 in 1000.

Waardenburg syndrome

Diagnosis. The combination of lateral displacement of inner canthi (dystopia canthosum), white forelock (50%), heterochromia iridis (20%) and deafness is characteristic.

Prognosis. Bilateral congenital severe sensorineural deafness (30–40%).

Genetics. Inherited as an autosomal dominant trait with locus heterogeneity (due to mutations in *PAX3* in some families).

Wilms' tumour

See p. 176.

Xeroderma pigmentosum

See p. 176.

Zellweger syndrome (cerebrohepatorenal syndrome)

Diagnosis. Marked hypotonia in infancy with hepatomegaly, seizures and dysmorphic facies (Fig. 14.16). Increased urinary pipecolic acid and dicarboxylic acids. Increased ratio of C26 to C22 chain fatty acids in plasma and skin fibroblasts. Reduced dihydroxyacetone phosphate acyltransferase (DHAP-AT) in skin fibroblasts and platelets.

Prognosis. Progressive course with death usual in the first year of life.

Genetics. Autosomal recessive trait due to defects in PMP70 transporter which results in defective numbers and function of hepatic peroxisomes. Prenatal diagnosis possible by assay of the ratio of fatty acids or DHAP-AT in chorionic villus samples (or amniocytes).

CHAPTER 15

Immunogenetics

CONTENTS

GENETICS OF THE NORMAL IMMUNE SYSTEM 150
INHERITED IMMUNODEFICIENCY 151
Genetic susceptibility/resistance to particular infections 151
BLOOD GROUPS 152
ABO blood group 152
Rhesus blood group system 153
HAEMOLYTIC DISEASE OF THE NEWBORN 153

NEONATAL ALLOIMMUNE
  THROMBOCYTOPENIA 154
MAJOR HISTOCOMPATIBILITY COMPLEX
  (MHC) 154
TRANSPLANTATION 155
Blood transfusion 156
Other tissues 156

GENETICS OF THE NORMAL IMMUNE SYSTEM

The prime function of the immune system is to recognize and attack foreign (non-host) antigens which include most proteins, some polysaccharides and some nucleic acids. The immune response has two components, cellular and humoral, which are shown in a simplified form in Fig. 15.1. In the humoral response, specific antibodies are produced from 20 weeks of gestation onwards by stimulated B-lymphocytes or plasma cells. Antibodies are immunoglobulins and are important in the response to bacterial infections. The cellular immune response is effected by T-lymphocytes which, when specifically stimulated, become T-effector cells. T-lymphocytes have subsets to enhance (T-helper, CD4+) or reduce (T-suppressor, CD8) the immune response and to destroy cells (T-cytotoxic, CD8+). This cellular response is important in the reaction to malignant cells, transplanted tissues, intracellular microbes including viruses, bacteria and fungi.

Each immunoglobulin molecule is a protein composed of two identical light and two identical heavy chains held together by disulphide bonds (Fig. 15.2). Two types of light chain, kappa (κ) and lambda (λ), occur. The light chains are alike in all classes of immunoglobulin, but each class has its own characteristic heavy chain (Table 15.1). Each immunoglobulin chain has three regions, a variable

(V) region at the N-terminal end, which is part of the antibody combining site, a junctional (J) region and a constant (C) region. In the heavy chains a short diversity (D) region is present between the V and J regions.

The heavy chain gene cluster consists of about 200 V genes, about 50 D genes; six J genes and one or more genes for the C region of each class of immunoglobulin (Fig. 15.3). In each plasma cell, by a process of somatic recombination, one V, one D, one J and one C gene are juxtaposed and transcribed into a single contiguous molecule of

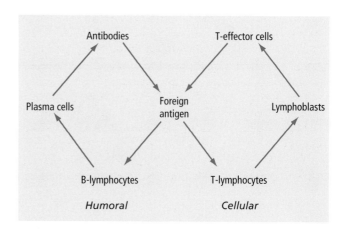

Fig. 15.1 Components of the immune response.

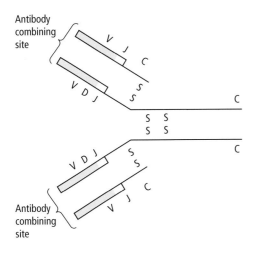

Fig. 15.2 Model of the immunoglobulin molecule.

mRNA. The remaining DNA of the cluster is excised, and this acts as a useful marker for lymphocytes of B-cell origin.

Any combination may occur, and this results in at least 12 000 possible VDJ combinations. Additionally, extra nucleotides may be inserted at the junctions and these genes are prone to undergo somatic mutation after being created, which results in even more diversity. Although the VDJ combination usually remains constant for that plasma cell and all its descendants, class switching of the C gene is possible, for example from IgM to IgG, but the antigenic specificity remains unchanged. This is achieved initially by differential mRNA splicing and subsequently by DNA rearrangement. The B-cell receptor is the antibody (usually IgM), and thus a plasma cell which responds to a different antigen will be expressing a different VDJC combination.

The kappa and lambda light chain gene clusters have a similar structure with about 200 V genes and four J genes, but in contrast have but a single C gene and no D genes (Fig. 15.4). Each plasma cell produces only one VJC light chain combination and produces either kappa or lambda light chains, but not both. This ability of each gene cluster to produce a host of different polypeptides is an important exception to the one gene–one polypeptide rule.

T-lymphocytes recognize foreign antigens (when processed and presented to them on the surface of another cell where it is recognized along with molecules of the major histocompatibility complex, p. 154) by a receptor. The T-cell receptor of most T-cells is very similar in structure to the immunoglobulins and consists of two chains, alpha and beta. Each has a structure analogous to the immunoglobulin clusters with at least 50 V and 50 J genes for the alpha chain and at least 80 V, one or two D and 13 J genes for the beta chain.

INHERITED IMMUNODEFICIENCY

Inherited defects may occur in either or both components of the immune response. The symptoms and signs depend upon the residual defence mechanisms, but generally include early onset of undue susceptibility to infections and failure to thrive. As outlined in Table 15.2 these conditions, although rare, show genetic heterogeneity. Antibody defects are most common (50%) followed by defects in cellular immunity (40%) and defects in the phagocytic system (6%) and complement system (4%). The most prevalent disorders are opsonic defect (5–7%) and selective IgA deficiency (1 in 570) but most of these patients are asymptomatic with a 1 in 10 000 combined frequency for the significant symptomatic antibody defects, a 1 in 15 000 combined frequency for phagocytic defects and a 1 in 70 000 frequency for severe combined immunodeficiency.

Genetic susceptibility/resistance to particular infections

There is likely to be a genetic contribution in many infections but at present this has been identified for relatively few conditions. Heterozygous carriers of sickle cell disease are more resistant to falciparum malaria than normal individuals as are carriers of beta-thalassaemia, glucose-6-phosphate dehydrogenase deficiency and perhaps alpha-thalassaemia (p. 98). A heterozygous advantage has also been demonstrated for carriers of congenital adrenal hyperplasia in respect of haemophilus influenzae type B infection and is suspected for Tay–Sachs carriers in respect of tuberculosis.

Leprosy may produce depigmented and anaesthetic patches (tuberculoid type) or diffuse infiltration (lepromatous type). Identical twins show increased concordance as compared with dizygotic twins (60–20%) and concordant

Table 15.1 Classes of immunoglobulin.

Class	Molecular weight	Heavy chain	Light chain	Comment
IgG	150 000	γ	κ or λ	Abundant, only class to cross placenta; appears late in immune response
IgM	900 000	μ	κ or λ	Precedes IgG in immune response
IgA	160 000	α	κ or λ	Surface immunity
IgD	185 000	δ	κ or λ	Function unknown
IgE	200 000	ε	κ or λ	Allergic response

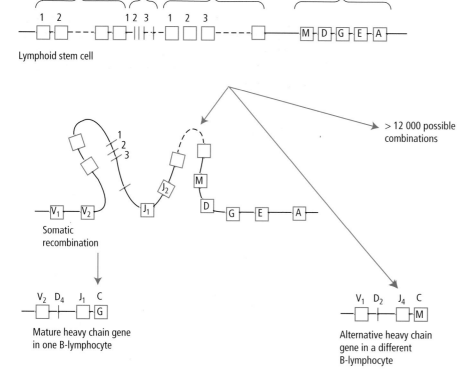

Fig. 15.3 Immunoglobulin heavy chain gene and the creation of different antibody sequences by somatic recombination.

Table 15.2 Inherited immunodeficiency.

Disease	Mode(s) of inheritance
Severe combined immunodeficiency	AR, XR
Agammaglobulinaemia	XR (several types), occ. AR
Wiskott–Aldrich syndrome	XR
Chronic granulomatous disease	XR, occ. AR
Chediak–Higashi syndrome	AR
Ataxia telangiectasia	AR
DiGeorge syndrome	Chromosomal microdeletion
Properdin deficiency	XR
Lymphoproliferative syndrome	XR
Opsonic defect	AD

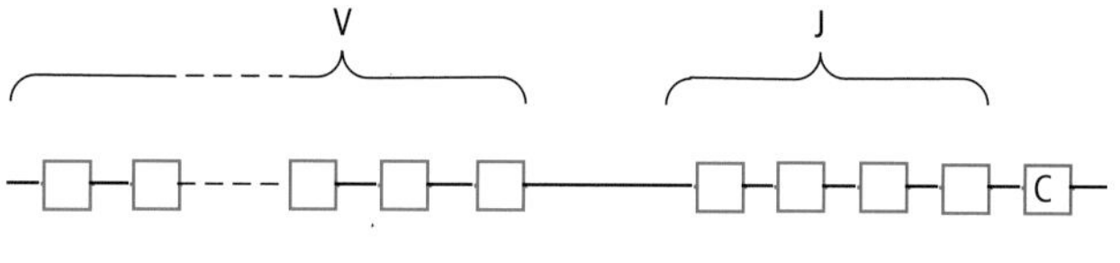

Fig. 15.4 Immunoglobulin light chain gene.

twins are usually concordant for type of leprosy. Furthermore, Orientals usually develop the lepromatous type whereas the tuberculoid type is commoner in Whites and Blacks.

Similarly the response to immunization appears to be genetically determined with, for example, poor responsiveness to hepatitis B (HBsAG) vaccination in HLA-B8, DR3 homozygotes (p. 155).

BLOOD GROUPS

Blood groups are determined by antigenic surface proteins on red cells. So far about 400 blood group antigens have been described and of these the best known are the ABO and Rhesus blood group systems.

ABO blood group

There are four major ABO phenotypes, O, A, B and AB, which are determined by the reaction of an individual's red cells with specific anti-A and anti-B antibodies (Table 15.3). The ABO antigens are also present on most other body cells, including white blood cells and platelets. Group A individuals possess antigen A on their red cells, group B possess antigen B, group AB have both and group O neither. Group A individuals have IgM anti-B (isoagglutinins) in their serum, group B have anti-A and group O have both.

Table 15.3 ABO blood group phenotypes.

Red cell phenotype	Reaction with specific antisera	
	Anti-A	Anti-B
O	–	–
A	+	–
B	–	+
AB	+	+

+ Agglutination.
– No agglutination.

Table 15.4 Genotypes and phenotypes at the ABO locus.

Genotype	Phenotype	UK frequency	Red cell antigens	Serum antibodies
OO	O	0.46	Neither	Anti-A and anti-B
AA AO	A	0.42	A	Anti-B
BB BO	B	0.09	B	Anti-A
AB	AB	0.03	A,B	Neither

In the *ABO* gene, three major alleles are identified, O, A and B. There are thus six possible genotypes, OO, AA, AO, BB, BO and AB. A and B are inherited as codominant traits, with O recessive to both (Table 15.4). It is not possible on blood grouping to distinguish AA from AO or BB from BO, but this may, however be possible from pedigree information or by DNA analysis.

The ABO alleles determine the activity of a glycosyl-transferase which modifies the cell surface H antigen (Fig. 15.5). The O allele has a single base deletion (G at nucleotide position 258) which causes a frameshift with an inactive protein product. The A allele adds *N*-acetylgalactosamine and the B allele adds D-galactose to the H antigen. The A and B alleles differ at several nucleotide positions.

Rhesus blood group system

There are two main Rhesus phenotypes, Rhesus-positive and Rhesus-negative, which are determined by the reaction of an individual's red cells with anti-D Rh antibody. Rhesus-positive persons possess the RhD antigen on their red cells and other tissues, whereas Rhesus-negative persons do not.

Rhesus phenotype is determined by the products of two contiguous homologous genes, one encoding both Cc and Ee polypeptides and the other encoding the D protein. Rhesus-negative persons lack the D gene whereas Rhesus-positive persons are heterozygous or homozygous for D. The E allele differs from the e allele by a C→G substitution at position 676 of the *RHCE* gene.

HAEMOLYTIC DISEASE OF THE NEWBORN

Haemolytic disease of the newborn is an acquired haemolytic anaemia due to the transplacental passage of maternal immunoglobulin. There are two main causes: ABO incompatibility and Rhesus incompatibility. ABO incompatibility between mother and fetus is relatively frequent, but as anti-A and anti-B are predominantly IgM, which cannot cross the placenta, the clinical disease tends to be mild. In contrast, haemolytic disease due to Rhesus incompatibility, although less frequent, is usually severe, as anti-D antibodies are IgG, which can freely cross the placenta.

Normally during pregnancy small amounts of fetal blood reach the maternal circulation. If mother and fetus are both Rhesus-negative or both Rhesus-positive then this is of no significance. However, when the mother is Rhesus-negative and the fetus is Rhesus-positive, the fetal cells may stimulate the formation of maternal anti-Rh (D) antibody. Once a Rhesus-negative woman has mounted such an immune response she is said to be sensitized. The small transplacental bleeds during pregnancy may be sufficient to cause sensitization, but a more significant bleed occurs at the time of delivery, and this is the commonest time for sensitization to occur. Sensitization is more likely if the mother and fetus are ABO compatible, as this allows the fetal cells to persist in the maternal circulation, thus increasing the immune stimulus. A Rhesus-negative woman can also be sensitized by a Rhesus-positive blood transfusion, by an abortion (either spontaneous or thera-

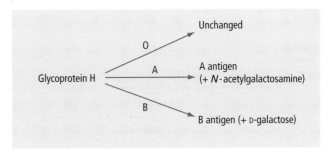

Fig. 15.5 Biosynthesis of ABO blood group substances.

peutic) or occasionally by amniocentesis or chorionic villus sampling.

If a sensitized woman has another Rhesus-positive fetus, maternal anti-Rh will cross the placenta and combine with the Rhesus-positive fetal cells. This results in a shortened red cell survival with an increased demand for production. Marrow hyperplasia and enlargement of the liver and spleen occur. Severe anaemia produces cardiac failure with generalized oedema (hydrops fetalis), and fetal death may ensue despite intrauterine blood transfusion. *In utero* the excessive production of unconjugated bilirubin from lysed cells is excreted by the placenta. After birth serum bilirubin levels rapidly rise and can produce brain damage (kernicterus) unless treated by repeated exchange transfusion.

Prevention

In Caucasian populations haemolytic disease of the newborn formerly affected 1% of all births. Typically the first-born was unaffected, as this pregnancy caused sensitization. The disease severity then increased with successive pregnancies until intrauterine death became inevitable.

A means of prevention was introduced in 1970. Anti-Rh gammaglobulin (anti-D immunoglobulin) is administered by intramuscular injection within 72 h to each Rhesus-negative non-sensitized woman who delivers a Rhesus-positive child. This antibody removes the fetal cells before they can cause sensitization. Anti-Rh antibodies are also given after a Rhesus-negative woman has an abortion, an amniocentesis or chorionic villus sampling.

With this technique the incidence of Rhesus haemolytic disease of the newborn has fallen, as reflected by its mortality rate in England and Wales, which was 0.52 in 1000 total births in 1968 but only 0.054 in 1000 in 1983. However, some women still become sensitized by small bleeds during pregnancy, rarely some women are sensitized to other Rhesus components, such as c or E, and unfortunately some women at risk are not given anti-Rh gammaglobulin or are sensitized by an inappropriate blood transfusion.

NEONATAL ALLOIMMUNE THROMBOCYTOPENIA

Maternal–fetal platelet incompatibility is very common but only rarely does a mother become sensitized to produce IgG which results in thrombocytopenia in the fetus and neonate. This occurs in 1 in 1500 births and is usually (75%) due to incompatibility for the platelet antigen Zwa, and less often for the Bra antigen. Sensitization may occur during the first pregnancy (50%) and is usually unsuspected until the neonate develops purpura or an intracranial haemorrhage. This complication occurs in 10–20% of affected infants (especially those sensitized to Zwa) and may occur before birth. Affected infants can be treated with maternal platelet infusions and with intravenous immunoglobulin. By comparison with the index case subsequently affected sibs are usually similarly or more severely affected. Prenatal diagnosis of fetal thrombocytopenia is possible by fetal blood sampling and *in utero* treatment with platelet transfusions or maternal immunoglobulin and/or dexamethasone has been attempted.

MAJOR HISTOCOMPATIBILITY COMPLEX (MHC)

The major histocompatibility complex is a dense gene cluster on the short arm of chromosome 6 which contains about 80 genes in a 4 Mb length of DNA (Fig. 15.6). These genes are subdivided into three classes. The class III genes include several components of the complement system (e.g. *C2*, *C4A*, *C4B*, *Bf*) and the gene (*CYP21B*) whose deficiency causes congenital adrenal hyperplasia (p. 134). The products of classes I and II are involved in the presentation of processed antigen to T-cells and hence play a vital role in regulation of the immune response. In general, class I genes present antigens to CD8+ T-cells which are primarily involved in cell-mediated cytotoxicity of virus infected cells and class II genes present antigen to CD4+ T-cells which help B-cells to produce appropriate immunoglobulins. The class I, gene products are present

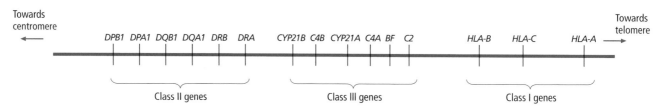

Fig. 15.6 Diagram of the major histocompatibility complex (MHC) (only some loci shown).

on the cell surface of all nucleated cells (except some trophoblast cells, choriocarcinoma cells and sperm) and platelets but the class II gene products are only found on the surface of B-lymphocytes, activated T-lymphocytes and on antigen-presenting cells such as macrophages. Most class I and class II genes have multiple alleles which can be defined by a combination of immunological tests and DNA analysis. Any combination of these alleles may occur and in view of the number of alleles involved it is unlikely that unrelated individuals will have the same pattern of alleles. These genes are physically close together and thus the alleles on each chromosome tend to be inherited together as a haplotype. Within a family, each parent's haplotypes can be distinguished and on average 1 in 4 of their children will have identical MHC genotypes and this has implications for tissue transplantation (Fig. 15.7).

The close linkage of genes within the MHC cluster has also resulted in extensive linkage disequilibrium (p. 86). Thus the frequencies of particular combinations of alleles often do not reflect their individual frequencies (e.g. DR3 is found more often with B8 than expected). Hence, if one MHC allele predisposes to a disease, an association will be found not only with that allele but also with other MHC alleles which are in linkage disequilibrium. The strength of the association is indicated by the relative risk which is a measure of the frequency of the disease in individuals with the allele versus the frequency in those without. Thus, in one study on autoimmune hepatitis, 46 of 96 patients had HLA B8 as did 23 of 100 controls. This gives a relative risk of 3.1 (46/23)/(50/77). In the same study, 48 of 92 patients had DR3 as did 21 of 100 controls. The relative risk for DR3 is 4.1 and this suggests that DR3 has a stronger influence on the occurrence of autoimmune hepatitis and that linkage disequilibrium of B8 and DR3 accounts for the dual association. Table 15.5 illustrates further example of associations of MHC alleles with disease.

Many of the diseases in Table 15.5 are autoimmune disorders and these are believed to reflect an aberrant response to a non-self antigen (e.g. an infectious agent) in

Table 15.5 Examples of MHC allele associations with disease.

Disease	MHC allele	Relative risk
Ankylosing spondylitis	B27	77–90
Autoimmune hepatitis	B8	3.1
	DR3	4.1
Coeliac disease	DPB4.2	10.8
Diabetes mellitus	DR3	5
	DR4	7
	DQB1 non-Asp/non-Asp at position 57	107
Multiple sclerosis	DQB1B	36
Narcolepsy	DR2	250–350
Psoriasis	DR7	43
Rheumatoid arthritis	DR4	3–6
Systemic lupus erythematosus	DR3	2
Systemic lupus erythematosus, hydralazine-induced	DR4	5.6
Thyrotoxicosis	DR3	5

a genetically susceptible host. The MHC genes (types I and II) are normally involved in the presentation of antigens to T-cells and the MHC encoded predisposition to disease is believed to reflect individual variation at these loci with protein products which vary in their ability to bind and present particular antigens.

TRANSPLANTATION

Tissue of one individual (the donor) may be transferred to another (the recipient). This transfer is known as a transplant and is further classified according to the relationship of the donor and recipient (Table 15.6).

The transplanted tissue in autografts and isografts is genetically identical to the recipient, and so rejection by cell-mediated immunity is not a problem. In contrast, grafts between different species are always rejected, and those between different members of the same species will usually be rejected in the absence of tissue matching and immune suppression therapy.

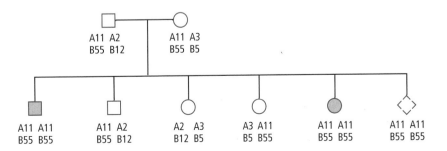

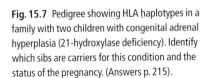

Fig. 15.7 Pedigree showing HLA haplotypes in a family with two children with congenital adrenal hyperplasia (21-hydroxylase deficiency). Identify which sibs are carriers for this condition and the status of the pregnancy. (Answers p. 215).

Table 15.6 Types of tissue transplant.

Type	Donor–recipient relationship
Autograft	Self
Isograft	Identical twins
Allograft	Same species
Xenograft	Different species

Table 15.7 Likelihood of adverse reactions in non-identical blood transfusions.

Blood group of recipient	Blood group of donor			
	O	A	B	AB
O	–	+	+	+
A	–	–	+	+
B	–	+	–	+
AB	–	–	–	–

+ Agglutination.
– No agglutination.

Blood transfusion

Blood transfusion is the commonest type of tissue transplant. Prior to transfusion, the ABO and Rhesus types of donor and recipient are determined and a screen for atypical antibodies is made. Donor cells are also mixed with the recipient's serum *in vitro* (cross-matching).

Generally blood of the same ABO group is given where possible, but in an emergency it is possible to give a different type, as indicated in Table 15.7. An ABO antibody present in the plasma of the recipient will cause agglutination of donor cells if they have the corresponding antigen but the donor antibodies are not important, as they are rapidly diluted in the recipient's circulation.

Other tissues

A wide variety of other tissues may be transplanted. Donor selection is critical, as host and donor need to be as antigenically similar as possible. Hence relatives provide the best chance of a match as determined by ABO group and MHC tissue type. Compatibility is also tested directly by mixing immune-competent lymphocytes from both host and donor (mixed lymphocyte culture test). If the match is accurate then rejection will not occur. If the match is poor then rejection will occur despite immunosuppression.

The fetus is antigenically different from the mother (an allograft), and yet rejection does not occur. The absence of MHC antigens from the outer layer of placental cells may be involved in this, as may the presence of fetal white cells in the maternal circulation (p. 203).

Genetics of Common Diseases

CONTENTS

Diseases discussed in this chapter are arranged in
alphabetical order

As indicated in Chapter 10 twin concordance and family correlation studies show that many common diseases have multifactorial inheritance whereby a gene or genes predispose individuals to particular environmental agents. Genes are also likely to be involved in the differences shown amongst patients with a particular disease with respect to prognosis, frequency and type of complications and response to different therapies. Hence in trying to answer the questions 'Why does this patient have this disease at this time and what is the prognosis?' the role of genetic factors cannot be ignored.

Although twin and family studies confirm a genetic contribution to susceptibility, they do not identify the number or nature of the genes involved. Advances in this area have, however, been made using population association studies, sib pair analysis, linkage analysis and mutational analysis of candidate genes.

So far, the most frequently utilized approach has been population association studies in which the frequency of polymorphisms of genes of interest are compared between affected and unaffected patients. Thus for example in insulin-dependent diabetes mellitus 95% of patients have DR3 or DR4 MHC alleles whereas the combined frequency in unaffected persons is 50%. This and other associations of this nature are believed to reflect linkage disequilibrium between the disease susceptibility locus and the candidate locus in question (see p. 155). Sib pair analysis compares the frequency of polymorphisms among those affected. Each sib has a 1 in 2 chance of receiving each allele at a locus from each parent and thus the presence of the disease can be compared with the frequency with which each sib has either (expected 50%),

neither (expected 25%) or both (expected 25%) alleles in common at the test locus. Routine linkage analysis using polymorphic markers (p. 82) can also be used if the trait is discontinuous. If any of these approaches suggest a particular candidate gene then this can be tested by mutational analysis in affected patients. Further research is required to define all contributing loci for each condition, to discover whether different contributing loci occur in different families (genetic heterogeneity) and to understand how the genotype interacts with environmental factors in the production of the final phenotype.

Alcoholism

Alcohol abuse or dependence occurs in 19% of men and 4% of women and a hereditary contribution has been demonstrated by adoption, twin and half-sib studies. Relatively little is known of the nature of the genetic contribution and genetic heterogeneity is suspected both for predisposition to aberrant drinking behaviour and for organ damage. About 50% of Orientals are deficient in activity of the mitochondrial aldehyde dehydrogenase 2 enzyme and this leads to unpleasant flushing with alcohol ingestion. These individuals are less prone to alcohol abuse than those with normal activity of this enzyme.

Alzheimer disease

Alzheimer disease is a common progressive form of dementia with characteristic neuropathology. The lifetime risk is 5–10% with a family history consistent with autosomal dominant inheritance in 10% of patients. Familial Alzheimer disease tends to have an earlier onset (<60 years) and is most commonly (75%) caused by mutations in presenilin 1 (*PS1*). In other families mutations in other loci, e.g. presenilin 2 and amyloid precursor protein, are found.

Late onset Alzheimer disease is associated with particular apolipoprotein E (apoE) genotypes. The apoE allele 4 is found in 64% of patients as compared with 31% of the general population (relative risk 4). ApoE 4 also shows a dosage effect as the average age of onset is lower in apoE 4 homozygotes (<70 years) and the disease course more rapid compared with other genotypes (e.g. average age of onset >90 years in apoE 2/3).

Aneurysm of the abdominal aorta

Abdominal aortic aneurysms occur most commonly in people older than 55 years and are commoner in men than women. Lifetime risks to sibs are increased to 60% compared with a general population risk of 15% and routine ultrasound surveillance can be considered to allow presymptomatic detection.

Ankylosing spondylitis

Ankylosing spondylitis may be isolated or complicate inflammatory bowel disease and overall 2 in 1000 men and 0.2 in 1000 women are symptomatically affected. Whether isolated or secondary, 77–95% of those affected have HLA B27, as compared with 7% of the normal population. However, not all with this allele develop the disease and the nature of the environmental factor(s)/ other genetic factor(s) involved and the mechanism of their interaction are unknown.

For sibs of a patient with HLA B27 the risk of ankylosing spondylitis is 9% if they too have HLA B27 whereas those without this allele have a risk of less than 1%. The risk of ankylosing spondylitis in individuals with HLA B27 but without an affected relative is 2%.

Atherosclerosis

Coronary atherosclerosis is the commonest cause of death in adults. By 55 years of age 1 in 60 males and 1 in 90 females will have evidence of ischaemic heart disease, and the prevalence rises rapidly thereafter and overall accounts for 1 in 2 deaths in adults in Europe, the USA and Japan.

The aetiology is heterogeneous but undisputed risk factors include cigarette smoking, abnormal lipid profiles (monogenic, multifactorial and environmental), hypertension, diabetes mellitus and a family history of premature (<55 years) ischaemic heart disease. Overall with premature ischaemic heart disease one-third will have abnormal lipids, of which one-half are monogenic in origin. If patients with monogenic causes of hyperlipidaemia are excluded the overall risk of premature ischaemic heart disease is doubled in first-degree male rel-

atives. Identical twin concordance ranges from 14 to 90% with the highest figures for males with premature disease.

The monogenic causes of hyperlipidaemia include elevated lipoprotein (a) (Lp(a)), familial combined hyperlipidaemia and familial hypercholesterolaemia (p. 141). Elevated levels of Lp(a) are found in 20% of the population and account for 28% of premature coronary heart disease. Levels of Lp(a) are constant for an individual and are genetically determined as an autosomal codominant trait. This variation correlates with the number (range 15–40) of plasminogen-like repeats in the gene for apolipoprotein (a) (small numbers of repeats associated with low Lp(a) and *vice versa*). Familial combined hyperlipidaemia with increased levels of cholesterol and triglyceride occurs in 0.5–2% of the population and accounts for 10% of premature coronary heart disease. This condition shows autosomal dominant inheritance and linkage to the apolipoprotein gene cluster on 11q has been described.

Association analysis has also suggested a role for the gene for angiotensin converting enzyme in the occurrence of myocardial infarction.

Atopic diathesis

Atopic individuals are characterized by a propensity to produce prolonged exuberant IgE responses to minute amounts of antigens. One in four of the population respond in this fashion and they may be asymptomatic or develop allergic rhinitis (1 in 5 of the population), atopic eczema (1 in 25 of the population), extrinsic bronchial asthma (1 in 25 of the population) or any combination of these.

Atopic diathesis is often inherited as an autosomal dominant trait with incomplete penetrance as defined by the presence of symptoms. Linkage analysis in these families indicates that a locus for atopy lies on chromosome 11q and that genomic imprinting appears to be involved to account for the higher risk of atopy in children of atopic mothers than in the children of atopic fathers in these families.

Attention deficit hyperactivity disorder

This affects 1–10% of the population and shows an increased monozygotic twin concordance. It may be secondary to the fragile X syndrome or untreated phenylketonuria or be unexplained. The risk is increased for first-degree relatives and may be as high as 30% in sibs.

Autoimmune hepatitis

Autoimmune hepatitis is associated with HLA B8 and DR3 at the major histocompatibility complex. DNA sequencing studies have revealed a specific amino acid motif LLEQKR (Table 2.3, p. 13) at positions 67–72 of *DRB* in 94% of patients (relative risk 9x). This region lies in the peptide binding groove of DR and can interact with bound peptide and the T-cell receptor and the variant form is believed to predispose to disease by aberrant response to an exogenous antigen.

Autism

Autism affects 1 in 500–2000 and is characterized by onset in early childhood of impaired social, language and cognitive development and stereotyped patterns of interests and activities. Mental handicap coexists in 75% and epilepsy in 30%. Monozygotic twin concordance varies from 40 to 90% and is higher if lesser degrees of cognitive impairment are taken as affected. Fragile X syndrome and tuberous sclerosis need to be excluded and the empiric recurrence risk for sibs is then 3–5%, with low risks to second (0.13%) and third degree relatives.

Diabetes mellitus—insulin-dependent (IDDM)

Diabetes mellitus is a heterogeneous condition with at least three clinical subtypes: insulin-dependent (IDDM, juvenile-onset type) and non-insulin-dependent (NIDDM, maturity-onset type), which both show multifactorial inheritance, and maturity-onset diabetes of youth (MODY). The latter is usually inherited as an autosomal dominant trait and in most families has been shown to be caused by mutations in the gene for glucokinase.

IDDM has an overall frequency of 1 in 500 with a 30–40% concordance in monozygotic twins as compared with 6% in dizygotic twins. The overall risk to sibs is 6.6%. For a child the risk is 4.8% if the father is affected but only 2% if the mother is affected.

A clue to the genetic contribution to IDDM first came from association studies with the major histocompatibility complex. The original associations were described with HLA B8 or B15 (about 60% of patients) and these were clues to DR3 and DR4 respectively which are in linkage disequilibrium. Ninety-five per cent of patients have DR3 or DR4 as compared with the combined frequency of these antigens of 50% in the normal population. This association was also supported by sib pair analysis which showed that affected sibs had the same MHC haplotypes in 57% (25% expected), had one haplotype in common in 38% (50% expected) and had no haplotype in common in only 5% (expected 25%). The association and relative risk increased still further when DNA polymorphisms at the neighbouring *DQB1* locus were studied and sequencing studies at this locus revealed consistent changes at amino acid position 57 which is part of the antigen binding cleft. If alanine, valine or serine was present at this site then individuals were susceptible whereas aspartate conferred resistance. Overall 90–96% of IDDM patients are aspartate-negative homozygotes and the remainder

are heterozygous as compared with the general population frequency of aspartate-negative homozygotes of 19.5% (relative risk 107). These changes are believed to account for 60–70% of the genetic predisposition to IDDM with some evidence for another important contributing locus on 14q and at or near the insulin gene on 11p and minor loci on other chromosomes.

This information has relevance for genetic counselling. Sibs of a patient with IDDM have a 12% risk if HLA identical, a 5% risk if only one haplotype is in common and a 1% risk if neither haplotype is shared. There is a curious unexplained reduced rate of transmission of the DR4 haplotype from the mother as compared with the father and this presumably correlates with the lower risk when the mother is affected as compared with the father (see earlier). For individuals who are aspartate-negative homozygotes with no family history of IDDM the overall risk of IDDM is 1 in 50.

The nature of the environmental trigger has also been investigated. About 30% of newly diagnosed patients have IgM antibodies to Coxsackie B4 or B5 and evidence for cytomegalovirus infection is present in some patients. In yet other patients no clear environmental agent has been identified and the need for a specific insult has been questioned.

Diabetes mellitus non-insulin-dependent (NIDDM)

NIDDM affects 3–7% of adults in most western countries. The concordance in monozygotic twins is close to 100% as compared with 10% in dizygotic twins and 10% in other first-degree relatives. In contrast to IDDM there is no HLA association and the nature of the genetic contribution is under investigation.

Epilepsy

Over 200 monogenic disorders include epilepsy as a component but these are individually rare and collectively account for <1% of patients with epilepsy. They generally have additional features and these and the pedigree are important clues.

Multifactorial epilepsy is more common and accounts for up to 20% of patients with epilepsy. There are usually no associated features and empiric risks are available for genetic counselling.

Febrile convulsions occur in 2–5% of children in Europe and the USA. The sib risk is 10–20% and for offspring of an affected individual, the risk is 10%.

Idiopathic generalized (grand mal) epilepsy affects 1 in 200 of the population and carries a 1 in 25 recurrence risk for first-degree relatives (8.7% by age 25 years if the mother is affected, 2.4% if the father is affected). This risk rises to 1 in 10 if two first-degree relatives are affected.

Childhood absence (petit mal) epilepsy affects 1 in 15 000 children and carries a risk to offspring of 8–10% and a risk to sibs of 5–10%.

Glaucoma

Primary open-angle glaucoma affects 1 in 200 elderly people and carries a risk to first-degree relatives of 1 in 10.

Gluten enteropathy (coeliac disease)

Malabsorption syndrome secondary to gluten intolerance affects 1 in 2000 individuals in Europe. The recurrence risk in sibs and offspring is 1 in 33 for symptomatic disease, although 1 in 10 have an abnormal jejunal biopsy. The risk for symptomatic disease is less than 1 in 100 for second-degree relatives.

The environmental trigger is the protein alpha-gliadin which is a component of wheat gluten, and susceptible individuals show a population association with HLA DR3 and DR7. DNA analysis has shown the associations with DPB4.2 and DPB3 to be particularly important. Polymorphic residues in the DP molecule at positions 69, 56 and 57 are believed to be critical in conferring susceptibility.

High blood pressure

Within the general population the distributions of systolic and diastolic blood pressures follow a normal or Gaussian distribution, but by convention young adults with values persistently above 140/90 are considered to be hypertensive. Blood pressure, especially the systolic, tends to increase with age and so upper normal limits are age-dependent. With standard upper normal limits at least 10% of the population are or will become hypertensive and the best predictors of this are the current centiles of an individual's own blood pressure and his or her parental blood pressure centiles.

Twin and family studies indicate that both genes and environmental factors are involved in the determination of blood pressure but the nature of these and their mechanism of interaction are currently obscure. Genes may also be important with regard to choice of antihypertensive therapy. For example, high blood pressure is associated with a better response to beta blockers in Blacks than Whites. If one parent is hypertensive, the risk to offspring is 30% and if both parents are hypertensive, the risk to offspring is 40%.

Inflammatory bowel disease

Two common subtypes of non-infectious inflammatory bowel disease are recognized: ulcerative colitis (frequency 1 in 1500) and Crohn's disease (frequency 1 in 5000). Twin and family studies suggest multifactorial inheritance and recurrence risks are increased for both. Thus for a patient with Crohn's disease the risk to first-degree relatives is increased 13-fold (30-fold in sibs) for Crohn's disease and 8- to 10-fold for ulcerative colitis. Similarly for a patient with ulcerative colitis the risk to first-degree relatives is increased 15-fold for ulcerative colitis and 3.5-fold for Crohn's disease.

Manic depression (bipolar affective disorder)

Severe cyclical depression and/or mania affects 1 in 100 of the population. Multifactorial inheritance is apparent with a monozygotic twin concordance of 70% as compared with 15% in dizygotic twins and a similar 15% frequency in other first-degree relatives.

Genetic heterogeneity is apparent with as yet no consensus from linkage analyses in affected families.

Motorneurone disease

Motorneurone disease affects 1 in 20 000 and in 5–10% of cases (which tend to have an earlier age of onset) appears to be inherited as an autosomal dominant trait. In familial motorneurone disease, 15–20% is caused by mutations in superoxide dismutase 1 and in these families, presymptomatic testing can be considered.

Multiple sclerosis

Multiple sclerosis shows an increased concordance in identical twins (25–30% monozygotic twin concordance versus 2–5% in dizygotic twins) and an increased risk for first-degree relatives (1–2%) which support multifactorial inheritance. Sib pair analysis shows distortion for the MHC with 40% sharing two, 47% sharing one and 13% with no haplotypes in common (compared with the expected frequencies of 25%, 50% and 25%). Association analysis shows a relative risk of 36 for DQB1B. The nature of the environmental influence is obscure and presumably accounts for the increasing prevalence with increasing latitude. If two first-degree relatives are affected, the recurrence risk rises to 5%.

Narcolepsy

Narcolepsy affects 1 in 2000 and has a 10–50% risk for first-degree relatives. A strong association is apparent with HLA DR2 which are present in 90–95% of patients (as compared with 20% of the general population – relative risk 250–350).

Parkinson's disease

The characteristic lesion in Parkinson's disease is depletion of the dopamine neurones in the substantia nigra. In normal subjects the levels decline with age, and clinical symptoms occur with depletion to about 30% of normal. The prevalence of Parkinson's disease is 1% at 50 years rising to 2–3% by 85 years. Amongst these patients there is an excess of slow metabolizers of debrisoquine (p. 135) which suggests an individual susceptibility in respect of the metabolism of environmental toxins.

For an isolated case the risks to relatives are probably little if at all increased above the general population risk but if two first-degree relatives are affected or for early-onset disease there is a risk of 30% to first-degree relatives by 75 years.

Pre-eclampsia/eclampsia (pregnancy-induced hypertension)

Pre-eclampsia occurs in 2–3% of pregnancies (4–6% of first pregnancies) with a diastolic blood pressure greater than 90 mmHg and proteinuria of over 0.25 g l^{-1} on two or more occasions after the 26th week of pregnancy in a previously and subsequently normotensive woman. Family studies support a genetic predisposition with 4- to 5-fold increased risks in first-degree relatives.

Psoriasis

Psoriasis affects 1–2% of the population and has a high identical twin concordance (70% concordance for monozygotic twins versus 23% concordance in dizygotic twins) and increased risks for first-degree relatives. With one parent affected the risk to a child is 25% (rising to 60–75% if both parents are affected) and for normal parents with one affected child, the sib risk is 17%. Association analysis reveals a relative risk of 43 for DR7 and in some families linkage with chromosome 17 markers has been demonstrated.

Rheumatoid arthritis

Rheumatoid arthritis affects 1% of the population and shows an increased concordance in identical twins (30% monozygotic twin concordance versus 5% in dizygotic twins) and increased risks (5%) for first-degree relatives.

Association analysis reveals a relative risk of 3–6 with DR4 and DNA sequencing of DRB shows specific amino acid patterns at position 67 to 74 (LLEQKRAA or LLEQRRAA). This portion of the DRB protein is adjacent to the peptide binding groove and probably comes into contact with the T-cell receptor and this probably influences the immune response which underlies the condition.

Schizophrenia

There are several clinical subtypes of schizophrenia which have a collective lifetime population frequency of 0.8%. Multifactorial inheritance is apparent with a pooled concordance rate in monozygotic twins of 45% as compared with 12–14% in dizygotic twins and a frequency in other first-degree relatives of 10–15% and in second-degree relatives of 3%. If both parents are affected the risk to a child is 40%. Recurrences within a family tend to be subtype-specific.

Genetic heterogeneity is apparent with as yet no consensus from linkage analyses in affected families.

Specific reading disability (dyslexia)

This is characterized by difficulty in learning to read despite conventional instruction, a normal IQ and adequate sociocultural opportunity. Five to ten per cent of the population are affected with an increased monozygotic twin concordance and an increased risk for first-degree relatives (sib risk of 20% if parents unaffected rising to 30–60% if one is affected).

Systemic lupus erythematosus (SLE)

SLE may be idiopathic, drug-induced or secondary to an inherited deficiency of complement components. The idiopathic form is commonest and shows an increased concordance rate in identical twins. In the idiopathic group the relative risk is 2- to 5-fold increased in association with the haplotype HLA A1 B8 DR3 and this is believed to reflect linkage disequilibrium with a C4 null allele which predisposes to SLE.

The drug-induced variant was the first described example of a human two gene–one environmental factor interaction. The drugs which can cause this include isoniazid and hydralazine, and slow acetylators (recessive homozygotes, p. 130) are especially at risk. The increased serum levels in these individuals have a direct inhibitory effect on complement C4, which is involved in the clearance of immune complexes from the circulation. However, not all slow acetylators on such treatment are affected, and a clue to the second genetic component came from the association in affected individuals with HLA DR4, which suggested that a certain C4 allele in linkage disequilibrium with DR4 is unduly susceptible to inhibition by these drugs.

C H A P T E R   1 7

Cancer Genetics

C O N T E N T S

TUMOUR SUPPRESSOR GENES. 162
ONCOGENES. 163
GENES INVOLVED IN DNA-REPAIR
  MECHANISMS 165
OTHER GENES 166

CLINICAL RELEVANCE OF GENETIC STUDIES
  IN CANCER 167
GENETIC COUNSELLING ASPECTS OF CANCER 169
SINGLE GENE CAUSES OF CANCER. 171

In contrast to the other types of genetic disorder, for most cancers the genetic mutations are not inherited and arise in somatic cells during adulthood as a result of exposure to environmental carcinogens. Multiple mutations are usually involved and this cumulation results in multiple steps which are reflected by the histopathological progression. In 5–10% of common cancers (e.g. breast cancer and colon cancer) and a higher percentage of certain rare cancer syndromes the first mutation is inherited and in these conditions there is a high risk of cancer in relatives. These mutations (inherited and acquired) commonly involve three types of genes: tumour suppressors, oncogenes and genes involved in DNA-repair mechanisms. Tumour suppressors and oncogenes are normally involved in the control of cellular growth and proliferation and disruption of such control is a consistent feature of cancer.

TUMOUR SUPPRESSOR GENES

Tumour suppressor genes were first discovered as a result of studies on the rare inherited forms of cancer as exemplified by retinoblastoma. Retinoblastoma is the commonest malignant eye tumour of childhood and in 20–30% of cases both eyes are affected. All of these bilateral cases and 15% of the unilateral cases are inherited as an autosomal dominant trait. The gene for this trait is localized to the proximal long arm of chromosome 13 (13q14) and in the tumour tissue this gene's functional protein product is absent. An autosomal dominant trait implies a mutation in only one member of a pair of genes and for a tumour to occur a person who inherits a mutant gene must also develop a fault in the partner gene within a retinal cell.

In the non-inherited cases of retinoblastoma two separate mutations have to occur *de novo* in each copy of chromosome 13 in a single retinal cell (Fig. 17.1). Hence in contrast to familial cases, bilateral involvement is most unlikely and the age at presentation is generally older.

The first retinoblastoma mutation in either familial or non-inherited retinoblastoma is usually a point mutation (nonsense, frameshift or splicing error) which results in a truncated or no protein product. In contrast the second retinoblastoma mutation usually involves loss of chromosome 13 either in whole or part following mitotic nondisjunction or partial deletion respectively (Fig. 17.2).

This second mutation thus often (60%) produces a variable loss of chromosome 13 alleles (Mechanisms 1, 2, 3 and 5) including the retinoblastoma locus and this can be readily demonstrated by DNA analysis which shows loss of heterozygosity (LOH) for probes within the deleted region when compared with normal somatic tissues (Fig. 17.3).

Many tumour types have been studied for loss of heterozygosity of chromosome 13 and elsewhere in order to identify the location of other tumour suppressor genes (Table 17.1). Over 20 tumour suppressor gene loci have been identified in this fashion and many including the

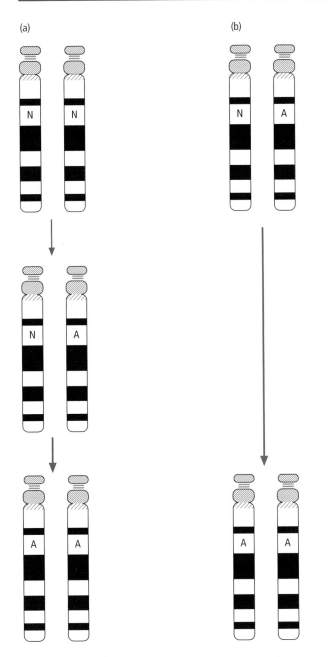

(a)

(b)

Fig. 17.1 (a) Sporadic and (b) inherited retinoblastoma. Copies of chromosome 13 are shown with either a normal (N) or an abnormal (A) gene.

retinoblastoma, p53 and adenomatous polyposis coli genes have been cloned.

Mutations in the p53 gene on chromosome 17p appear to be the most common genetic change in cancers. In colon cancer, for example, 75–80% of tumours show loss of heterozygosity for p53 and adjacent loci and it is also involved in other tumours including lung cancer, breast cancer, brain tumours, hepatocellular carcinoma and chronic myeloid leukaemia in blast crisis. The first p53

mutation in colon cancer is usually a point mutation due to a C to T transversion at a CpG dinucleotide (especially at positions 175, 248, 273 and 282). In other tumours the positions and type of mutation differ. For example in aflatoxin-induced hepatocellular carcinomas mutation of GpC to TpC at position 249 is prominent and in lung cancer CpN to ApN p53 mutations are generally found. Patients with inherited mutations of p53 have been described and as might be expected they develop multiple primary cancers at diverse sites (Li–Fraumeni syndrome, p. 172).

For retinoblastoma two inactivating mutations in the retinoblastoma locus can produce cancer but for the majority of tumours multiple stages are expected with involvement of several loci. Such multistage progression is currently best understood for colon cancer where at least three tumour suppressor loci and one oncogene locus are involved (Fig.17.4).

ONCOGENES

Oncogenes were first discovered by molecular analysis of oncogenic retroviruses which cause cancer in mice, cats

Table 17.1 Examples of loss of heterozygosity in human cancers.

Tumour (alphabetical order)	Site(s) of allele loss
Acoustic neuroma	22
Astrocytoma	17p
Bladder carcinoma	11p
Breast carcinoma	3p, 7q, 11p, 13q, 16q, 17p, 17q
Colon carcinoma	5q, 17p, 18q, 22, others
Hepatoblastoma	11p
Hepatocellular carcinoma	4q, 11p, 17p
Insulinoma	11
Lung carcinoma	
Small cell	3p, 13q, 17p
Other types	3p (occ. 13q, 17p)
Medullary thyroid carcinoma	1p
Melanoma	Various
Meningioma	22
Osteosarcoma	13q
Ovarian carcinoma	17p, 17q
Phaeochromocytoma	1p, 22
Renal carcinoma	3p
Retinoblastoma	13q
Rhabdomyosarcoma	11p
Stomach carcinoma	13q
Wilms tumour	11p

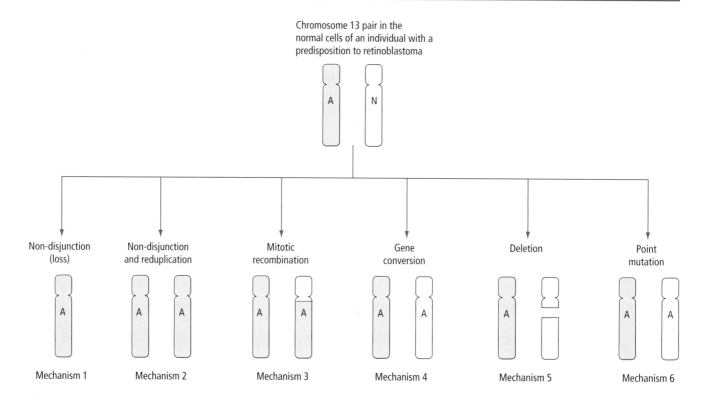

Chromosome 13 pair in the
normal cells of an individual with a
predisposition to retinoblastoma

Non-disjunction (loss)

Non-disjunction and reduplication

Mitotic recombination

Gene conversion

Deletion

Point mutation

Mechanism 1   Mechanism 2   Mechanism 3   Mechanism 4   Mechanism 5   Mechanism 6

Six possible chromosome 13 pairs that might be seen in a
retinoblastoma tumour arising in the individual shown above

Fig. 17.2 Mechanisms of loss of second retinoblastoma allele. (N, Normal; A, mutant gene.)

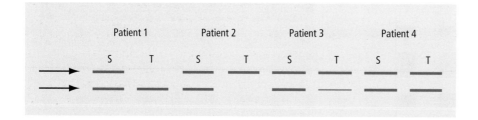

Patient 1   Patient 2   Patient 3   Patient 4

S   T   S   T   S   T   S   T

Fig. 17.3 Loss of heterozygosity for a DNA polymorphic marker with two arrowed alleles. Complete loss of one allele in patients 1 and 2, partial loss in patient 3 and no loss indicating another mechanism in patient 4. S, Somatic tissue; T, tumour tissue.

and monkeys. For example, the *ras* oncogene is derived from the Rous avian sarcoma virus which causes a sarcoma in chickens. Each of these viral oncogenes (v-onc) was actually derived from a normal host gene (which is not normally oncogenic) by recombination between it and the ancestral viral genome. Over 100 normal cellular copies of the oncogenes, the c-onc, have now been isolated and mapped to human chromosomes. These c-onc can be activated to cause cancer by point mutation, as a result of chromosome rearrangement or secondary to gene amplification.

Comparison of the DNA sequence in c-oncogenes in tumour tissue with the other somatic tissues has revealed that specific point mutations can lead to different tumour types. For example, in the *HRAS* gene a glycine residue is normally present at position 12 but in some patients with bladder cancer, lung cancer or melanoma the tumour tissue shows a point mutation (GGC to GTC) with substitution of valine at position 12. This change is not inherited but is a somatic mutation within the cells which originate the cancer. Specific point mutations have also been identified at other critical positions (e.g. 13, 61 and 119) within *HRAS* and within other c-oncogenes. The presence of an activated oncogene can be demonstrated by showing that extracts of tumour DNA have the ability to transfect a susceptible rodent cell line and produce malignant clones.

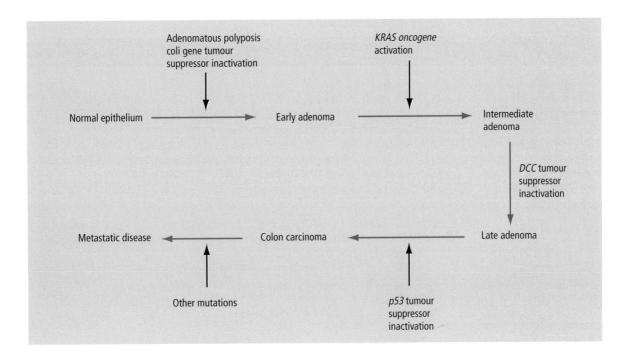

Fig. 17.4 Stages in progression from normal colonic epithelium to metastatic cancer.

Human oncogenes can also be activated as a result of chromosome rearrangement (Table 17.2). This is exemplified by chronic myeloid leukaemia (CML) and the Philadelphia chromosome. The majority of affected patients show this chromosome (a smaller than normal chromosome 22) within the malignant bone marrow (but not in the unaffected somatic tissues). It is actually a reciprocal translocation between chromosomes 9 (usually the paternal copy) and 22 (usually the maternal copy) (Fig. 17.5). As a result of this translocation the *ABL* oncogene is translocated from its normal site in 9q34 to chromosome 22q11 where it rearranges with a specific sequence called the breakpoint cluster region (*BCR*). As a result the hybrid gene produces a novel protein in CML cells which is believed to be responsible for the neoplastic transformation. Another important example is found in Burkitt's lymphoma. This is a B-cell malignancy characterized by specific chromosomal translocations involving 8q24 and either 14q32, 2p11 or 22q11. An oncogene *MYC* which is normally located at 8q24 is transferred to 14q32 in the majority of cases and it appears that the *MYC* gene is activated by enhancers of the heavy chain immunoglobulin gene located in 14q32. In the other translocations it has been shown that parts of the light chain genes (kappa at 2p11 and lambda at 22q11) have been transferred to activate the *MYC* locus on 8q24. T-cell lymphomas can also be caused by rearrangement of the T-cell receptor alpha chain gene from 14q11 to the locus of the immunoglobulin heavy chain genes on 14q32 by paracentric inversion.

These studies illustrate the importance of recognizing specific chromosomal rearrangements in tumour cells. However, for many tumours with specific cytogenetic findings (Table 17.2) no oncogenes or tumour suppressor genes have yet been identified at the appropriate chromosomal site and the disease mechanism remains obscure. Further, as with allele loss revealed by DNA analysis similar chromosomal abnormalities may occur in tumours of different types and the reason for this is unknown.

GENES INVOLVED IN DNA-REPAIR MECHANISMS

DNA-repair mechanisms exist to correct DNA damage due to environmental mutagens (p. 21) and accidental base misincorporation at the time of DNA replication. Inherited defects of either system result in an increased frequency of cancer and whilst the former group are generally rare autosomal recessive disorders (e.g. xeroderma pigmentosum, p. 176 and Plate 1), the latter are common and are inherited as autosomal dominant traits. In this latter group four gene loci have been identified (*MSH2*,

Table 17.2 Some malignancies associated with specific chromosomal abnormalities.

Tumour type	Chromosomal abnormality
Acute non-lymphocytic leukaemia (ANLL)	
M1 Acute myeloblastic leukaemia	inv(3) (q21,q25–27), del 3p, –5, 5q-(q13q31), t(6;9) (p22;q34), –7, 7q-, +8, t(9;22) (q34;q11), –17, +21
M2 Acute myeloblastic leukaemia	inv(3) (q21,q25–27), t(3;5) (q26;q22), del 3p, +4, –5, 5q-(q13q31), t(6;9) (p22;q34), –7, 7q-, +8, t(8;21) (q22;q22), t(9;11) (p22;q23), t(9;22) (q34;q11), inv(16) (p13q22), 16q-(q22)
M3 Acute promyelocytic leukaemia	t(15;17) (q22;q11), i(17q)
M4 Acute myelomonocytic leukaemia	+4, –5, 5q-(q13q31), t(6;9) (p22;q34), –7, 7q-, +8, t(9;11) (p22;q23), t(9;22) (q34;q11), inv(16) (p13q22), 16q-(q22)
M5 Acute monocytic leukaemia	–5, 5q-(q13q31), +8, [5a] t(9;11) (p22;q23), [5b] inv(16) (p13q22), [5b] 16q-(q22)
M6 Acute erythroleukaemia	dup(1), –5, 5q-(q13q31), –7, 7q-, +8
Acute lymphatic leukaemia	
L1	t(1;19) (q21–q23;p13), 9p-, *t(9;22) (q34;q11), t(11;14) (q13,q32), 14q+(q32), 14q-(q11), near haploid
L2	*t(4;11) (q21;q23), del(6) (q21q25), 7p-, +8, *t(9;22) (q34,q11), t(11;14) (p13–14;q11–13), 11q-, 12p-, 14q+(q32), 14q-(q11), i(17q), +21
L3	1q+, t(2;8) (p11–13;q24), 6q-, +8, *t(8;14) (q24;q32), t(8;22) (q24;q11), 14q+
Bladder carcinoma	i(5p), +7, –9
Bronchial carcinoma	del(3) (p14–p23)
Burkitt's lymphoma	t(2;8) (p12;q24), *t(8;14) (q24;q32), t(8;22) (q24;q11)
Chronic lymphatic leukaemia (B cell)	+12, del(14) (q22–q24), 14q+
Chronic lymphatic leukaemia (T cell)	inv(14) (q11q32)
Chronic myeloid leukaemia	+7, –7, +8, *t(9;22) (q34;q11), i(17q), +21
Colonic adenocarcinoma	+7, +12
Ewing's sarcoma	t(11;22) (q24;q12)
Follicular lymphoma	t(14;18) (q32;q21)
Lipoma	t(12) (q13–14)
Liposarcoma	t(12,16) (q13;p11)
Lung small cell carcinoma	del(3) (p14p23)
Malignant lymphoma	6q-, t(14;18) (q32.3;q21.3), 14q+, i(17q)
Malignant melanoma	del(1) (p12–p22), i(6p)
Meningioma	–22
Neuroblastoma	del(1) (p32–p36)
Ovarian carcinoma	t(6;14) (q21;q24)
Parotid mixed tumour	t(3;8) (p21;q12), t(9;12) (p13–22;q13–15)
Polycythaemia rubra vera	20q-
Prostatic adenocarcinoma	del(10) (q24), del(8p), del(7q)
Renal carcinoma	del(3) (p21)
Retinoblastoma	del(13) (q14.1)
Rhabdomyosarcoma	t(2;13) (q37;q14)
Synovial sarcoma	t(X;18) (p11;q11)
Testicular carcinoma	i(12p)
Uterine adenocarcinoma	1p–, duplq
Wilms' tumour	del(11) (p13)

* Most frequently observed abnormality.

MLH1, *PMS1* and *PMS2*) and these gene products normally interact to effect mismatch repair. With somatic loss of the second normal allele the cell becomes prone to accumulate genetic mutations and one consequence of this is that the pattern of microsatellite repeats at a polymorphic locus can differ from the surrounding normal tissue (also called RER[+], replication error positive). Figure 17.6 shows an example where the tumour tissue shows instability of a microsatellite repeat due to loss of function of *MSH2*.

OTHER GENES

Other genes are also involved in the predisposition to cancer by virtue of their role in metabolism of carcinogens. For example, the risk of bladder cancer is increased in

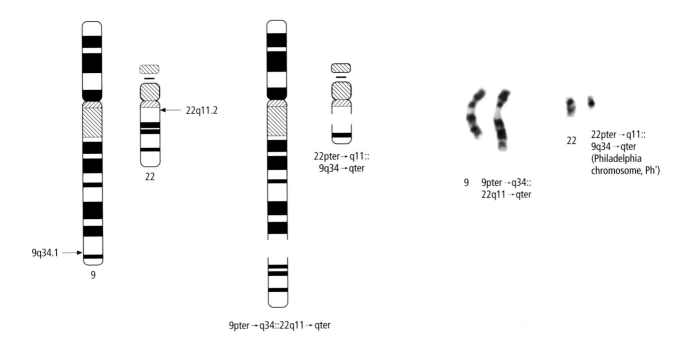

9pter→q34::22q11→qter

Fig. 17.5 Philadelphia chromosome (Ph') resulting from a reciprocal translocation between chromosomes 9 and 22 [t(9;22) (q34;q11)].

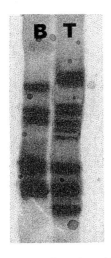

Fig. 17.6 DNA analysis of a microsatellite polymorphism to show new alleles in tumour (T) as compared with blood (B).

aniline dye workers who are slow metabolizers of isoniazid (p. 130).

Additional chromosomal changes frequently occur during the evolution of a cancer, increasing its malignancy. These changes are often associated with amplification of oncogenes or involvement of new oncogenes. The number of copies of a particular oncogene can be increased by the generation of multiple repeats, often in the form of homogeneously stained chromosomal regions (HSRs) or a series of tiny fragments called double minutes (small paired extrachromosomal elements lacking centromeres, Fig. 17.7). These double minutes may also contain genes which have a selective advantage for the tumour such as dihydrofolate reductase in patients on methotrexate chemotherapy. They tend to be lost once the selective pressure is removed unless incorporated into the cell's chromosomes as HSRs.

CLINICAL RELEVANCE OF GENETIC STUDIES IN CANCER

Genetic studies (chromosomal and DNA analysis) are of value in a growing number of tumours for diagnostic classification and determination of prognosis (Tables 17.1 and 17.2). To date, leukaemias have been studied most, and certain general conclusions are possible. First, the primary chromosomal event appears to determine the basic biology of the disease. Thus, for example, the FAB type 2 of acute myeloid leukaemia (AML) may be associated with three different tumour translocations. AML patients with t8;21 usually have Auer bodies in the leukaemic cells, a ready response to therapy with long complete remissions and a relatively long survival (Fig. 17.8). In contrast AML patients with t9;22 (Philadelphia chromosome) appear to have a rather poor prognosis and those with t6;9 have an intermediate outlook. Amongst patients with ALL, translocations are seen in about one-third and these patients have a poorer prognosis than those with normal

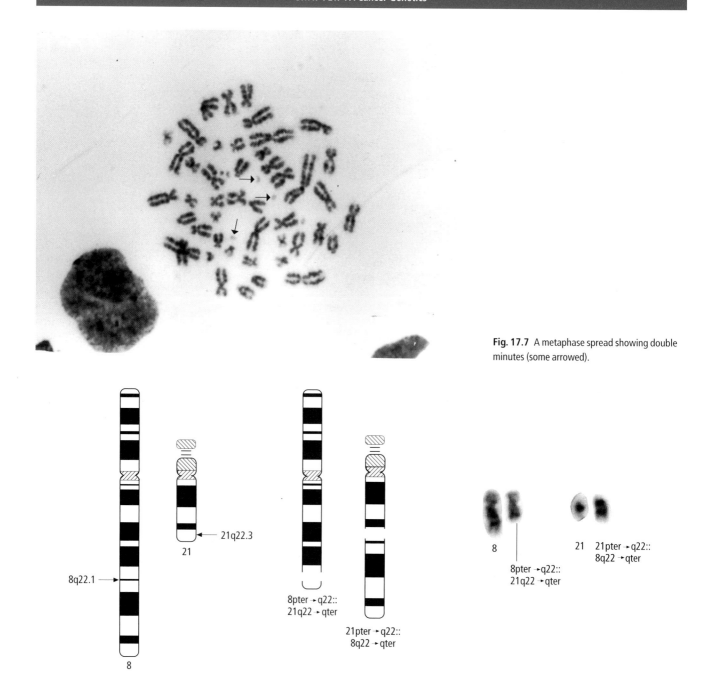

Fig. 17.7 A metaphase spread showing double minutes (some arrowed).

Fig. 17.8 Reciprocal translocation between chromosomes 8 and 21 [t(8;21) (q22;q22)] in a patient with acute myeloid leukaemia.

karyotypes or numerical abnormalities and amongst the translocations the t4;11 and t9;22 carry a particularly poor prognosis. Leukaemia secondary to chemotherapy, irradiation or toxic exposure is characterized cytogenetically by changes involving chromosomes 5 (5q– or –5), 7 (7q– or –7), 17, 12 and 3 and patients with monosomy 5 or 7 appear to have the worst prognosis within this group.

Most patients with CML have the Philadelphia chromosome (p. 165) but 10% do not. These negative patients may have a masked Philadelphia translocation (mosaic or more complex translocation) or may be truly Philadelphia-negative. The former group has the *BCR/ABL* product and has the same disease as cytogenetically positive patients whereas the true Philadelphia-negative patients have no *BCR/ABL* product and have a worse prognosis.

Second, additional chromosomal changes usually herald a worse prognosis. Thus, for example, in AML patients with t8;21 the disease has a benign course until secondary changes usually consisting of loss of a sex chromosome, an additional 8 or other abnormalities appear in the leukaemic cells. The disease then becomes more aggressive with resistance to chemotherapy and difficulty in obtaining complete or long-lasting remissions. Further, in general the number of additional changes correlates with an increasingly poor prognosis.

Third, karyotypic abnormalities may precede clinical evidence of relapse/disease acceleration. Thus, for example, the appearance of secondary chromosomal changes (especially isochromosome 17q, trisomy 8, trisomy 19, loss of the Y or an extra Philadelphia chromosome) in Philadelphia-positive CML usually heralds the existence of the acute blastic phase and such changes may appear weeks to months before clinical or other evidence of such a phase (Fig. 17.9).

GENETIC COUNSELLING ASPECTS OF CANCER

In the following sections the key points for genetic counselling of patients with common cancers and their families are summarized and additional information is provided under 'Further Reading' on p. 216. In general the recurrence risk for other relatives is low for the common tumour types provided there is no relevant family history and if the proband has a unifocal late-onset tumour. A cancer family syndrome (site-specific or non-specific) should be suspected with a positive family history or if the proband has early-onset, multifocal or multiple primary tumours. Similarly a high risk single gene disorder should be suspected if other features co-exist and information on the commoner and clinically most important of these is provided later in this chapter.

Brain tumours

Primary brain tumours are uncommon with a frequency of 1 in 10 000. In children they tend to occur in the posterior fossa and in adults most are supratentorial. Most are sporadic with a low risk to relatives but single gene disorders should be excluded if there are associated features (e.g. neurofibromatosis types 1 and 2, p. 174; tuberous sclerosis, p. 175; von Hippel–Lindau disease, p. 176; and Li–Fraumeni syndrome, p. 172).

Breast cancer

The female lifetime risk of breast cancer is 1 in 12 and the disease is hereditary in 5–10% (>35% of cases under 30

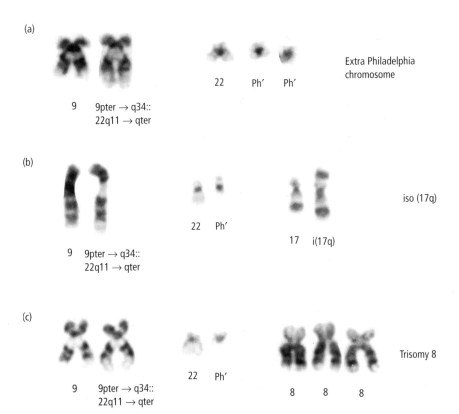

(a)

22   Ph'   Ph'   Extra Philadelphia chromosome

9   9pter → q34::
     22q11 → qter

(b)

22   Ph'

9   9pter → q34::
     22q11 → qter

17   i(17q)   iso (17q)

(c)

22   Ph'

9   9pter → q34::
     22q11 → qter

8   8   8   Trisomy 8

Fig. 17.9 Additional abnormalities in three patients with Philadelphia chromosome [t(9;22)(q34;q11)]-positive chronic myeloid leukaemia indicating acute blastic crisis: (a) additional Philadelphia chromosome, (b) isochromosome of 17q and (c) trisomy 8.

years of age but <1% of cases over 80 years of age). Most inherited breast cancer is due to mutations in *BRCA1* (60%, p. 172) or *BRCA2* (35%, p. 172) with a small minority due to ataxia telangiectasia (carriers, p. 171), Li–Fraumeni syndrome (p. 172) and other rare single gene disorders. Inherited breast cancer should be suspected if there is an early age of onset (under 40 years), bilateral disease, co-existent ovarian cancer or a family history of breast cancer or ovarian cancer.

Carcinoma of the cervix

Carcinoma of the cervix affects about 1% of women and environmental factors (especially an association with E6 and E7 papilloma virus proteins) appear to be the primary determinants. A genetic susceptibility may be involved as 88% of patients are HLA DQw3 compared with the general population frequency of 50% but for counselling purposes the risk for relatives is not increased beyond the general population risk and routine cervical cytology screening can be offered.

Carcinoma of the stomach/oesophagus

Environmental factors appear to be particularly important in the causation of carcinoma of the stomach or oesophagus with consequent low recurrence risks for relatives. One important exception is a rare single-gene disorder where thickening of the skin on the palms and soles (tylosis) and a predisposition to oesophageal carcinoma are inherited as an autosomal dominant trait.

Colorectal cancer

The population risk for colorectal cancer is 1 in 50 in the UK and the disease is hereditary in 5–15%. Most hereditary colorectal cancer is due to hereditary non-polyposis colon cancer (HNPCC, p. 172) and intestinal polyposis (p. 171) accounts for under 1%. Inherited colon cancer should be suspected if the tumour shows microsatellite instability (a characteristic feature of HNPCC), if multiple polyps are present, if there is an early age of onset or multifocal disease and if there is a family history of colorectal or other related cancers. If no information on the proband is available, the risk to first degree relatives is 1 in 17 rising to 1 in 10 if the proband was under 45 years of age at presentation. If a first- and a second-degree relative are affected, the risk is 1 in 12 and if two first-degree relatives are affected the risk is 1 in 6.

Leukaemia

The proportion of leukaemia with a heritable component has been variously estimated as 0–25%. Monozygotic twin concordance is about 25% but this must be accepted with reservation since concordance beyond 5 years of age is rare, the twins tend to be affected within weeks to months of each other and they usually share cytogenetic abnormalities, suggesting the possibility of cross-transfusion of a single malignant clone through the common placental circulation. Risks to sibs in childhood leukaemia are 2–4 times higher than the population incidence, but the absolute risk under these circumstances is low (1 in 100–300). In addition certain chromosomal (e.g. trisomy 21) and single gene disorders (e.g. Bloom syndrome and Fanconi syndrome) carry an increased risk for acute leukaemia.

Lung cancer

Environmental factors appear to be of primary importance in the causation of the commonest types of lung cancer. In the UK it has been estimated that habitual smoking of 25 cigarettes per day gives a 12% risk of death due to lung cancer. Genetic susceptibility to environmental factors may also be involved (e.g. a disputed lower risk of lung cancer in slow metabolizers of debrisoquine, p. 135).

Lymphoma

The risk of a relative developing Hodgkin's disease has been estimated to be sevenfold higher than the basic age-adjusted population risk if diagnosis is made under 45 years of age but with no increase for later diagnosis. Sib pair analysis shows a statistically significant excess of HLA sharing suggesting a role for this locus in the genetic susceptibility.

Osteosarcoma

Osteosarcoma is a rare tumour which is generally sporadic with low risks to relatives. The risk is higher in patients with retinoblastoma (p. 175) and patients with multiple exostoses (p. 173).

Ovarian cancer

The female lifetime risk for ovarian cancer is 1 in 50–100 in Europe and the USA and the disease is hereditary in 5–10%. Mutations in *BRCA1* (inherited breast cancer type 1) cause 35–50% of hereditary ovarian cancer and this and other hereditary causes should be suspected with early age of onset (under 50 years), bilateral disease or a family history of ovarian or breast cancer.

Pancreatic cancer

Most pancreatic cancer is sporadic but some cases occur as one of the associated tumours in HNPCC (p. 172) or as a complication of autosomal dominant hereditary pancreatitis.

Prostatic cancer

Prostatic cancer is the most common malignancy in males

with a male lifetime risk of 1 in 11 in the USA. The relative risk is increased 3–11-fold in first-degree relatives.

Renal cell carcinoma

Renal cell carcinoma is uncommon and about 1% is inherited as an autosomal dominant trait (where it may be the only feature or a component of von Hippel–Lindau disease, p. 176).

Skin cancer

Single gene disorders can cause each of the three main types of skin cancer although overall environmental factors are more important. Five to ten per cent of malignant melanoma is heritable as an autosomal dominant trait (familial atypical malignant melanoma, p. 172); basal cell carcinomas may be due to the naevoid basal carcinoma syndrome (p. 173) or xeroderma pigmentosum (p. 176); and squamous cell carcinoma may be due to Fanconi anaemia, xeroderma pigmentosum or multiple self-healing squamous epithelioma syndrome (p. 173).

Testicular cancer

The risk to male sibs is increased 9.8-fold and to sons is increased 4-fold. Familial cases tend to have an earlier age at diagnosis and an increased risk of bilaterality and show autosomal dominant inheritance with male limitation.

Thyroid cancer

Cancer of the thyroid is histologically subdivided into papillary (50%), follicular and other rarer types which include medullary tumours. The last are associated with multiple endocrine neoplasia (p. 173) but for the non-medullary types, the overall risk is increased fivefold (compared with the general population prevalence of 0.7/100 000 males and 1.9/100 000 females).

SINGLE GENE CAUSES OF CANCER

Over 300 single gene traits have cancer as a recognized complication but in this section only the commoner and clinically most important of these are outlined, and additional information can be sought from the 'Further Reading' references on p. 216.

Ataxia telangiectasia

Diagnosis. Childhood onset of progressive cerebellar ataxia, recurrent infections and oculocutaneous telangiectases. Increased serum alphafetoprotein, non-random chromosomal rearrangements (especially involving 14q, pericentric inversion of 7 and end-to-end fused chromatids), hypersensitivity of fibroblasts and lymphocytes (and patients) to X-rays.

Prognosis. Increased risk of lymphoreticular malignancy (10–20%), especially leukaemias and lymphomas under 16 years of age with mainly carcinomas later. Increased risk of breast cancer in female heterozygotes.

Genetics. Autosomal recessive trait due to mutations in *ATM*. Prenatal diagnosis possible by DNA analysis or demonstration of increased chromosomal breakage. Frequency 1 in 40 000.

Bloom syndrome

Diagnosis. Low birth weight, short stature and a photosensitive facial rash. Increased (10-fold) rate of sister chromatid exchange with formation of quadriradials due to somatic recombination between homologues.

Prognosis. Increased risk (20%) of neoplasia at all ages. Acute leukaemia and lymphoid neoplasia predominate before 25 years and subsequently carcinomas at a variety of sites may occur.

Genetics. Autosomal recessive trait with a higher carrier frequency in Ashkenazi Jews. Prenatal diagnosis possible by demonstration of sister chromatid exchanges.

Familial adenomatous polyposis (FAP, polyposis coli, Gardner syndrome)

Diagnosis. Multiple (>100) intestinal polyps (especially in the colon) from early childhood, congenital hyperplasia of the retinal pigment epithelium (CHRPE, 80% of families), epidermoid cysts (in two-thirds, especially on scalp) and osteomas on the mandible (90%).

Prognosis. Malignant transformation of the colorectal polyps (100%) with consequent need for prophylactic surgery. Increased risk of upper gastrointestinal tract cancer (12%).

Genetics. FAP is inherited as an autosomal dominant trait and is caused by mutations in the adenomatous polyposis coli (*APC*) tumour suppressor gene. Multiple different mutations are found but commonly they result in protein truncation and a 5 bp deletion of AAAGA at nucleotides 3927–3931 accounts for 10% of all mutations. The penetrance is high (almost complete by 40 years of age) but there is intrafamilial variability in respect of age of onset. Presymptomatic detection is possible by demonstration of CHRPEs (in families which show this feature) and by direct and indirect DNA analysis. Mutant gene carriers need regular endoscopy and consideration of prophylactic surgery. FAP has a frequency of 1 in 8000.

Familial atypical malignant melanoma (FAMM)

Diagnosis. Multiple dysplastic pigmented naevi with increased risk of malignant melanoma.

Prognosis. Variable.

Genetics. Autosomal dominant trait with evidence suggestive of genetic heterogeneity.

Fanconi syndrome

Diagnosis. Pancytopenia (progressive from 5 to 10 years), skin pigmentation, congenital malformations (especially radial limb defects) and short stature. Undue sensitivity to DNA cross-linking agents such as mitomycin C and to diepoxybutane-induced chromosome breakage.

Prognosis. Increased risk of acute non-lymphatic leukaemia (5–10%), hepatocellular carcinoma and squamous cell carcinomas.

Genetics. Autosomal recessive trait with genetic heterogeneity. Prenatal diagnosis possible by DNA analysis or chromosomal breakage studies.

Hereditary non-polyposis colon cancer (HNPCC, includes Lynch syndromes I and II)

Diagnosis. Familial clustering of colorectal and related tumours (see Prognosis). DNA analysis of tumours shows microsatellite instability (p. 167).

Prognosis. Colorectal tumours are commonest (60%) and tend to be right-sided (65% compared with 25% of sporadic tumours). Other common tumour types are endometrial carcinoma and cancer of the breast, stomach and pancreas. Less common tumour types in HNPCC families are cancer of the ovary or kidney and brain tumours.

Genetics. HNPCC shows genetic heterogeneity and can be caused by mutations in four gene loci (*MSH2* (60%), *MLH1* (30%), *PMS1* and *PMS2*). Each shows autosomal dominant inheritance with incomplete (75–90%) penetrance (especially in females). Colorectal tumours from affected individuals show microsatellite instability and overall 10–17% of colorectal tumours show such instability (many due to HNPCC, some due to somatic mutations). Mutant gene carriers can be identified by direct or indirect DNA analysis and these gene carriers can be offered regular colonoscopy. The combined frequency of HNPCC gene mutations is believed to be 1 in 200 of the general population.

Inherited breast cancer type 1 (BRCA1)

Diagnosis. Familial clustering of breast and/or ovarian cancer.

Prognosis. Female carriers of *BRCA1* mutations have a high risk of both breast cancer (50% by 50 years, 80% by 70 years) and ovarian cancer (23% by 50 years, 63% by 70 years). *BRCA1* mutant gene carriers are also at increased risk for colorectal cancer and cancer of the prostate.

Genetics. Inherited breast cancer type 1 is inherited as an autosomal dominant trait and is caused by a variety of mutations (which commonly result in loss of function) in *BRCA1*. One common mutation is 185delAG which is found in 1% of Ashkenazi Jews. Presymptomatic gene carriers can be detected using direct DNA analysis (or indirect DNA analysis in extensive families) and offered regular tumour surveillance. Overall inherited breast cancer type 1 accounts for 60% of inherited breast cancer (over 80% of families with breast and ovarian cancer, 45% of families with breast cancer alone) and 1 in 200–500 of the population carry a mutation in *BRCA1*.

Inherited breast cancer type 2 (BRCA2)

Diagnosis. Familial clustering of breast cancer.

Prognosis. Carriers of *BRCA2* mutations have a high risk of breast cancer in both females (80% by 70 years) and males (5% by 70 years).

Genetics. Inherited breast cancer type 2 is inherited as an autosomal dominant trait and is caused by a variety of mutations in *BRCA2*. Presymptomatic gene carriers can be detected by DNA analysis and offered regular tumour surveillance. Inherited breast cancer 2 accounts for 35% of inherited breast cancer (45% of families with breast cancer alone but not involved in the families with breast and ovarian cancer).

Li–Fraumeni syndrome

Diagnosis. Multiple early-onset primary malignant tumours. Sarcomas, adrenal carcinomas, leukaemias and brain tumours are recognized in childhood. Later high frequency of breast cancer, astrocytoma, carcinoma of the lung, carcinoma of the pancreas, prostatic carcinoma, melanoma and gonadal germ cell tumours.

Prognosis. Variable depending upon the number and location of tumours.

Genetics. Autosomal dominant trait due to mutations in the *p53* tumour suppressor gene in some families.

Multiple endocrine neoplasia type 1 (MEN1, Werner syndrome)

Diagnosis. Hyperparathyroidism (95%), pancreatic islet tumours (80%, most functional, usually as gastrinomas) and pituitary adenomas (50%).

Prognosis. Patients also have an increased risk of carcinoid tumours, multiple lipomas, adrenal tumours and thyroid tumours.

Genetics. MEN1 is inherited as an autosomal dominant trait which shows intrafamilial variability and age-related penetrance using clinical and biochemical evaluation of 44% by 20 years, 74% by 35 and 91% by 50 years. Presymptomatic gene carriers can be detected by biochemical testing and indirect DNA analysis. MEN1 accounts for 20% of patients with primary hyperparathyroidism and 50% with Zollinger–Ellison syndrome.

Multiple endocrine neoplasia type 2 (MEN2)

Diagnosis. There are two allelic subtypes. MEN2A (Sipple syndrome) includes medullary thyroid carcinoma (100%), phaeochromocytoma (50–75%), prominent corneal nerves (57%) and hyperparathyroidism (25%). MEN2B also includes medullary thyroid carcinoma, prominent corneal nerves and phaeochromocytoma (25%) but hyperparathyroidism is rare and patients have additional features with neuromas of mucous membranes, a marfanoid habitus and megacolon.

Prognosis. Variable depending upon malignancy or hyperfunction of the tumours.

Genetics. MEN2A and MEN2B are inherited as autosomal dominant traits and are both caused by mutations in *RET*. In MEN2A most mutations occur at codon 634 and if this cysteine is replaced with arginine the patient usually has parathyroid disease. In MEN2B most mutations occur at codon 918 and M918T is the single commonest mutation. Presymptomatic diagnosis can be offered by biochemical and direct DNA analysis. MEN2A and MEN2B account for 25% of patients with medullary thyroid carcinoma.

Multiple exostoses (diaphyseal aclasis)

Diagnosis. Multiple cartilage-capped exostoses (Fig. 17.10).

Prognosis. Involved bones may be shortened or bowed. Malignant change occurs in 1–2% and should be suspected with growth of an exostosis after puberty.

Genetics. Multiple exostoses is inherited as an autosomal dominant trait with a high penetrance (67–100%) and a

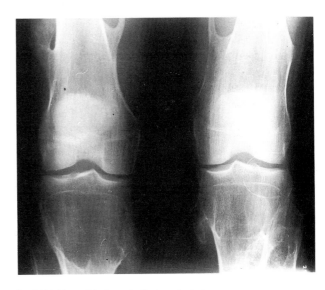

Fig. 17.10 X-ray of the knees in diaphyseal aclasis.

frequency of 1 in 2000. Genetic heterogeneity is apparent with loci on chromosomes 8 (commonest, due to mutations in *EXT1*), 19 (occasional, due to mutations in *COMP*) or 11.

Multiple self-healing squamous epithelioma (MSSE)

Diagnosis. Multiple well-differentiated squamous cell epitheliomas (keratoacanthomas) which each resolve spontaneously over several months.

Prognosis. Self-limiting (grow over 2–3 weeks, ulcerate then regress over 2–3 months) but heal with scarring and cosmetic surgery is often required. No tumours before puberty.

Genetics. MSSE is inherited as an autosomal dominant trait.

Naevoid basal cell carcinoma syndrome (Gorlin–Goltz syndrome)

Diagnosis. Skin naevi (pink or brown papules) from around puberty, multiple basal cell carcinomas with an early age of onset (75%), recurrent jaw odontogenic keratocysts (85%), palmar and plantar pits on the hands and feet (65%), hypertelorism and frontal and parietal skull bossing.

Prognosis. Variable. Patients are at increased risk of medulloblastoma and are also unduly sensitive to irradiation.

Genetics. Caused by mutations in the human patched (PTC) gene. Inherited as an autosomal dominant trait with a high (97%) penetrance but very variable expression. Frequency is 1 in 57 000 and this syndrome accounts for 1 in 200 patients with one or more basal cell carcinomas.

Neuroblastoma

Diagnosis. Present with an abdominal mass in early childhood.

Prognosis. Variable depending upon tumour staging.

Genetics. Mostly sporadic with autosomal dominant inheritance evident in <1%. Empiric risk to sibs or offspring in the absence of a family history is <6%. These relatives can be offered screening with serial assays of urinary catecholamines from birth to six years.

Neurofibromatosis type 1
(NF1, von Recklinghausen disease)

Diagnosis. Multiple café au lait patches in early childhood (more than six 15 mm or larger in an adult or 5 mm or larger in a child), skin neurofibromata from adolescence onwards (Fig. 17.11) and iris hamartomas (Lisch nodules, evident on slit-lamp examination in 90%).

Prognosis. An estimated 65% of patients have none of the complications which include: learning difficulties (30%), moderate-to-severe mental handicap (3%), plexiform neurofibromas (25%), optic pathway gliomas (10–15% on computed tomography (CT) scan but usually asymptomatic), other CNS tumour (1–2%), malignant change in a neurofibroma (1.5%, almost invaribly a plexiform neurofibroma), phaeochromocytoma (1–3%), hypertension (2%), seizures (3–4%), scoliosis (5%), pathological fracture of the tibia (1%) and spinal cord or root compression (hence operation scar in Fig 17.11). NF1 accounts for about one-third of patients with optic gliomas and about 5% with phaeochromocytomas.

Genetics. NF1 is inherited as an autosomal dominant trait with almost full penetrance but very variable expression. A variety of mutations are found in the tumour suppressor gene neurofibromin (*NF1*). Prenatal and presymptomatic diagnosis are possible by DNA analysis. Prevalence 1 in 3500 with 50% of cases due to new mutations (usually paternal in origin).

Neurofibromatosis type 2
(NF2, bilateral acoustic neurofibromas)

Diagnosis. Bilateral acoustic schwannomas, resulting in unilateral or bilateral tinnitus, deafness and vertigo; skin plaques (neurilemmomas); occasional café au lait patches; lens opacities (30–50%); spinal schwannomas or meningiomas; falx meningioma; parenchymal astrocy-

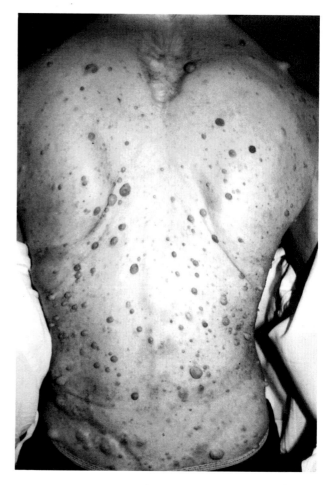

Fig. 17.11 Neurofibromatosis with scar from spinal cord decompression.

toma or ependymoma; onset of symptoms most often in teens or early 20s (range 5–70 years). NF2 accounts for virtually all patients with bilateral acoustic neurofibromas.

Prognosis. Variable depending upon the number and type of tumours.

Genetics. Type 2 neurofibromatosis is inherited as an autosomal dominant trait with full penetrance by 60 years and is caused by a variety of mutations in the tumour suppressor, schwannomin (*NF2*). Presymptomatic and prenatal diagnosis using direct or indirect DNA analysis. Frequency 1 in 35 000–40 000. Gene carriers can be offered screening with MRI (brain and spinal), audiology with attention to speech discrimination and brain stem auditory evoked responses.

Peutz–Jeghers syndrome

Diagnosis. Multiple intestinal polyps together with melanin spots on the lips and fingers (95% but tend to fade after 25 years).

Prognosis. Increased risk of colonic and small bowel cancer, intussusception and ovarian granulosa cell tumour.

Genetics. Inherited as an autosomal dominant trait. At risk relatives can be offered regular screening by endoscopy.

Retinoblastoma

Diagnosis. Onset is usually in the first five years with a white cat's eye reflex or squint; 20–30% are bilateral and these tend to have an earlier onset.

Prognosis. Ninety per cent are cured if unilateral and small. In inherited cases 11–20% develop a further primary tumour, especially osteosarcoma in childhood, or melanoma or cancer of the bladder, lung or pancreas as an adult.

Genetics. Incidence 1 in 18 000–20 000 births. Familial cases (which include all bilateral cases and 15% of unilateral cases) are inherited as an autosomal dominant trait with 90% penetrance and are caused by a variety of mutations in the *RB1* tumour suppressor gene.

Prenatal and presymptomatic diagnosis is possible in familial cases by direct or indirect DNA analysis. For a sporadic unilateral case the risk to sibs is 0.8% and to offspring is 7.5% and these children should have regular ophthalmological screening. Rarely, spontaneous regression may occur, leaving a retinal scar, and this should be excluded in apparently isolated cases by ophthalmological evaluation of the parents. For normal parents of a child with bilateral disease, the risk to sibs is 5%.

Tuberous sclerosis

Diagnosis. White skin patches which may only be apparent under ultraviolet light (Wood's lamp) (82% by five years); facial fibroangiomatous rash (adenoma sebaceum, Fig. 17.12; 50% by five years); skin fibromatous plaques (shagreen patches, 20–40%); enamel pits (70%); phalangeal cysts; ungual fibromas (15–50%); whitish retinal phakomata (50%); intracranial calcification or periventricular hamartomas on CT scan (Fig. 17.13); glial pathway high signal on MRI; evidence of complications.

Prognosis. Epilepsy (90%); mental handicap (50%); variable lifespan which depends upon the severity of the mental handicap. Renal angiomyolipomata (60%) and cardiac rhabdomyomata (most infants, 30% of adults) may occur. Malignant brain tumours, usually giant cell astrocytomas, occur in <3%.

Genetics. Autosomal dominant trait with genetic heterogeneity, one locus (*TSC1*) in 9q and one (*TSC2*) on 16p;

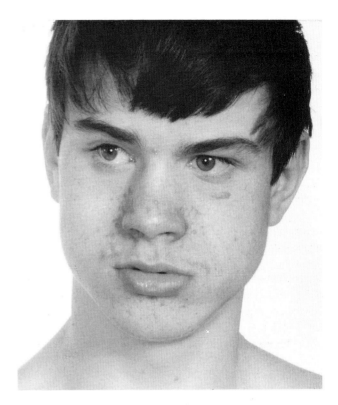

Fig. 17.12 Facial fibroangiomata (adenoma sebaceum) in tuberous sclerosis.

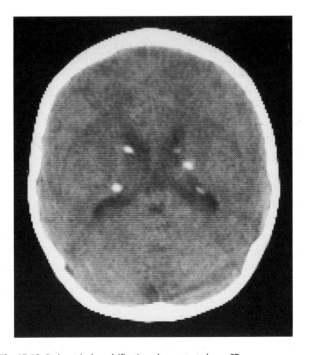

Fig. 17.13 Periventricular calcifications demonstrated on a CT scan.

60–70% of cases represent new mutations. However, before concluding that a child has a new mutation it is vital to examine both parents for mild disease stigmata and to consider parental CT scans. If all investigations on parents of an isolated case are normal the recurrence risk is about 2% due to gonadal mosaicism. Direct (for *TSC2*) or indirect DNA analysis may be considered for presymptomatic and prenatal diagnosis in familial cases.

Tuberous sclerosis has a birth frequency of 1 in 10 000 and accounts for 10–20% of patients with infantile spasms.

von Hippel–Lindau disease

Diagnosis. Features include: retinal haemangiomas (60%), cerebellar haemangioblastomas (60%), spinal haemangiomas and brain stem haemangiomas (18%).

Prognosis. Renal carcinoma (28%), phaeochromocytoma (7%) and renal, pancreatic, hepatic and epididymal cysts.

Genetics. Inherited as an autosomal dominant trait due to a variety of mutations (especially of codon 238) in the tumour suppressor gene *VHL*. Penetrance is age-related (52% by 25 years, 91% by 45 years and 99% by 65 years). Presymptomatic diagnosis possible by direct or indirect DNA analysis. Gene carriers need regular surveillance for tumours. von Hippel–Lindau disease has a frequency of 1 in 35 000 and accounts for all patients with multiple CNS or ocular haemangiomas and about 30% of patients with single cerebellar haemangioblastomas and about 40% of single ocular haemangiomas.

Wilms tumour (nephroblastoma)

Diagnosis. Usually present in early childhood with a renal mass which has characteristic histology.

Prognosis. Variable depending upon delay to diagnosis; 5–10% bilateral.

Genetics. Frequency 1 in 10 000; mostly sporadic; about 1% familial (autosomal dominant), usually bilateral. May be associated with microdeletions at 11p13 and some of these patients have coexistent aniridia; genito-urinary malformations and mental and growth retardation (WAGR syndrome). About 30% of all tumours show loss of heterozygosity for 11p and in these cases with loss of heterozygosity there is preferential (over 90%) loss of the maternal allele. Surprisingly, familial cases show no evidence of linkage to 11p.

Patients with Beckwith–Wiedemann syndrome (p. 191) show an increased risk of Wilms tumour.

Xeroderma pigmentosum

Diagnosis. Defective DNA excision repair after exposure to ultraviolet light.

Prognosis. Multiple skin cancers and corneal scarring (see Plate 1).

Genetics. At least nine subtypes each inherited as autosomal recessive traits. Prenatal diagnosis may be possible by assay of DNA repair capacity or by indirect DNA analysis. Combined frequency 1 in 70 000.

CHAPTER 18

Congenital Malformations

C O N T E N T S

Incidence 177
Aetiology 178
MINOR CONGENITAL MALFORMATIONS **178**
MAJOR CONGENITAL MALFORMATIONS **178**
Central nervous system 179
Heart 184
Gastrointestinal tract 184

Kidney and urinary tract 186
Limbs 188
Thyroid 189
**MULTIPLE CONGENITAL MALFORMATIONS
    AND DYSMORPHIC SYNDROMES** **189**
Multiple malformations due to known teratogens 194

Incidence

A malformation is a primary error of normal development or morphogenesis of an organ or tissue. All malformations are thus congenital or present at birth, although they may not be diagnosed until later, especially if microscopic or if internal organs are involved. Malformations may be single or multiple and may be of minor or major clinical signficance. About 14% of newborns have a single minor malformation, 3% of newborns have a single major malformation and 0.7% of newborns have multiple major malformations (Table 18.1). The frequency of major malformations is even higher at conception (10–15%), but the majority of these fetuses are spontaneously aborted (Fig. 18.1).

A disruption (or secondary malformation) is a morphological defect due to breakdown of a previously normal organ or tissue. Disruptions can arise at any stage of gestation after initial morphogenesis. Similarly, deformations arise after the embryonic period and are alterations in shape caused by unusual mechanical forces. About 2% of newborns are affected, with multiple deformations in one-third. Malformations and deformations may coexist, and there is an increased risk of deformation (8%) in the presence of a major congenital malformation, especially of the central nervous system or urinary tract.

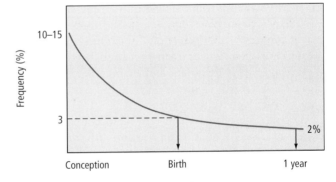

Fig. 18.1 Frequency of major congenital malformations.

Table 18.1 Classification and birth frequency of congenital malformations and deformations.

Classification		Frequency
Minor malformations	Single	140 in 1000
	Multiple	5 in 1000
Major malformations	Single	30 in 1000
	Multiple	7 in 1000
Deformations	Single	14 in 1000
	Multiple	6 in 1000

Table 18.2 Aetiology of major congenital malformations.

Idiopathic	60%
Multifactorial	20%
Monogenic	7.5%
Chromosomal	6%
Maternal illness	3%
Congenital infection	2%
Drugs, X-ray, alcohol	1.5%

Table 18.3 Causes of congenital deformation.

Intrinsic	Neuromuscular disease, connective tissue defects, CNS malformations
Extrinsic	Primigravidae, small maternal stature, oligohydramnios, breech presentation, uterine malformation, multiple pregnancy

Table 18.4 Examples of congenital deformation.

Talipes
Congenital dislocation of the hip
Congenital postural scoliosis
Plagiocephaly
Torticollis
Mandibular asymmetry

Aetiology

Table 18.2 indicates the identifiable causes of congenital malformations. Multifactorial inheritance is the commonest identifiable cause followed by monogenic and chromosomal disorders. Thus genetic conditions account for at least one-third of all congenital malformations of known aetiology.

Visible duplication or deficiency of any of the autosomes is almost invariably associated with mental handicap, postnatal growth deficiency and dysmorphic features. Multiple malformations and intrauterine growth retardation are also commonly seen and roughly correlate in severity with the extent of the chromosomal imbalance. The phenotypes of over 250 single gene disorders include major congenital malformations (including tissue dysplasias) as a consistent or frequent feature. Recognition of these single gene disorders and of inherited structural chromosome rearrangements is of clinical importance in view of their high recurrence risks.

Maternal illnesses which are associated with an increased risk of fetal malformation include insulin-dependent diabetes mellitus, epilepsy, alcohol abuse and phenylketonuria. There is a 5–15% risk of congenital malformation (especially congenital heart disease, neural tube defect and sacral agenesis) for the offspring of a diabetic mother in proportion to the quality of her diabetic control (but no increase if the mother has gestational or non-insulin-dependent diabetes). The risk is also increased (to about 6%, especially for cleft lip and congenital heart disease) for a mother with epilepsy, although here it is difficult to separate the risk due to the disease and that due to her medications. Untreated maternal phenylketonuria carries a high risk to the fetus for mental retardation, microcephaly and congenital heart disease (25%).

Deformations are caused by any factor which restricts the mobility of the fetus and so causes prolonged compression in an abnormal posture. Causes may be intrinsic or extrinsic (Table 18.3). Deformations are correctible by

pressure, and complete resolution is usual in the newborn period (Table 18.4).

Congenital dislocation of the hip (CDH)

Four to seven in 1000 livebirths have temporarily unstable or clicking hips; actual dislocation is found in 1 in 1000. The sex ratio is 6 females to 1 male. The risk of recurrence for sibs is 1 in 20 (3% for male sibs, 8% for female sibs) and for offspring is 1 in 8. The risks are slightly but not significantly greater for male probands.

Talipes equinovarus (club foot)

Five in 1000 livebirths have talipes equinovarus and this is severe in 1 in 1000. The sex ratio is 2 males to 1 female with a sib risk of 1 in 50 for a male proband but 1 in 20 for a female proband. For an affected parent of either sex the risk of recurrence is 1 in 33.

MINOR CONGENITAL MALFORMATIONS

Table 18.5 lists some common minor congenital malformations. These are of no functional significance but should alert the clinician to the possibility of an associated major malformation which coexists in about 20% of infants with multiple minor malformations.

MAJOR CONGENITAL MALFORMATIONS

Single major congenital malformations are present in 3% of neonates and Table 18.6 indicates the relative frequencies for each organ.

Table 18.5 Examples of minor congenital malformations.

Epicanthic folds
Mongoloid or antimongoloid slant
Coloboma
Ear tag or pit
Bifid uvula
Simian crease
Fifth-finger clinodactyly
Soft-tissue syndactyly
Mongolian spot
Haemangioma
Umbilical hernia
Minor hypospadias
Single umbilical artery

Table 18.6 Birth incidence of major congenital malformations.

Organ	Incidence/1000 births
Brain	10
Heart	8
Kidney	4
Limbs	2
Other	6
Total	30

Central nervous system

The neural groove appears at 20 days from conception and is mostly closed by 23 days. The anterior neuropore closes at 24 days and the posterior neuropore at 28 days. Although the most active period of CNS embryogenesis is from the third to 12th weeks, neuronal proliferation, migration, development of synapses and myelination continue throughout the whole pregnancy and up to 2–3 years of age. The brain thus has a longer period of developmental organization than any other organ. This and its complexity account for its relatively high frequency of malformations. Some of the commoner of these are outlined in this section, but it should be emphasized that only a small proportion of these malformations produce any external change and, for example, those contributing to idiopathic mental handicap are difficult to diagnose without detailed neuropathology.

Holoprosencephaly

In holoprosencephaly there is failure of the development of the forebrain and associated midface. This results in hypotelorism, bilateral cleft lip with an absent philtrum and severe mental handicap. In the most severe cases only a single central eye is present (cyclops, Fig. 18.2). Death within 6 months is usual.

One-third of cases are due to trisomy 13 or other chromosomal abnormalities, but the rest are unexplained, with a 2–6% empiric recurrence risk for sibs, and parental reassurance by detailed ultrasound scanning in future pregnancies is indicated.

Isolated hydrocephalus

Hydrocephalus may be secondary to a neural tube defect or isolated (0.4/1000 livebirths). Identifiable causes of isolated hydrocephalus include intracranial haemorrhage, fetal infection and multifactorial, X-linked recessive or autosomal recessive inheritance. Less than 1% of cases are inherited as an X-linked recessive trait, and these boys have characteristic hypoplastic flexed thumbs (Fig. 18.3), aqueductal stenosis and absence of the pyramids from sections of the medulla. In the absence of an X-linked pedigree or these clinical features (aqueductal stenosis alone is not diagnostic as it occurs in one-third of cases of isolated hydrocephalus) the empiric recurrence risk of an unexplained case of hydrocephalus is 3–4%.

Prenatal diagnosis of hydrocephalus is often but not always possible in the second trimester by serial ultrasound scanning and for the X-linked form may be possible by direct or indirect DNA analysis.

Lissencephaly

Defective neuronal migration during the third to fifth months results in a smooth brain (lissencephaly), few broad thick gyri (pachygyria) or many small plications (polymicrogyria). These changes may coexist in different areas of the same brain and result in epilepsy and mental handicap. The changes may be due to autosomal recessive traits such as the Smith–Lemli–Opitz syndrome (p. 194) or be due to a 17p microdeletion (Miller–Dieker syndrome). For a couple with one child affected with isolated unexplained lissencephaly the recurrence risk is under 10%.

Macrocephaly

Macrocephaly is an abnormally large head (head circumference >3 SD above the mean for the patient's age and sex). In contrast to hydrocephalus the ventricles are of normal size. Patients may be asymptomatic (e.g. benign familial macrocephaly inherited as an autosomal dominant trait), have non-progressive mental handicap (e.g. Sotos syndrome (p. 194), neurofibromatosis type 1, (p. 174)) or have progressive dementia (e.g. Tay–Sachs disease (p. 147)). Recurrence risks depend upon the aetiology.

Microcephaly

Microcephaly is an abnormally small head (head circum-

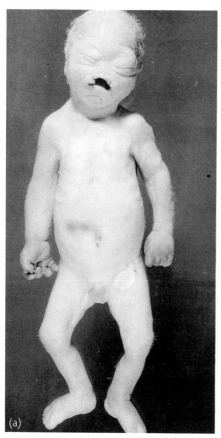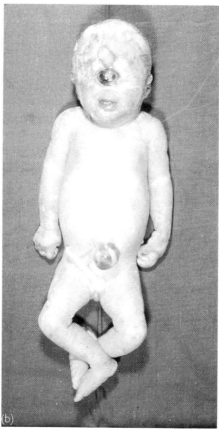

Fig. 18.2 (a, b) Holoprosencephaly of variable severity.

ference <3 SD below the mean for the patient's age and sex) which reflects defective brain growth. Identifiable causes include congenital infection (with rubella, cytomegalovirus or toxoplasmosis), birth trauma, chromosomal imbalance, maternal phenylketonuria, fetal alcohol syndrome, severe postnatal insult and several autosomal recessive traits.

The recurrence risk depends upon aetiology. If the parents are consanguineous, or if two children are affected, autosomal recessive inheritance is likely (Fig. 18.4), and for an unexplained isolated case of microcephaly the empiric recurrence risk is up to 20%, which suggests that recessive inheritance is a major contributing factor.

Prenatal diagnosis may be possible in a future pregnancy by serial ultrasound scanning, but not infrequently the delay in head growth is not apparent until the last trimester.

Neural tube defect

Defective closure of the neural tube may occur at any level. Failure at the cephalic end (anterior neuropore) produces anencephaly or an encephalocele, and failure lower down produces spina bifida. Overall anencephaly (with or without spina bifida) accounts for 40% of neural tube defects, spina bifida alone for 55% and encephaloceles for 5%. Other malformations, particularly exomphalos and renal malformations, coexist in 25%.

In anencephalics the skin and cranial vault are missing (i.e. open lesions) and the exposed nervous tissue degenerates (Fig. 18.5). The hypothalamus is defective, and this leads to fetal adrenal atrophy with low maternal oestriols. Polyhydramnios may complicate the pregnancy. Stillbirth or neonatal death is invariable.

Spina bifida is most commonly lumbosacral with paralysis of the legs and sphincters. About 15–20% have a covering of intact skin (closed lesions) and these tend to cause less neurological disability than the open lesions. Hydrocephalus occurs in 80% (with aqueductal stenosis in about one-third). Without surgical therapy only 20% survive to 2 years. With surgery within 24 h 40% survive more than 7 years but only 8% have little or no handicap with 10% moderately handicapped and 82% severely handicapped. Patients with gross paralysis of the legs, thoracolumbar or thoraco–lumbar–sacral lesions, kyphoscoliosis, hydrocephalus at birth or associated abnormalities have a particularly poor prognosis. In contrast 60% of patients with closed lesions survive to 5 years and one-third are free of

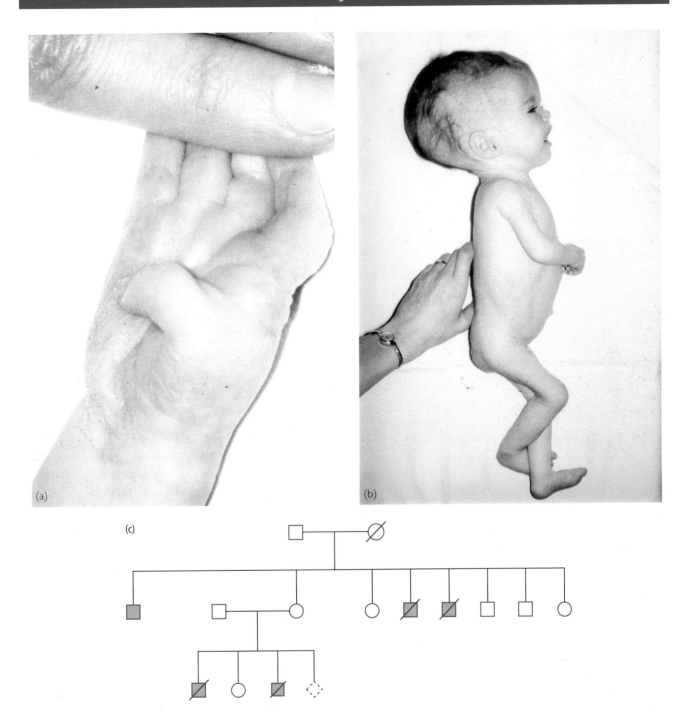

Fig. 18.3 (a–c) Pedigree of a family with X-linked hydrocephalus. Note characteristic flexed hypoplastic thumb in an affected male.

handicap with one-third moderately handicapped and one-third severely handicapped.

Encephaloceles are usually (95%) covered with intact skin (i.e. closed lesions). The degree of disability varies and depends upon the extent of nervous tissue involvement.

The frequency of neural tube defects shows geographical and secular variation. In the USA, Africa and Mongolia 1 in 1000 births are affected. In south-east England in the 1970s, 3 in 1000 births were affected and at that time the frequency was even higher (5 to 8 in 1000) in Ireland, Wales and the west of Scotland. Subsequently the frequency has fallen throughout the UK and the current frequency in the west of Scotland is 2 in 1000 (see Fig. 21.4). The reasons for this secular fall in the UK are unknown.

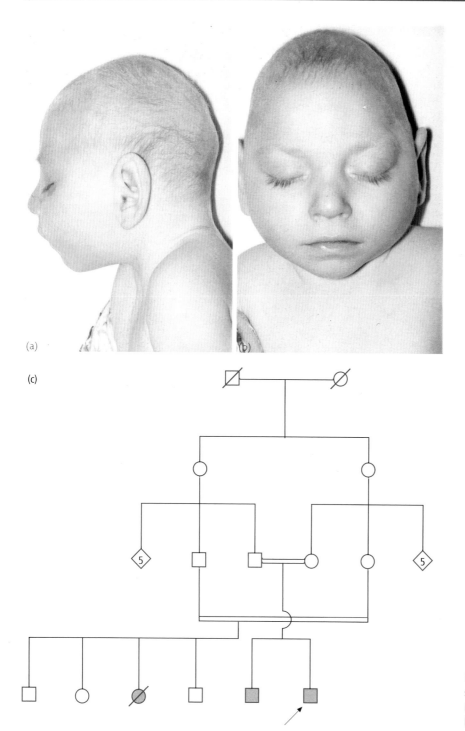

(a)

(b)

(c)

Fig. 18.4 (a–c) Autosomal recessive microcephaly showing an affected child (indicated as the proband) in a consanguineous family. The ears look relatively large as the head is so small.

Epidemiological evidence and genetic analysis favour multifactorial inheritance with important environmental components. One environmental component, maternal levels of folic acid, has been identified and supplementation with folic acid can reduce the recurrence risk in subsequent high risk pregnancies.

In the UK the recurrence risk after an affected pregnancy is 1 in 25–33 and this risk is reduced to 1 in 100 by periconceptional folic acid supplementation introduced *prior* to conception (5 mg folic acid per day). The risk for offspring of an affected patient is also 1 in 25–33.

For second-degree relatives the risk is 1 in 70 and for

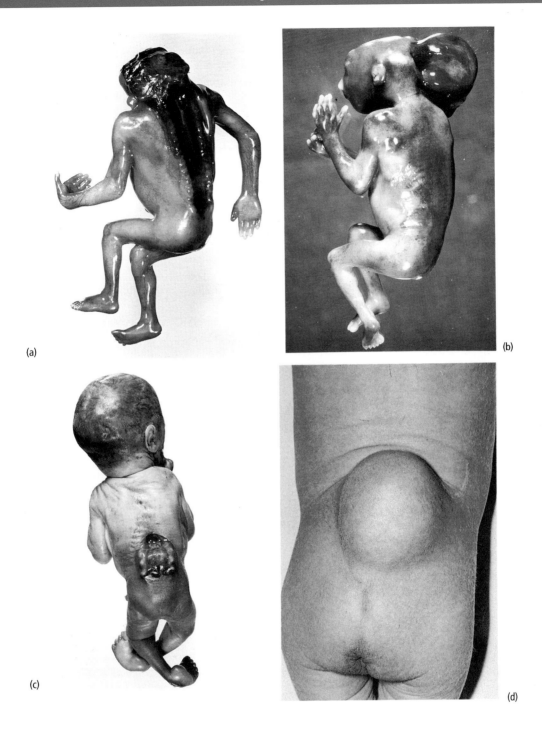

(a)

(b)

(c)

(d)

Fig. 18.5 Neural tube defects. (a) Anencephaly. (b) Encephalocele. (c) Open spina bifida. (d) Closed spina bifida.

third-degree relatives it is 1 in 150. After two or more affected children the recurrence risk rises to 1 in 10. The recurrence risk is lower in countries with a lower incidence, and in general is about 10 times the incidence for first-degree relatives. Prenatal diagnosis is possible by a combination of detailed ultrasound scanning and amniotic fluid biochemistry (alpha-fetoprotein assay and acetylcholinesterase pattern). This will detect 100% of anencephaly and 98% of open spina bifida. In view of the frequency of this serious condition, screening by assay of maternal serum alpha-fetoprotein is commonly offered in high risk populations (Chapter 20).

Isolated neural arch defects (spina bifida occulta) of one or two vertebrae (especially S1, S2 or L5) occur in about 23% of normal individuals. These localized defects are asymptomatic (but may be associated with an overlying hairy patch). They do not appear to increase the risk for sibs with a major neural tube defect but if three or more neural arches are involved the lesion would be termed a closed spina bifida and would carry the usual recurrence risk.

Although most neural tube defects are multifactorial as outlined, some are secondary to teratogenic influences (sodium valproate, maternal diabetes mellitus) and some are secondary to chromosomal or rare single-gene disorders. Trisomy 18 should be excluded if other congenital malformations coexist, and the combination of encephalocele, polydactyly and cystic kidneys is characteristic of an autosomal recessive trait—Meckel syndrome (p. 188).

Heart

The period of active cardiac organogenesis extends from the third to the eighth weeks.

Many different congenital heart lesions have been described and the commoner are outlined in Table 18.7, together with the recurrence risks for family members if no cause can be identified. Overall congenital heart lesions affect 8 in 1000 births, with 2% due to environmental factors, 10% due to chromosomal disorders (including 22q11 microdeletions which account for 5% of congenital heart disease), 3% due to single gene disorders and 80% multifactorial in aetiology. Diagnosis of the latter group is by exclusion and overall the risk to sibs is 1 in 50 and to

offspring 1 in 25 (1 in 20 for mothers, 1 in 30 for fathers). However, for second-degree relatives the risk is less than 1 in 100. If two first-degree relatives are affected the recurrence risk rises to 1 in 10. Recurrence is only specific to the type of heart lesion in 50% and congenital heart disease is also unusual for a multifactorial disorder as the recurrence risks are not higher when the rarer sex is affected and are not higher with commoner as compared with rarer lesions. The prognosis varies with the lesion and improvements in cardiac surgery have meant that some previously lethal lesions are now curable.

Prenatal diagnosis is possible for the more serious of these defects by detailed fetal echocardiography at 18–20 weeks of gestation.

Gastrointestinal tract

The period of active organogenesis of the gastrointestinal tract extends from 3 to 8 weeks of pregnancy. The intestinal loops have usually returned to the abdomen by the 12th week.

Anterior abdominal wall defects

Failure of the intestines to return to the abdomen occurs in 1 in 6000 pregnancies. Three types of lesion are identified (Table 18.8; Fig. 18.6). Exomphalos and gastroschisis may be surgically correctible in the absence of chromosomal abnormality or other malformations. Prenatal diagnosis by ultrasound is possible, and as these malformations may cause elevation of amniotic fluid and maternal serum alpha-fetoprotein they may be detected by a screening programme for neural tube defects (Chapter 20).

Table 18.7 Incidence and recurrence risks for various types of congenital heart disease.

Lesion	Birth incidence	Recurrence risk		
		For sibs (at birth)	For sibs at (prenatal diagnosis)	For offspring
Ventricular septal defect	1 in 400	1 in 25		1 in 25
Atrial septal defect	1 in 1000	1 in 33		1 in 33
Patent ductus arteriosus	1 in 830	1 in 33		1 in 25
Coarctation of aorta	1 in 1600	1 in 50	1 in 15	1 in 50
Aortic stenosis	1 in 2000	1 in 50	1 in 28	1 in 33
Common atrioventricular canal	1 in 2500	1 in 50		?
Total anomalous pulmonary venous drainage	1 in 5000	?		?
Transposition of the great vessels	1 in 16 000	1 in 50		?
Tetralogy of Fallot	1 in 1000	1 in 33		1 in 25
Truncus arteriosus	1 in 6500	1 in 80	1 in 13	—
Complex cyanotic heart disease			1 in 11	—
Hypoplastic left heart	1 in 5000	1 in 50		

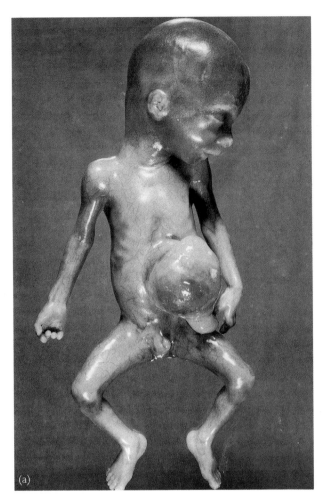

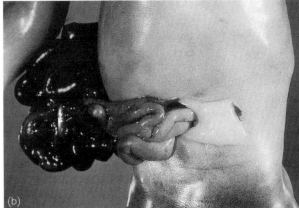

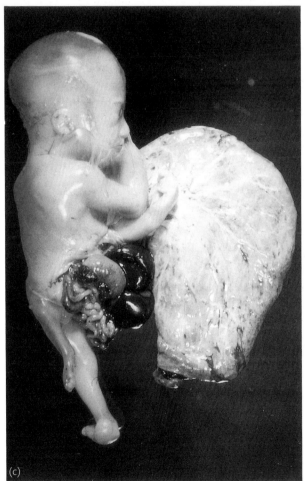

Fig. 18.6 Anterior abdominal wall defects. (a) Exomphalos. (b) Gastroschisis. (c) Body stalk anomaly.

Cleft lip and/or palate

The lip is usually fused by day 35. If this fails it may impair closure of the palatal shelves, which occurs at 8–9 weeks (see Fig. 10.4, p. 95).

Cleft lip with or without cleft palate occurs in 1 in 1000 births and is most often due to multifactorial inheritance, although it may be a feature of over 230 single gene traits (e.g. Treacher Collins syndrome (p. 148) or the van der Woude syndrome (p. 186)), chromosomal abnormalities (e.g. trisomy 13) or dysmorphic syndromes (e.g. holoprosencephaly, amniotic bands sequence). Surgical repair without sequelae is usual.

Table 18.8 Classification of anterior abdominal wall defects.

Type	Comments
Exomphalos	Umbilical cord attached to apex of sac; sac may contain liver and/or intestines; chromosomal abnormality in 30%; congenital heart disease (10%)
Gastroschisis	No sac and umbilical cord not involved in defect: may be associated areas of atretic intestine and congenital heart disease (20%)
Body stalk anomaly	Very short umbilical cord attached to apex of sac; severe spinal deformity; cloacal exstrophy; hypoplastic legs

For the multifactorial lesion the recurrence risk for normal parents with a child who has a unilateral cleft lip alone is 1 in 50, which rises to 1 in 20 if the child has bilateral cleft lip and palate. For second-degree relatives the overall risk is 1 in 150, and it is 1 in 300 for third-degree relatives. Periconceptional multivitamins including folic acid may help to reduce (by 25–50%) these risks.

Cleft palate without cleft lip also shows multifactorial inheritance but is distinct from cleft lip with or without cleft palate. Isolated cleft palate affects 1 in 2000 births with a recurrence risk of 1 in 50 for sibs and offspring.

van der Woude syndrome

This is inherited as an autosomal dominant trait and is characterized by paramedian pits on the lower lip, and cleft lip or cleft palate. Non-penetrance occurs and expression is variable, hence the importance of examining the parents when a child has apparently isolated cleft lip or cleft palate. This syndrome accounts for 1–3% of all cleft lip and palate.

Hirschsprung disease (colonic aganglionosis)

Rectal biopsy confirms the absence of submucosal and myenteric ganglion cells which results in neonatal constipation and abdominal distension. A short or long segment may be involved, starting from the rectum.

One in 5000 neonates is affected, with a 3–5 to 1 male excess. Overall, for a male proband the risk to sibs is 1 in 25 but is less than 1 in 100 for offspring. For a female proband the risk to sibs is 1 in 8 but again is less than 1 in 100 for offspring. The risk also varies somewhat in proportion to the extent of the aganglionic segment.

Genetic heterogeneity is apparent with mutations in *RET* in some families, mutations in endothelin β receptor in some families and other loci involved in other families.

Congenital pyloric stenosis

Affected infants present in the first few weeks of life with persistent vomiting, and the hypertrophic pylorus may be palpable. Surgical treatment is curative.

The incidence in males is 1 in 200 and in females 1 in 1000. The empiric recurrence risks support multifactorial inheritance and are detailed in Table 10.10 (p. 96).

Intestinal atresia

Atresia may occur at any level of the intestine with resulting symptoms and signs of obstruction. One in 330 neonates is affected. The lesion is usually sporadic with no increased recurrence risk. The rare apple-peel syndrome is an exception as it is inherited as an autosomal recessive trait. It derives its name from the characteristic appearance at surgery with agenesis of the mesentery and twisting of the distal small bowel around the marginal artery.

Duodenal atresia presents with a characteristic double-bubble appearance on an ultrasound scan either after birth or antenatally. In 60–70% the lesion is isolated but trisomy 21 should be excluded.

Oesophageal atresia

Oesophageal atresia and/or tracheo-oesophageal fistula affects 1 in 3000 livebirths. The specific recurrence risk is 0.6%, but in addition an unexplained threefold increase over the population risk for a neural tube defect is apparent.

Kidney and urinary tract

The period of active urinary tract organogenesis extends from the fourth to the seventh weeks. The overall frequency of renal and urinary tract malformations is 4 in 1000.

Bilateral renal agenesis

Absence of the kidneys results in oligohydramnios, which in turn produces Potter sequence with large low set ears, a squashed facies, talipes, pulmonary hypoplasia and amnion nodosum (Fig. 18.7). Neonatal death is invariable. Potter sequence may also result from other causes of severe oligohydramnios with cystic dysplasia (50%), obstructive uropathy (25%) and bilateral renal agenesis (20%) most commonly found.

The incidence of bilateral renal agenesis is 1 in 3000 births, and the empiric recurrence risk for the parents of an affected child is 1 in 33. Prenatal diagnosis is possible with detailed ultrasonography.

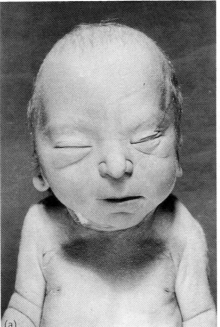
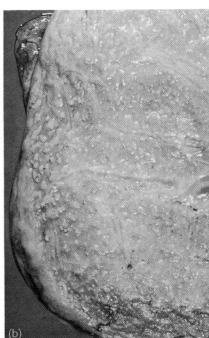

Fig. 18.7 Potter sequence due to bilateral renal agenesis. (a) Characteristic facies. (b) Amnion nodosum.

Renal hypoplasia and dysplasia

Congenitally small disorganized kidneys which may result in renal failure are aetiologically heterogeneous. A few cases are monogenic (e.g. branchio-oto-renal syndrome, below), some are part of a dysmorphic syndrome (e.g. Noonan syndrome, (p. 193), Klippel–Feil syndrome (p. 192) or Turner syndrome (p. 121)), but the majority are unexplained and have a low empiric recurrence risk.

Obstructive uropathy

Fetal obstructive uropathy is most commonly secondary to urethral valves and shows a marked male excess (20 males to 1 female). The prognosis depends upon the severity of the obstruction, and ranges from Potter sequence due to oligohydramnios to survival with a dilated urinary tract, renal impairment and evidence of fetal abdominal distension (the prune belly appearance, Fig. 18.8). The dilated urinary tract is apparent on ultrasound, and attempts have been made to decompress the kidneys *in utero*. The recurrence risk is low for this group of conditions.

Hypospadias

Hypospadias affects 1 in 5000 males and has a recurrence risk of 6–10% for male sibs and offspring.

Branchio-oto-renal syndrome (BOR syndrome)

The BOR syndrome is an autosomal dominant trait with variable expression including pre-auricular pits, cup-

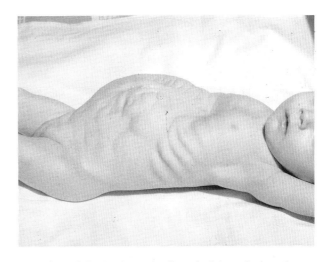

Fig. 18.8 Prune belly appearance secondary to fetal obstructive uropathy.

shaped ears, branchial sinuses and fistulae, childhood deafness (of variable type) and renal hypoplasia (resulting in chronic renal failure in 6%). The frequency is 1 in 40 000 and this syndrome is found in 2% of profoundly deaf children.

Infantile polycystic disease

This autosomal recessive trait results in cysts in the liver, kidneys and pancreas which interfere with function and so result in death in early childhood. Prenatal diagnosis is possible by detailed ultrasonography.

Meckel syndrome

Meckel syndrome is inherited as an autosomal recessive trait and is characterized by abdominal enlargement due to polycystic kidneys, post-axial polydactyly and an encephalocele (Fig. 18.9). Prenatal diagnosis in at-risk pregnancies can be offered by means of detailed ultrasound scanning.

Adult polycystic kidney disease

This common autosomal dominant trait affects 1 in 1000 of the population and results in cysts in the kidneys, liver, pancreas and spleen (Fig. 18.10). The renal cysts are usually asymptomatic until renal failure or hypertension ensues in the fourth decade. Although about one-half of affected individuals will not have reached end-stage renal disease by 70 years, it accounts for 7–15% of all adults with chronic renal failure.

Offspring of an affected person can be screened with ultrasound and nearly 100% of gene carriers will be positive on ultrasound by 30 years of age. Genetic heterogeneity is apparent with most families (86%) due to mutations in polycystin (*PKD1*) on chromosome 16 (see Fig. 3.5, p. 27) and a second locus on chromosome 4. Presymptomatic detection by direct (for PKD1) or indirect DNA analysis may be possible.

Limbs

The period of active limb formation extends from 4 to 7 weeks of pregnancy. The overall birth frequency of major limb malformations is 2/1000. The commoner types of limb defect are illustrated in Fig. 18.11.

Extra digits may occur on the thumb or big toe side (preaxial) or on the little finger side (postaxial). One in every 2000 Caucasians has one or more extra digits. Extra digits may be features of chromosomal disorders (e.g. trisomy 13), single gene disorders (e.g. autosomal dominant polydactyly) or be of unknown aetiology. If the extra digit(s) is the only feature and there is no family history the recurrence risk for normal parents is low.

Fusion of digits may affect the bones or only the soft tissues. If minor degrees of soft-tissue syndactyly between toes two and three are excluded, the incidence is 1 in 1000. The aetiology is again heterogeneous, but if parents are normal the recurrence risk for isolated syndactyly is low.

The incidence of transverse limb defects is 1 in 5000. Most if not all are due to *in utero* amputations by strands of amnion produced by premature rupture of the amnion. If the chorion is also involved, there may be a history of leakage of liquor and the child might also show congenital deformations due to oligohydramnios. The amniotic bands may produce a variety of other defects, including asymmetric facial clefts. The recurrence risk is low, and reassurance in a future pregnancy can be offered by ultrasound scanning.

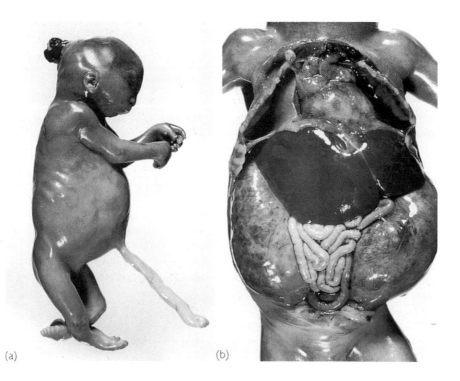

(a)   (b)

Fig. 18.9 (a, b) Meckel syndrome showing polycystic kidneys, polydactyly and encephalocele.

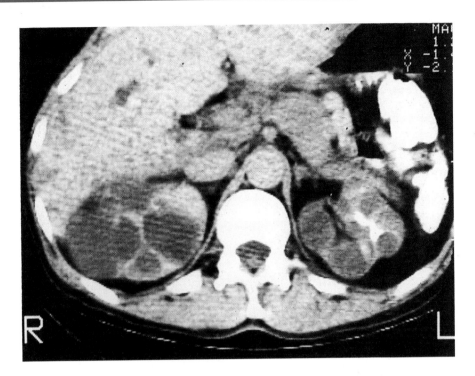

Fig. 18.10 Multiple cysts in the kidneys and liver on abdominal CT scan in adult polycystic kidney disease.

Radial aplasia may be isolated but can also be a feature of several syndromes, including trisomy 18, the autosomal dominant hand–heart syndrome (Holt–Oram syndrome) where variable limb defects and congenital heart disease coexist, Fanconi syndrome (p. 172) or the TAR syndrome (autosomal recessive thrombocytopenia with absent radii but intact thumbs).

Split hands or feet (ectrodactyly) occur in 1 in 90 000 births. Heterogeneity is marked, but many families show autosomal dominant inheritance with variable expressivity.

Absence of the limb (amelia) or a seal-like extremity (phocomelia) are rare. Thalidomide is the classic environmental cause, but limb defects of this severity can also be seen in the hand–heart syndrome or as a result of maternal diabetes mellitus.

Arthrogryposis or congenital multiple joint contractures shows marked heterogeneity as it can result from any process which limits movement at a fetal joint. Four broad categories are recognized: myopathic (e.g. amyoplasia), neuropathic (e.g. neural tube defect or chromosomal disorder), connective tissue disorders and extrinsic limitation of fetal movements (e.g. from oligohydramnios in Potter sequence). If neural tube defects, chromosomal abnormalities and the Potter sequence are excluded about one-third of patients have amyoplasia with symmetric fibrous replacement of multiple muscles. In cases where the cause is unknown the empiric recurrence risk is 5% (15% if neuropathic). Prenatal diagnosis by demonstration of reduced fetal movements on ultrasound is not completely reliable.

Thyroid

The thyroid gland develops from an outpouching of the floor of the pharynx during weeks 3–4 which descends into the neck, reaches its final position by the seventh week, and begins to function by the end of the third month.

Thyroid dysgenesis

The thyroid is absent or severely hypoplastic in 1 in 3500 livebirths. The sex ratio is 4 females to 1 male. Birth weight and length are normal, and symptoms are vague and not invariably present in the first few months of life (see Table 20.5, p. 208). Without therapy mental handicap and extremely short stature occur, so now this condition is included in neonatal screening programmes (Chapter 20).

The defect is sporadic with no increased recurrence risk.

MULTIPLE CONGENITAL MALFORMATIONS AND DYSMORPHIC SYNDROMES

Multiple malformations, often a combination of minor and major, are present in 0.7% of newborns. In the

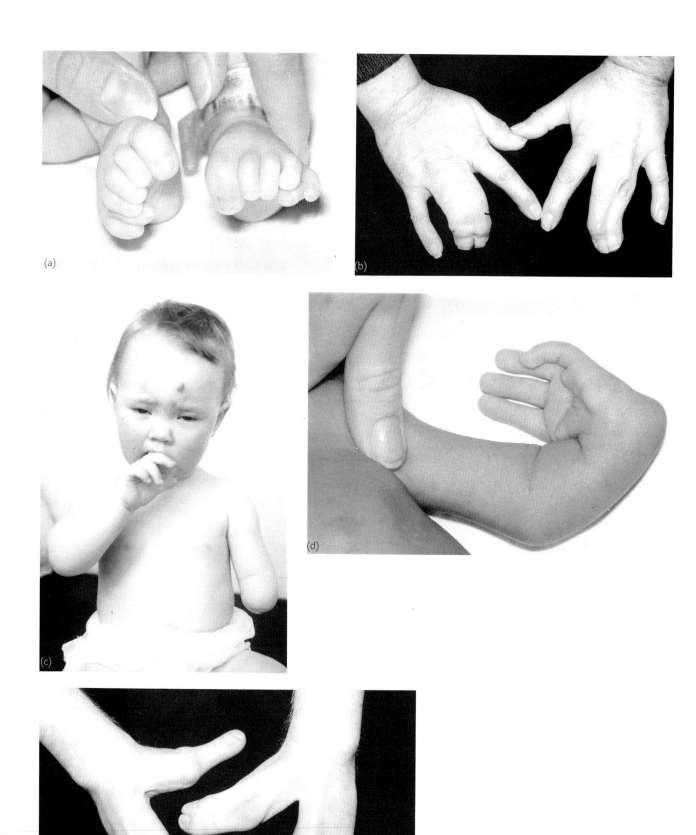

Fig. 18.11 (*and facing page.*) Examples of limb defects. (a) Postaxial polydactyly. (b) Syndactyly. (c) Transverse limb amputation due to an amniotic band. (d) Radial aplasia. (e) Ectrodactyly. (f) Phocomelia. (g) Amelia.

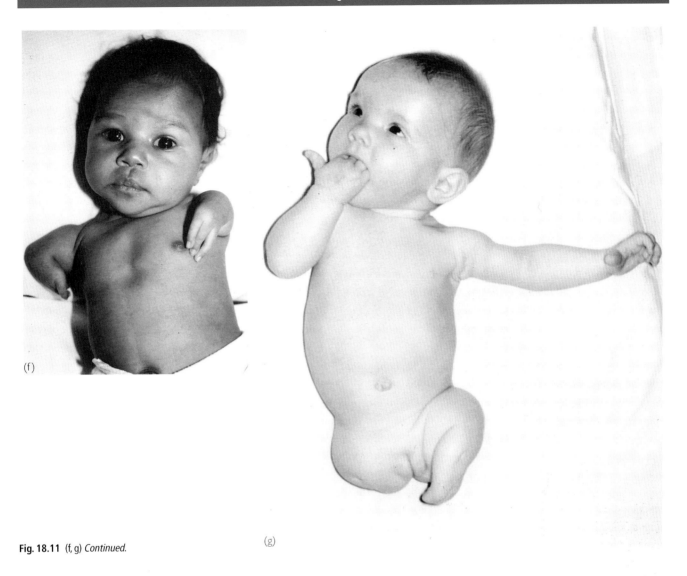

Fig. 18.11 (f, g) *Continued.*

majority the combination is random, but for some the pattern is non-random and one of over 2000 dysmorphic syndromes can be identified. Sequences and associations are subtypes of dysmorphic syndromes. In a sequence the series of abnormalities can be causally related to a primary malformation (e.g. Potter sequence secondary to renal agenesis, p. 186) and in an association there is a non-random combination of two or more structural defects which are not due to a single localized defect of embryogenesis (e.g. VATER association, p. 194). Recognition of these dysmorphic syndromes is important, as for many accurate recurrence risks and prenatal diagnosis can be provided. Searching the medical literature on rare syndromes is greatly facilitated by the computerized databases which are now available.

Undoubtedly some idiopathic dysmorphic syndromes and cases of random multiple congenital malformations are due to submicroscopic chromosomal lesions, since they share so many features with known chromosomal syndromes. In the following section some dysmorphic syndromes not covered in Chapter 13 (chromosomal disorders) or Chapter 14 (single gene disorders) are outlined.

Beckwith–Wiedemann syndrome

The clinical features are: macroglossia (90%), anterior, abdominal wall defect (90%), high birth weight, ear lobe grooves and hemihypertrophy (15%) (Fig. 18.12). Neonatal hypoglycaemia may occur and result in mental handicap if untreated. Neoplasia, especially Wilms' tumour, hepatoblastoma, rhabdomyosarcoma or adrenal cortical carcinoma, occurs in 10% (40% if hemihypertrophy is present, 3% if not), and merits serial abdominal ultrasound examination for the first three years. One in 14 000 births is affected, and it may be aetiologically hetero-

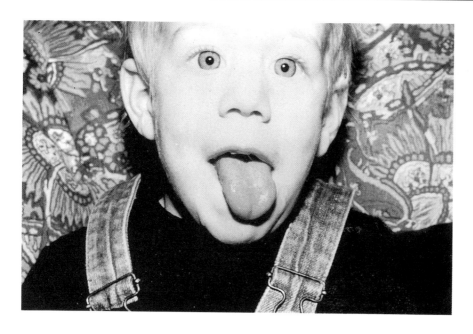

Fig. 18.12 Beckwith–Wiedemann syndrome.

geneous, as a small paternal duplication of chromosome 11p15 has been found in some patients and in occasional families autosomal dominant inheritance with variable expression is apparent. For normal parents the sib recurrence risk is low, and prenatal reassurance by detailed ultrasound scanning can be provided.

CHARGE association

This is a sporadic non-random association of malformations: coloboma (80%), heart defects, choanal atresia (58%), retarded growth and development (87%), genital abnormalities (78%) and abnormal ears (88%). The name is an acronym from the features.

de Lange syndrome (Amsterdam dwarfism)

Clinical features include: severe mental handicap, growth retardation, limb malformations, congenital heart disease (29%), cleft palate (20%) and a characteristic facies with thin lips, synophrys and anteverted nostrils (Fig. 18.13). Death in early childhood is usual.

One in 30 000 births is affected with an empiric sib recurrence risk of 2–6%. Prenatal diagnosis may be possible by assay of pregnancy-associated plasma protein A in maternal serum which is very low in affected pregnancies.

DiGeorge syndrome

Clinical features include: neonatal seizures secondary to hypoparathyroidism, recurrent viral and fungal infections secondary to thymic aplasia, failure to thrive, aortic arch anomalies and dysmorphic facies with hypertelorism, down-slanting palpebral fissures and a fish-like mouth.

A visible microdeletion at 22q11 is seen in 15–20% of patients and in the remainder a deletion can be demonstrated using DNA probes. This deletion may be maternal or paternal in origin (i.e. no evidence for imprinting in this region).

Goldenhar syndrome (oculo-auriculo-vertebral spectrum)

This syndrome is usually sporadic with an incidence of 1 in 25 000 births. Clinical features include facial asymmetry with mandibular hypoplasia, small malformed ears with conductive deafness, epibulbar dermoids (35%), cervical vertebral fusion (20–25%), cleft lip or palate, congenital heart disease (35%) and mental handicap (5–15%).

Hypomelanosis of Ito

Affected patients have whorled or streaked skin hypopigmentation with mental handicap (in 60%) and seizures. Inconsistent features include macrocephaly, hemihypertrophy and dental anomalies. Autosomal dominant inheritance has been seen in some families and some patients have chromosomal mosaicism.

Klippel–Feil syndrome

Klippel–Feil syndrome is characterized by a short stiff neck with a low hairline secondary to malformed cervical vertebrae. Other malformations may coexist: congenital heart disease (25%), renal malformations (30%), congenital scoliosis and an elevated hypoplastic scapula (Sprengel shoulder).

This is a sporadic condition with an incidence of 1 in 42 000.

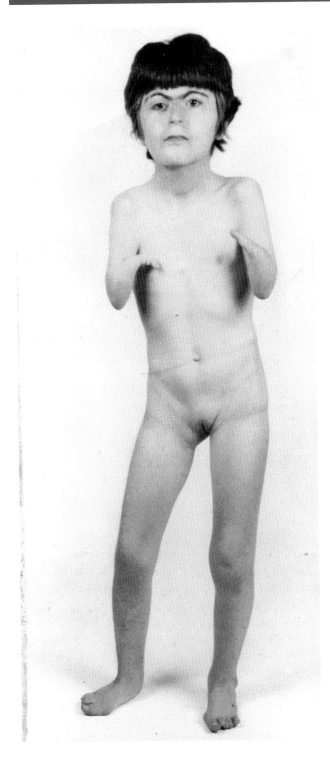

Fig. 18.13 de Lange syndrome.

Noonan syndrome

Noonan syndrome is characterized by proportionate short stature (72%), variable hypogonadism, mild to moderate mental handicap (61%), congenital heart disease, espe-

cially pulmonary stenosis (55%), low set ears, hypertelorism, ptosis, neck webbing, chest deformity, cubitus valgus and urinary tract malformations (Fig. 18.14).

One in 2000 children are affected and although in some families autosomal dominant inheritance is apparent most patients appear to be sporadic with a low recurrence risk.

Rubinstein–Taybi syndrome

Patients with Rubinstein–Taybi syndrome typically show broad terminal phalanges of the thumbs and halluces, mental handicap and a characteristic facial appearance.

The condition is caused by point mutations or microdeletions (25%) which result in loss of function of CREB binding protein which is located on 16p 13.3. Most patients have been sporadic due to new mutations and hence a low recurrence risk is appropriate.

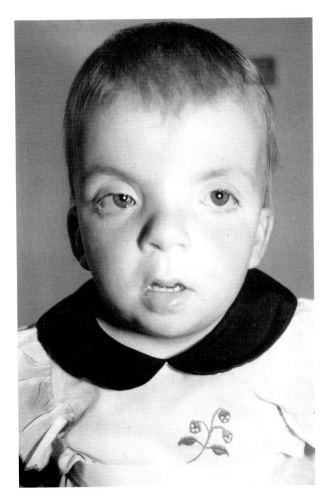

Fig. 18.14 Noonan syndrome.

Russell–Silver syndrome

This syndrome is characterized by short stature of prenatal onset, limb asymmetry, short incurved fifth fingers and a small triangular facies. Intelligence is normal and most cases are sporadic.

Smith–Lemli–Opitz syndrome

This syndrome is characterized by mental handicap, microcephaly, syndactyly of toes two and three, cryptorchidism, poor growth, a high frequency of digital whorls and a dysmorphic facies with ptosis, a broad nasal tip and anteverted nares.

Smith–Lemli–Opitz syndrome is inherited as an autosomal recessive trait and is caused by deficiency of 7-hydrocholesterol reductase. Prenatal diagnosis is possible by biochemical analysis in at-risk pregnancies.

Sotos syndrome (cerebral gigantism)

Excessive growth is apparent from before birth with acromegalic features (large hands and feet, prognathism), advanced bone age, clumsiness and mild mental handicap.

Most cases have been sporadic but occasional families have been described with inheritance consistent with an autosomal dominant trait.

Sturge–Weber syndrome

This sporadic syndrome results in a facial haemangioma with a trigeminal distribution and an ipsilateral pia-arachnoid haemangioma. Glaucoma, epilepsy, hemiplegia and mental handicap may supervene.

VATER association

This is a sporadic non-random combination of malformations: vertebral defects (70%); anal atresia (80%); tracheo-oesophageal fistula (70%); renal defects; radial limb dysplasia (65%); congenital heart disease; and a single umbilical artery (35%). The name is an acronym from the involved organs. Intelligence is normal.

Waardenburg syndrome

This autosomal dominant trait accounts for 2% of adult deafness. In addition to sensorineural deafness patients may show irises of different colours, a white forelock and lateral displacement of the inner canthi. This condition can be caused by mutations in *HUP2*.

Williams syndrome

Clinical features of this syndrome include: short stature, mental handicap, transient hypercalcaemia, supravalvular aortic stenosis and a characteristic facies with prominent lips and an anteverted small nose (Fig. 18.15). Many patients are sporadic but autosomal dominant inheritance

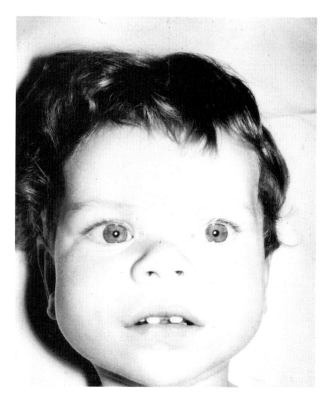

Fig. 18.15 Williams syndrome.

is apparent in some families and microdeletions in 7q11 are present in many patients. Overall frequency is 1 in 20 000.

Multiple malformations due to known teratogens

Several environmental factors, called teratogens, have been shown to cause malformations (Table 18.9). Numerous other agents are suspected to have teratogenic activity, but the difficulty lies in establishing the causal relationship, since animal experiments may not be directly informative (for example thalidomide is teratogenic in monkeys and rabbits, but not in rats or mice). Furthermore, retrospective studies are hampered by the facts that about 6% of all women experience a viral type of illness other than a cold during pregnancy and over 80% take one or more medications.

Malformations due to fetal infections with rubella, cytomegalovirus or toxoplasmosis are now uncommon in the UK. Each produces a distinctive pattern of malformations, and often there is evidence of active neonatal infection with jaundice, purpura and hepatosplenomegaly. The diagnosis is confirmed by the demonstration in the neonate of raised levels of specific antibodies, especially IgM. With the exception of cytomegalovirus infection

Table 18.9 Recognized human teratogens.

Teratogen	Critical period	Malformations
Rubella	Most affected if infection in first 6 weeks; very low risk >16 weeks	Congenital heart disease (especially patent ductus arteriosus), cataracts, microcephaly, mental handicap, sensorineural deafness, retinopathy, later insulin-dependent diabetes mellitus in 20%
Cytomegalovirus	Third or fourth month	Mental handicap or microcephaly occurs in 5–10% with congenital infection
Toxoplasmosis	12% risk at 6–17 weeks 60% risk at 17–28 weeks	Mental handicap, microcephaly, chorioretinitis
Alcohol	? First trimester	Mental handicap, microcephaly, congenital heart disease, renal anomaly, growth retardation, cleft palate, characteristic facies (Fig. 18.16)
Phenytoin (hydantoin)	First trimester; about 10% affected	Hypoplasia of distal phalanges, short nose, broad flat nasal bridge, ptosis, cleft lip and palate, mental handicap, later increased risk of malignancy, particularly neuroblastoma
Thalidomide	34–50 days from LMP	Phocomelia, congenital heart disease, anal stenosis, atresia of external auditory meatus
Warfarin	Exposure at 6–9 weeks results in structural abnormalities in 30%; after 16 weeks mental handicap alone may be seen	Hypoplastic nose, upper airway difficulties, optic atrophy, stippled epiphyses, short distal phalanges, mental handicap
Chloroquine		Deafness, corneal opacities, chorioretinitis
Lithium		Congenital heart disease
Sodium valproate		Neural tube defect (1–2%), hypospadias, microstomia, small nose, long thin fingers, developmental delay

where recurrent infection may involve the fetus, maternal immunity prevents recurrence in a future pregnancy. If a pregnant woman has evidence of seroconversion during the critical period then fetoscopic blood sampling to demonstrate evidence of fetal infection is of value in deciding whether termination of pregnancy is indicated.

Treatment with spiramycin reduces the risk of fetal toxoplasmosis when the mother is infected, and if fetal seroconversion still occurs then treatment (via the mother) with trimethoprim helps to reduce the incidence of sequelae.

Maternal alcohol ingestion of more than 150 g per day poses a substantial risk to the fetus, but lesser levels of intake may also be harmful. The facies in the fetal alcohol syndrome is characteristic with short palpebral fissures and a smooth philtrum (Fig. 18.16).

For all of these teratogenic agents a critical period has been identified beyond which no malformation is produced. The early embryo is apparently relatively resistant to the action of teratogens, and for most organs the period of vulnerability is from 4 to 8 weeks of gestation (from the LMP). There also appear to be individual differences in susceptibility to these agents. For example, only 10–40% of offspring of mothers on warfarin are affected. This

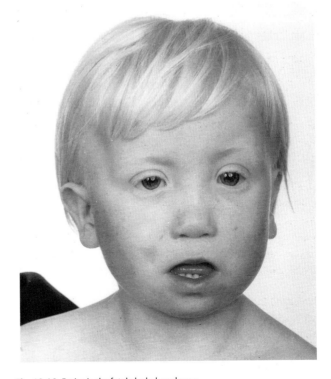

Fig. 18.16 Facies in the fetal alcohol syndrome.

susceptibility may reflect differences in fetal or maternal metabolism of the teratogen by the cytochrome P450 monooxygenases. Although a few drugs, including aspirin, paracetamol, cephalosporins and aminoglyco-sides, are considered non-teratogenic, for the majority of drugs their safety in pregnancy is unknown, and where possible they should be avoided.

CHAPTER 19

Prenatal Diagnosis

CONTENTS

AMNIOCENTESIS 197
Fetal sexing 197
Fetal karyotyping 198
Fetal enzyme assay 199
Amniotic fluid biochemistry 199
Fetal DNA diagnosis 200

Risks of amniocentesis 200
CHORIONIC VILLUS SAMPLING (CVS) 200
CORDOCENTESIS, FETAL SKIN BIOPSY, FETAL
  LIVER BIOPSY 202
ULTRASONOGRAPHY 202
FETAL CELLS IN THE MATERNAL CIRCULATION 203

Prenatal diagnosis includes all aspects of embryonic and fetal diagnosis. Prenatal diagnosis for genetic conditions is presently indicated in about 8% of all pregnancies, and for these couples at increased risk of serious genetic disease it provides the reassurance without which many would decline to undertake a pregnancy. In practice, 93% of prenatal tests provide reassurance for the couple concerned, and selective termination of pregnancy is necessary in only 7%. Termination of pregnancy for fetal indications that are not associated with a risk of serious fetal abnormality is not permitted by law. In particular, current practice does not permit the procedure to be used solely for choosing the sex of offspring by terminating pregnancies of the undesired sex.

At-risk pregnancies may be identified prior to or during a pregnancy (Table 19.1). Whatever the reason for the test, it is important to outline to the couple the limitations of the appropriate test or tests and to remind them that no single test or even a combination can exclude all abnormalities. In the event of a positive test resulting in termination of pregnancy it is important that the *complete* products of conception are sent to the laboratory for diagnostic confirmation.

Prenatal diagnostic techniques may be divided into two broad groups: invasive and non-invasive (Table 19.2).

AMNIOCENTESIS

Amniocentesis is the withdrawal of amniotic fluid. This is usually performed at 16–18 weeks of gestation when there is about 180 ml of liquor and the ratio of viable to non-viable cells is maximal. However, earlier amniocentesis between 12 and 15 weeks of gestation is being used increasingly. Under aseptic conditions, and after prior placental localization with ultrasound, a needle is introduced under ultrasound guidance into the amniotic cavity via the maternal abdomen. Ten to twenty millilitres of liquor is withdrawn and this can be used for several different tests (Table 19.3). The chance of maternal cell contamination is greatly reduced if a stilette is used in the needle and if the first few drops of amniotic fluid withdrawn are discarded.

Fetal sexing

This is required for female carriers of serious X-linked disorders, as a preliminary step before using DNA or biochemical analysis to identify the affected males.

Visualization of the Barr body (in 50–80% of cells) will usually permit fetal sexing within 3 h (Fig. 19.1). Y fluorescence may be confused with fluorescent autosomal heteromorphisms or be missed in patients with a heteromorphic small Y chromosome.

Table 19.1 Identification of at-risk pregnancies.

	CHR	SGD	MCM
Factors identifiable prior to a pregnancy			
Elevated maternal age	+	−	−
Parental consanguinity	−	+	+
Ethnic origin	−	+	(+)
Positive family history	+	+	+
Maternal illness or medication	−	−	+
Population carrier screening	−	+	−
Factors identifiable during a pregnancy			
Abnormal ultrasound appearance	(+)	(+)	+
Alphafetoprotein screening	(+)	(+)	(+)
Other biochemical screening tests	(+)	−	−
Polyhydramnios, oligohydramnios	(+)	(+)	(+)
Maternal exposure to teratogens	−	−	+

CHR, chromosomal disorders; SGD, single gene disorders; MCM, multiple congenital malformations.
+ Associated.
(+) May be associated.
− Not associated.

Table 19.2 Techniques for prenatal diagnosis.

Invasive	Amniocentesis
	Chorionic villus sampling
	Cordocentesis
	Fetal skin biopsy
	Fetal liver biopsy
Non-invasive	Ultrasonography
	Other types of imaging
	Fetal cells in the maternal circulation

Table 19.3 Tests on amniotic fluid cells and supernatant.

*Fetal sexing
*Fetal karyotyping
**(Fetal enzyme assay)
  Amniotic fluid biochemistry
**(Fetal DNA diagnosis)

*   Chorionic villus sampling may be preferred to amniocentesis (p. 200).
**   Chorionic villus sampling is usually preferred to amniocentesis.

Fetal karyotyping

Fetal karyotyping is indicated for an increased risk of aneuploidy on the basis of maternal age and prenatal screening tests (Chapter 20); a previous child with aneuploidy;

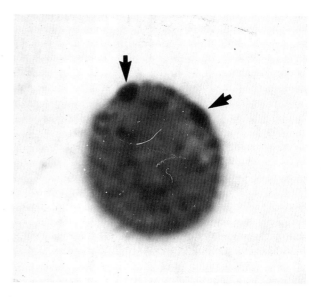

Fig. 19.1 Sexing amniotic fluid cells by demonstration of the Barr body. In this case two Barr bodies are present (arrowed) indicating the presence of three X chromosomes. Full chromosome analysis showed 47,XXX.

pregnancies where one parent has a balanced structural chromosomal rearrangement; and to confirm the fetal sex in X-linked conditions.

The amniotic fluid cells are grown in culture and a result is available in 2–3 weeks. About 1.5% of samples fail to grow, and this is especially likely if the fluid was heavily blood-stained, was less than 5 ml in volume, if transport to the laboratory was delayed or if local anaesthetic was used. In experienced laboratories contamination of the fetal amniotic cells with maternal cells is unlikely, but should be suspected if the cell cultures take longer than usual to grow and if fibroblasts rather than epithelioid cells predominate.

Chromosomal mosaicism can pose difficult diagnostic problems. In true mosaicism (i.e. mosaicism in the fetus or placenta) the abnormal cell line is usually present in several different cultures set up from the original sample, whereas in pseudomosaicism (i.e. *in vitro* artefact) only one culture is involved. In cases of doubt fetal blood sampling by cordocentesis or a repeat amniocentesis needs to be considered. Figure 19.2 shows an extra copy of chromosome 20 which was present in 25% of amniotic fluid cells. Fetal blood sampling showed a normal karyotype and the baby was normal, as in this case the mosaic cell line was confined to the placenta. True mosaicism is found in 0.25% of all amniocenteses and in about one-quarter of these the phenotype is abnormal. (46,XX/46,XY 'mosaicism' is an exception to this as it almost invariably represents maternal cell contamination.) Pseudomosaicism (in multiple cells) is found in about 1% of all amniocenteses. Repeat

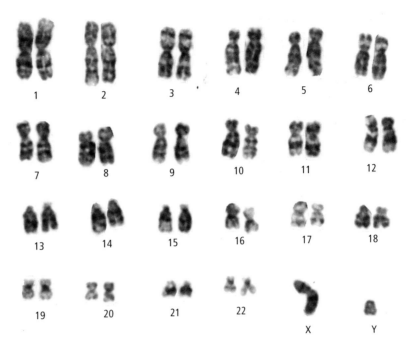

Fig. 19.2 Karyotype from amniotic fluid demonstrating an extra copy of chromosome 20 which was present in 25% of cells from several cultures (true mosaicism).

amniocentesis or fetal blood sampling may be required especially if few cells were available for analysis and if the abnormality is seen in liveborns.

Single-cell pseudomosaicism (excluding single-cell hypodiploidy) is found in about 3% of amniocenteses and as there is less than a 1% chance that this represents true mosaicism no further action is generally taken.

Fetal karyotyping is very labour-intensive and attempts have been made to circumvent this and to shorten the time to diagnosis. One of the most promising recent developments is interphase cytogenetics using *in situ* hybridization with non-radioactively labelled probes (Plate 13).

Fetal enzyme assay

Prenatal diagnosis is now possible for more than 100 inborn errors of metabolism and is indicated in at-risk pregnancies (Table 19.4). The amniotic fluid cells need to be grown in culture for 4–6 weeks in order to provide sufficient cells for the assay of the appropriate enzyme. The enzyme level in these cells is compared with data from known normal and homozygous deficient amniotic fluid cells and with fibroblasts from the proband and parents. Many of these enzymes are expressed in chorionic villi, and if so this permits earlier prenatal diagnosis, as not only is the test in the first trimester but it also yields sufficient material for assay without prior culture. However, for metabolic diseases where experience is limited, it is

Table 19.4 Examples of prenatally diagnosable inborn errors of metabolism.

Lipid metabolism
Tay–Sachs disease, Gaucher disease, Niemann–Pick, familial hypercholesterolaemia, adrenoleucodystrophy, metachromatic leucodystrophy

Mucopolysaccharidoses

Amino acid metabolism
Methylmalonic acidaemia, homocystinuria, cystinosis, maple syrup urine disease, arginosuccinicaciduria

Carbohydrate metabolism
Galactosaemia, glycogen storage disease (some types)

Others
Lesch–Nyhan syndrome, adenosine deaminase deficiency, xeroderma pigmentosum, urea cycle defects, organic acidurias

prudent to confirm fetal normality with subsequent amniocentesis.

Amniotic fluid biochemistry

Assay of alpha-fetoprotein (AFP) in amniotic fluid is indicated if there is an increased risk of a neural tube defect indicated by, for example, a previously affected child or a raised maternal serum AFP (Chapter 20).

Table 19.5 Current major indications for fetal DNA diagnosis.

Condition
Alpha-thalassaemia
Beta-thalassaemia
Cystic fibrosis
Fragile X syndrome
Haemophilia A
Huntington disease
Muscular dystrophy (Duchenne and Becker)
Myotonic dystrophy
Spinal muscular atrophy

The level of 17α-hydroxyprogesterone in amniotic fluid is measured in pregnancies at risk of salt-losing 21-hydroxylase deficient adrenogenital syndrome and two-dimensional electrophoresis of glycosaminoglycans can be used for the prenatal diagnosis of some types of mucopolysaccharidosis.

Fetal DNA diagnosis

The current major indications for fetal DNA diagnosis are listed in Table 19.5 and many more rarer single gene disorders are also diagnosable with this approach. DNA can be extracted from amniotic cells after culture for 3–4 weeks and the diagnosis may be through direct demonstration of the molecular defect or be established by indirect tracking of the mutant gene (Figs 19.3–19.6). As sufficient DNA can usually be extracted from a chorionic villus sample without prior culture, and as the test is performed earlier in pregnancy, chorionic villus sampling is usually the preferred technique to obtain fetal tissue for DNA analysis.

Risks of amniocentesis

Amniocentesis carries a small additional risk of miscarriage for the pregnancy. In one randomized controlled trial of over 4000 women, this risk was estimated to be 1.0%. In addition, for any pregnancy at 16 weeks gestation there is a 2.5% chance of spontaneous miscarriage. If the indication for amniocentesis is raised maternal serum alpha-fetoprotein then a spontaneous abortion rate of 7% is found, since AFP is raised in many non-viable pregnancies. Maternal risks are negligible.

A history of threatened abortion is not a contraindication to amniocentesis but an added indication. Twenty-six per cent of mothers of babies with trisomy 21 have a

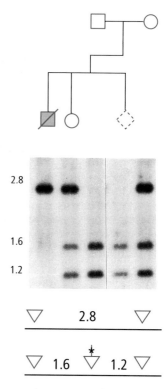

Fig. 19.3 Prenatal diagnosis in a family with Duchenne muscular dystrophy using an intragenic RFLP (87.15/*Xmn*I). The polymorphic site (*) gives alternative alleles of 2.8 kb and 1.6 kb + 1.2 kb at this locus. The mother is a carrier on the basis of elevated creatine kinase levels. Is the male pregnancy affected and is the daughter a carrier? (Answer p. 215.)

history of persistent first-trimester bleeding as compared with 1% of controls.

CHORIONIC VILLUS SAMPLING (CVS)

Sampling of chorionic villi from the fetus is performed from 10 weeks of gestation onwards and is now available in most major obstetric centres. The biopsy is usually taken under ultrasound guidance via a transabdominal approach. Each biopsy yields about 5–30 mg of tissue which can be used for fetal sexing, fetal karyotyping, biochemical studies and DNA analysis. A direct fetal chromosomal analysis is possible within 24 h but in view of the problem of mosaicism in CVS samples this should always be followed by chromosomal analysis on cultured cells from the sample 2–3 weeks later. (A sample of 5 mg should be adequate for chromosomal analysis.) DNA analysis or biochemical tests can be completed in 1–2 weeks, usually without need to culture the cells if the sample is 15–20 mg (or less if DNA analysis using PCR is applicable) and if ter-

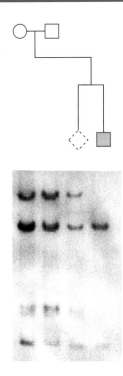

Fig. 19.4 Prenatal diagnosis in a family with Duchenne muscular dystrophy using a dystrophin cDNA probe. The affected son is deleted for two DNA fragments whereas the male pregnancy has a normal pattern and is hence unaffected.

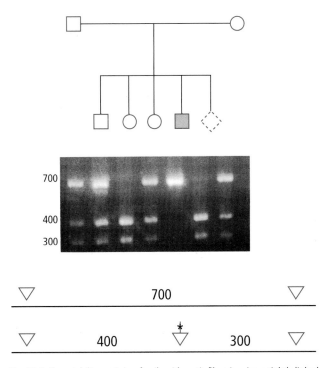

Fig. 19.5 Prenatal diagnosis in a family with cystic fibrosis using a tightly linked extragenic RFLP (XV-2c/*Taq*I). The polymorphic site (*) gives alternative alleles of 700 bp and 400 bp + 300 bp at this locus. Predict the genotypes of the sibs and the present pregnancy. (Answers p. 215.)

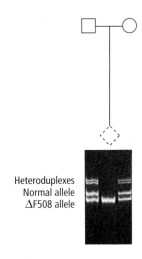

Heteroduplexes
Normal allele
ΔF508 allele

Fig. 19.6 Prenatal diagnosis for a couple who are both carriers of the common ΔF508 cystic fibrosis mutation. Each parent is heterozygous with a faster moving band representing the mutant allele (and bands above the normal allele representing heteroduplexes). The pregnancy has received both mutant alleles and is thus homozygous affected.

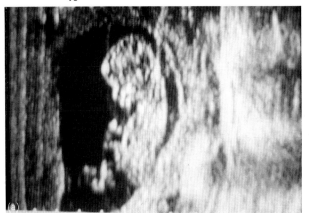

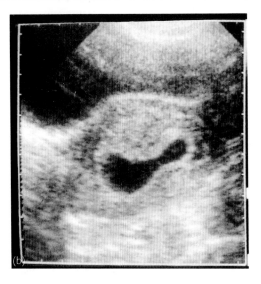

Fig. 19.7 (a) Normal fetus at 10 weeks gestation. (b) Anembryonic sac at 10 weeks gestation.

mination of pregnancy is necessary following any of these tests it can thus be performed in the first trimester. At this stage the abortion procedure is technically simpler than in the second trimester, there is less parental bonding to the fetus and only the couple and their medical attendants need know about the pregnancy. The spontaneous abortion rate at or beyond 10 weeks of pregnancy is 7%. In most of these pregnancies which are destined to abort the ultrasound reveals an anembryonic sac or dead fetus (Fig. 19.7). If the fetus is viable on ultrasound at this stage the subsequent spontaneous abortion rate is 1–2% if the mother is under 35 years of age. The added rate from the procedure is 2% and Rhesus isoimmunization should be avoided in Rhesus-negative unsensitized mothers by giving anti-D.

Where the indication for CVS is increased maternal age, a chromosomal abnormality is found in 4–6% as compared with 2% for non-chromosomal indications. These figures both reflect the high frequency of chromosomal disorders in early gestation (see Table 13.4, p. 118) and make it prudent to karyotype all CVS samples (if sample size permits) whatever the primary indication.

At the time of CVS 1 in 65 pregnancies reveal twins. This exceeds the delivery frequency (p. 91) and the discrepancy is believed to reflect spontaneous miscarriage of one or both twins. If one twin is chromosomally abnormal, this twin is liable to die *in utero* ('the vanishing twin') and CVS may reveal 'mosaicism'. Mosaicism is found in 0.66% of CVS cultures and 1.26% of direct analyses (as compared with a figure of 0.25% for true mosaicism at amniocentesis). Most of the CVS mosaics are confined to the placenta and do not reflect mosaicism in the fetus but subsequent amniocentesis will be required in 1–2% of patients who have CVS in order to help confirm this.

Table 19.6 Indications for fetal blood sampling.

Fetal infections
Suspected mosaicism
In utero transfusion for Rh isoimmunization
Unexplained hydrops
Failed amniotic cell culture or late booking
Potentially treatable congenital malformation
Unexplained severe fetal growth retardation
Haemophilia A and B*
Beta-thalassaemia*
Sickle cell disease*
Severe combined immunodeficiency

* In cases where DNA diagnosis not possible.

Table 19.7 Examples of congenital malformations which can be diagnosed by ultrasound.

CNS	Anencephaly, spina bifida, hydrocephalus*, microcephaly*, encephalocele
Limb	Severe short-limbed dwarfism, polydactyly, severe osteogenesis imperfecta, limb reduction deformity
Heart	Severe congenital heart disease
Kidney	Renal agenesis, bladder outflow obstruction, infantile polycystic disease
GIT	Duodenal atresia, anterior abdominal wall defect, diaphragmatic hernia

* May not be detectable in all cases before the last trimester.

CORDOCENTESIS, FETAL SKIN BIOPSY, FETAL LIVER BIOPSY

Under ultrasound guidance, a fine needle can be passed transabdominally into the fetal umbilical cord where it enters the placenta in order to take a fetal blood sample or to perform an *in utero* transfusion. The procedure is possible from 18 weeks of gestation onwards and the procedure-related fetal loss rate is about 1%. There is also a risk of feto-maternal haemorrhage with development or enhancement of Rhesus isoimmunization. Table 19.6 outlines the main indications for fetal blood sampling using this approach.

Some serious skin disorders (e.g. epidermolysis bullosa) can be diagnosed in a fetal skin biopsy taken via a fetoscope and in occasional metabolic disorders a fetal liver biopsy is necessary for diagnosis.

ULTRASONOGRAPHY

Visualization of the fetus by ultrasound carries no proven hazard for either mother or fetus. Over 280 different congenital malformations may be diagnosed by an experienced ultrasonographer (Table 19.7). Ultrasound is indicated for a pregnancy at increased risk for any of these disorders. Anencephaly may be detected on ultrasound as early as 10–12 weeks gestation but for most abnormalities 16–18 weeks is the optimal time. Serial scans may be required, especially to detect abnormal growth of, for example, the head or limbs.

Although fetal genitalia can be visualized from 16 weeks of gestation, this would not be adequate for fetal sexing for a serious genetic condition.

FETAL CELLS IN THE MATERNAL CIRCULATION

There is good evidence that small numbers of nucleated fetal cells enter the maternal circulation throughout pregnancy. These include fetal leucocytes, nucleated red cells and trophoblast cells. Attempts are in progress to obtain enrichment of fetal cells with the aim of achieving prenatal diagnosis using DNA analysis (by the polymerase chain reaction) or fluoresence *in situ* hybridization. The technique is not yet sufficiently reliable to attempt the diagnosis of aneuploidy, but progress is promising. A non-invasive method of prenatal diagnosis would have obvious advantages over current procedures.

CHAPTER 20

Population Screening

CONTENTS

PRENATAL SCREENING 204
Maternal AFP screening for neural tube defects 204
Screening for fetal chromosomal abnormalities 206
Ultrasound screening 206
NEONATAL SCREENING 207
Phenylketonuria 208
Congenital hypothyroidism 208

SCREENING FOR CARRIER DETECTION 208
Beta-thalassaemia 208
Sickle cell disease 209
Tay–Sachs disease 209
Cystic fibrosis 209
PRESYMPTOMATIC SCREENING OF ADULTS 209

Population screening entails the testing of a whole population in order to detect those at risk of a genetic disease for either themselves or their offspring. This approach is not appropriate for all genetic diseases as certain principles need to be observed (Table 20.1). Thus, although many genetic diseases are well-defined they are too rare to merit a whole population screening programme. There must be an advantage to early diagnosis, for example carrier detection permits genetic counselling and perhaps prenatal diagnosis in a future pregnancy. Prenatal diagnosis provides the option of selective termination, and neonatal diagnosis permits presymptomatic therapy. Any test used for population screening must be sensitive or cases will be missed, and yet it must be relatively specific or else re-testing of large numbers of false-positives will be necessary. The sensitivity of a screening test is measured by determining the proportion of affected persons detected, and its specificity from the proportion of unaffected persons testing as normal.

PRENATAL SCREENING

There are two major prenatal screening programmes at the present time in the UK: maternal alpha-fetoprotein (AFP) screening for neural tube defects and screening for fetal chromosomal abnormalities on the basis of maternal age and biochemical analytes. Ultrasound screening for congenital malformations is as yet generally restricted to at-risk pregnancies.

Maternal AFP screening for neural tube defects

As over 95% of all children with neural tube defects are born to couples with no relevant family history, it is clear that only by screening the pregnant population can most pregnancies at risk be identified. AFP is the major fetal plasma protein and has a similar structure and function to albumin in the adult. AFP is made initially by the yolk sac and later by the liver. It peaks in the fetal bloodstream at $2–3 \, g \, l^{-1}$ around 12–14 weeks of gestation and falls thereafter. Neonatal blood levels fall rapidly but basal levels of up to $25 \, \mu g \, l^{-1}$ persist into adult life.

AFP is also found in the amniotic fluid at one-hundredth the concentration found in fetal serum. Most of this is derived from fetal urine, and again the maximum concentration of $50 \, mg \, l^{-1}$ is attained at 14–15 weeks with a fall to below $10 \, mg \, l^{-1}$ by 22 weeks of gestation. Fetal AFP also reaches the maternal bloodstream and is detectable with levels 1000 times less than those found in amniotic fluid. The maternal serum AFP (MSAFP) rises from 13 weeks and peaks around 32 weeks at $500 \, \mu g \, ml^{-1}$ before falling towards term.

Table 20.1 Principles of a screening programme.

- Clearly defined disorder
- Appreciable frequency
- Advantage to early diagnosis
- Few false-positive (specificity)
- Few false-negative (sensitivity)
- Benefits outweigh the costs

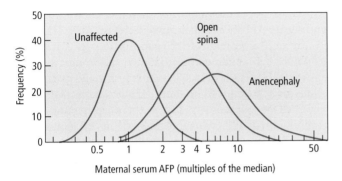

Fig. 20.1 MSAFP in normal pregnancies and pregnancies affected with neural tube defects (the distribution is log-Gaussian and hence medians rather than means are used).

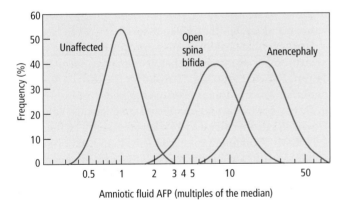

Fig. 20.2 Amniotic fluid AFP in normal pregnancies and pregnancies affected with neural tube defects.

In pregnancies where the fetus has a neural tube defect or certain other malformations, MSAFP and amniotic fluid AFP are elevated by leakage into the amniotic fluid from exposed fetal capillaries (Figs 20.1 & 20.2). Measurement of MSAFP is undertaken at 16–20 (optimum 17) completed weeks of gestation (Fig. 20.3). If the level is above the 95th centile (equivalent to two multiples of the median) a second blood sample is requested and ultrasound is advised to check the gestation and to exclude a missed abortion or a multiple pregnancy. If this sample also exceeds the 95th centile then fetal ultrasound (and perhaps amniocentesis) are indicated as there is a 2% positive predictive value for a neural tube defect.

The causes of elevated AFP in maternal serum and amniotic fluid are listed in Table 20.2. In differentiating these causes it is useful to look at the pattern of cholinesterases in the amniotic fluid by polyacrylamide gel electrophoresis (PAGE). Normal amniotic fluid produces only a single band of pseudocholinesterase. Open neural tube defects always have a faster second band of acetylcholinesterase (AChE), as do about 50% of anterior abdominal wall defects. Rarely a normal fetus may also have a second band, and thus this test must be interpreted in conjunction with the amniotic AFP level and information from fetal ultrasound. As false-negative AChE results are *not* found in open neural tube defects, the PAGE test is invaluable as a confirmatory test.

Unexplained elevations of MSAFP are associated with an increased risk of spontaneous miscarriage, premature labour, stillbirth, low birth weight and perinatal death.

The amniocentesis rate with such a screening programme is 1%, and the sensitivity is 100% for anencephaly and 88% for open spina bifida. The sensitivity of measurement of amniotic fluid AFP is 100% for anencephaly and >98% for open spina bifida. In the west of Scotland 75% of all pregnant women are tested for MSAFP at 16–20 weeks gestation. This has led to a 74% overall reduction of neural tube defect births in the region (see Fig. 21.4, p. 213).

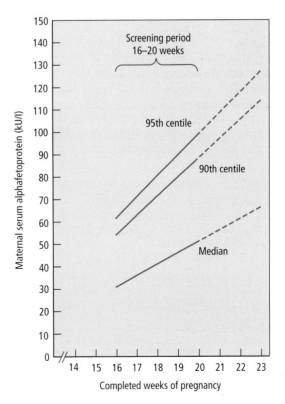

Fig. 20.3 MSAFP centiles for the screening period.

Screening for fetal chromosomal abnormalities

Formerly, screening for fetal chromosomal abnormalities, of which trisomy 21 is numerically the most important, was confined to mothers of 35 years and older in view of the rising incidence with maternal age (see Table 13.4, p. 118). Thus for example in the west of Scotland 30% of trisomy 21 births occurred to mothers of 35 years or older (who accounted for 6.7% of all pregnancies).

In recent years a new approach has been developed to combine information from maternal serum biochemistry with maternal age risk, and so extend screening to younger mothers. MSAFP levels are generally reduced to

Table 20.2 Causes of elevated maternal serum and amniotic fluid AFP.

Cause	MSAFP	Amniotic fluid AFP
Underestimated gestation	+	−
Overestimated gestation	−	+
Fetal blood in amniotic fluid	+/−	+
Multiple pregnancy	+	−
Threatened abortion	+*	−
Missed abortion	+	+
Anencephaly	++	++
Open spina bifida	+	+
Closed spina bifida	−	−
Isolated hydrocephalus	−	−
Anterior abdominal wall defect	+/−	+
Fetal teratoma	+/−	+/−
Maternal hereditary persistence of AFP	++	−
Congenital nephrotic syndrome	+	+
Skin defects	+	+
Placental haemangioma	+	+

* MSAFP returns to normal within a week after symptoms subside.
++, very elevated; +, elevated; −, not elevated.

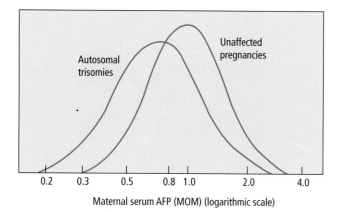

Fig. 20.4 MSAFP in MOM in normal pregnancies and pregnancies affected with autosomal trisomies.

Maternal serum AFP (MOM) (logarithmic scale)

an average of 0.7 multiples of the median (MOM) in pregnancies affected with trisomy 21 or other autosomal trisomies (Fig. 20.4). A risk (likelihood ratio) can be derived from the overlapping distributions of the affected and unaffected pregnancies. The likelihood ratio for any given AFP level is the height of the curve for affected pregnancies divided by the height of the curve for unaffected pregnancies. By multiplying the left hand side of the maternal age-specific risk by the likelihood ratio, an individual woman's risk, combining information from both her age and serum AFP level, can be obtained (Fig. 20.5). Thus, for example, if a woman of 30 years has an AFP value of 0.5 MOM her combined risk of Down syndrome from her age and AFP result is 1 in 230 (equivalent to the risk on age alone for a 36-year-old mother). Conversely, an AFP level of 1.5 MOM in a woman of 37 years of age would give a combined risk of Down syndrome of 1 in 700 (equivalent to the risk of age alone for a 30-year-old mother). This combination of maternal age and AFP is more sensitive than maternal age alone and results in a detection rate of 37% as compared with 30% for maternal age alone (with a small increase in specificity from an amniocentesis rate of 6.7% to one of 6.6%).

Appropriate population controls for MSAFP are required as levels are generally lower (by 6%) in Asian women and higher (by 15%) in Blacks.

Further enhancement of this approach is possible by the measurement of other biochemical analytes in maternal serum. For example, Fig. 20.6 shows the distributions of maternal serum human chorionic gonadotrophin (HCG) in Down syndrome and unaffected pregnancies. Values in Down syndrome tend to be elevated (with a mean of 2.2 MOM). Combination of HCG, AFP and maternal age enhances the sensitivity to 60–70% and enhances the specificity (i.e. amniocenteses required) to 5%. In the west of Scotland this screening programme has resulted in a reduction of over 50% in the birth frequency of Down syndrome in the region (see Fig. 21.3, p. 213).

The molecular mechanisms of these changes are not understood and the picture is further complicated when other chromosomal disorders are considered (Table 20.3).

Ultrasound screening

A wide variety of serious congenital malformations may be diagnosed prenatally by ultrasound scanning (see Table 19.7). Currently, in most centres, detailed scanning is confined to pregnancies at increased risk of one of these conditions, but if the efficacy in general screening practice can be demonstrated and hence the benefits versus costs determined this may become a routine component of antenatal care.

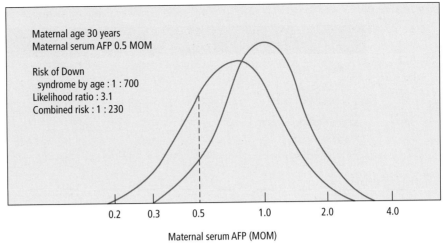

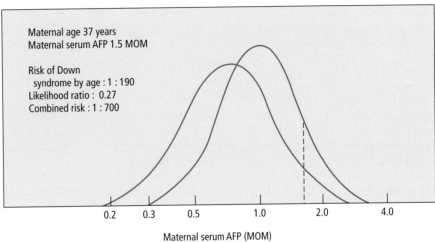

Fig. 20.5 Examples, likelihood ratio calculations.

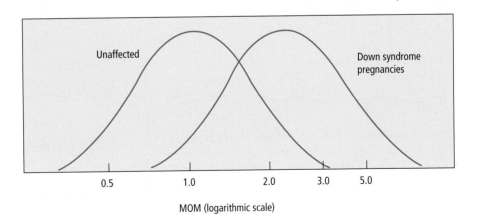

Fig. 20.6 Maternal serum human chorionic gonadotrophin in normal pregnancies and pregnancies with Down syndrome.

NEONATAL SCREENING

Neonatal screening was first introduced in 1961 (for phenylketonuria) and its success has encouraged the development of other neonatal screening tests, although the range of tests offered varies in different countries (Table 20.4). These tests are all performed on a dried blood spot which is collected from a heel prick within the first 2 weeks of life (Guthrie card). In the UK virtually all newborns are tested in this way.

Table 20.3 Variations in alpha-fetoprotein and human chorionic gonadotrophin levels in maternal serum and amniotic fluid in chromosomally abnormal pregnancies.

	Trisomy 21	Trisomy 18	Trisomy 13	X-chromosomal abnormalities
Alpha-fetoprotein				
Maternal serum	L	L	L	N
Amniotic fluid	L	N	N	N
Human chorionic gonadotrophin				
Maternal serum	H	L	N	N
Amniotic fluid	H	L	N	N

L, low; H, high; N, normal.

Table 20.4 Examples of conditions which may be included in neonatal screening programmes.

> Phenylketonuria
> Galactosaemia
> Congenital hypothyroidism
> Congenital adrenal hyperplasia
> Cystic fibrosis

Table 20.5 Signs in infants with congenital hypothyroidism at the time of diagnosis by newborn screening.

Prolonged jaundice	80%
Open fontanelles	60%
Poor feeding	60%
Large tongue	47%
Hypothermia	40%
Umbilical hernia	35%
Hoarse cry	18%
Increased TSH	100%

Phenylketonuria

Early diagnosis and therapy of phenylketonuria are mandatory if normal development is to occur. However, few if any physical signs are present in the neonate. The presence of an increased level of blood phenylalanine in the dried blood spot is detected by the Guthrie bacterial inhibition assay. Mild elevations of phenylalanine due to prematurity or delayed enzyme maturation are not uncommon and these can be excluded by repeat testing. False-negatives are rare.

Congenital hypothyroidism

Early diagnosis and therapy will permit normal development, yet few physical signs are present in the newborn (Table 20.5). Thyroid stimulating hormone (TSH) is measured on the dried blood spot. Neonates with primary hypothyroidism have elevated levels of TSH. The recall rate is 0.05% and false-negatives appear to be rare. The incidence of congenital hypothyroidism is 1 in 3000–4000 in the UK as compared with 1 in 900 in Asians and 1 in 20 000–30 000 in US Blacks. Although occasional cases are recessive enzyme defects (in which case there is usually a goitre) the majority are sporadic failures of normal thyroid development with a low recurrence risk.

Table 20.6 Indications for carrier screening.

Conditions	Ethnic group(s)
Beta-thalassaemia and glucose-6-phosphate dehydrogenase deficiency	Mediterraneans, Indians, Middle East populations, Thais, Chinese, Blacks
Sickle cell disease	US and African Blacks, West Indians, Asian Indians, Mediterraneans (especially Greeks) and Middle East populations
Tay–Sachs disease	Ashkenazi Jews

SCREENING FOR CARRIER DETECTION

At the present time screening for carrier detection is mainly focused on ethnic groups who are at high risk for particular single gene disorders (Table 20.6). Approaches to whole population screening for carriers of cystic fibrosis and fragile X syndrome amongst Caucasians are also being evaluated.

Beta-thalassaemia

The heterozygote frequency of beta-thalassaemia varies

widely in different populations but is especially high in Mediterranean countries and southeast Asia. Thus persons from these ethnic groups merit carrier screening. The carrier state is detected by the finding of microcytosis (MCV < 80 fl) with a low mean cell haemoglobin (less than 27 pg; normal range 27–30 pg) and an increased haemoglobin A_2 concentration (more than 3.5%; normal upper limit 2.5%). Carrier detection permits genetic counselling and prenatal diagnosis for couples who are both heterozygotes.

Sickle cell disease

Sickle cell disease is especially prevalent in Blacks but also occurs in individuals from the Mediterranean, India and the Middle East. Heterozygotes are screened by the demonstration of sickled cells on exposure of red cells *in vitro* to a very low oxygen tension (Sickledex test) (with confirmation by haemoglobin electrophoresis). Detection of heterozygotes permits genetic counselling and alerts the anaesthetist prior to general anaesthesia.

Tay–Sachs disease

The heterozygote frequency for this autosomal recessive trait is 1 in 30 for Ashkenazi Jews but only 1 in 300 for other ethnic groups. Carriers are detected by the measurement of serum-beta-*N*-acetylhexosaminidase A (leucocyte beta-*N*-acetylhexosaminidase A is more reliable during pregnancy) or by DNA analysis. Carrier detection permits genetic counselling and prenatal diagnosis for couples at risk.

Cystic fibrosis

Cystic fibrosis is the most common serious autosomal recessive disorder in northern Europe and the USA. From the birth frequency of 1 in 2500 a carrier frequency of 1 in 25 is predicted. Currently, prenatal diagnosis is confined to at-risk pregnancies as defined by the previous birth of an affected child but carrier screening offers the prospect of prior identification of all high-risk pregnancies.

Mutational heterogeneity is apparent (p. 134) with one common (ΔF508) and multiple rarer mutations. The impact of population screening depends upon the proportion of mutations which the programme can detect. For example if 75% of mutations can be detected then 56% of at-risk couples could be identified. In this situation if one partner is positive and one negative the residual risk is 1 in 400 (or 1 in 667 if 85% of mutations can be detected).

PRESYMPTOMATIC SCREENING OF ADULTS

At the present time, presymptomatic screening of adults mainly relates to family members for autosomal dominant conditions with a delayed onset of symptoms. This permits genetic counselling of presymptomatic individuals who are found to carry the mutant gene and may also be necessary for effective therapy, for example surveillance for tumours in carriers of genes for inherited forms of cancer (Chapter 17). In the future identification of the 'at-risk' genotype for the common chronic diseases of adulthood may be possible, and screening to identify these individuals might permit avoidance of the environmental trigger(s) and so prevent disease.

CHAPTER 21

Prevention and Treatment

CONTENTS

OVERALL IMPACT OF GENETIC DISEASE 210
TYPES OF GENETIC DISEASE 211
TREATMENT OF GENETIC DISEASE 211
Chromosomal disorders 211
Single gene disorders 211
Multifactorial disorders 212
Mitochondrial disorders 212
Somatic cell genetic disorders 212

SECONDARY PREVENTION OF GENETIC DISEASE . . . 212
Chromosomal disorders 212
Single gene disorders 214
Multifactorial disorders 214
PRIMARY PREVENTION OF GENETIC DISEASE 214
Chromosomal disorders 214
Single gene disorders 214
Multifactorial disorders 214

The old adage that prevention is better than cure applies as much to genetic as to acquired diseases. For diseases due to environmental agents, such as infections, the relationship between health and disease is outlined in Fig. 21.1. For genetic diseases the relationship is a little more complex since symptoms (i.e. disease) may not occur with an abnormal genotype until the person reaches adult life or until exposed to an environmental trigger. Primary prevention of the abnormal genotype would need to act prior to conception (Fig. 21.2). Prenatal diagnosis with selective termination (secondary prevention) alters the birth frequency of the condition but is really a holding measure pending the development of primary prevention of genetic disease. If prevention fails then therapy is required.

OVERALL IMPACT OF GENETIC DISEASE

Genetic diseases affect all populations and have been apparent since prehistory. The recent focus of attention upon this group of conditions reflects the declining importance of environmental factors, especially infectious diseases, as a cause of morbidity and mortality.

The infant mortality rate, IMR (number of babies dying during the first year of life per 1000 livebirths), exemplifies this trend. The IMR for England and Wales was 154 in 1000 in 1900 with 3.5 in 1000 of the total due to genetic disease. By 1991 the IMR had fallen to 7.4 in 1000 due largely to improved public health and the control of infectious disease, but the number due to genetic disease was unaltered. Thus the genetic contribution to the IMR has risen from 3% to nearly 50%. The same pattern is apparent for fetal wastage and also for diseases of later childhood and adult life.

At least 20% of all conceptions have a chromosomal abnormality, but the majority of these are lost as early spontaneous miscarriages. These early miscarriages also have a much higher rate (10–15%) of major congenital malformations than seen in the newborn (3%), with genetic causes accounting for at least one-third of all malformations. Nearly one-half of stillbirths and 20% of early neonatal deaths are attributable to major congenital malformations. Genetic disease now causes about one-half of all deaths in childhood and accounts for one-third of all paediatric hospital admissions. Between 0.3% and 0.4% of children are severely mentally handicapped, with mild mental handicap in a further 0.4% and significant physical handicap in 1–2%. Most of this handicap is genetic in aetiology. Finally, chronic diseases with a significant genetic component affect about 10–20% of the adult population and a further 25% will develop a somatic cell genetic

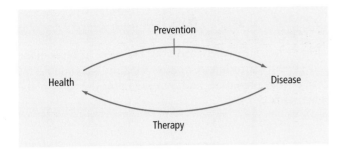

Fig. 21.1 Relationship between prevention and therapy for acquired disease.

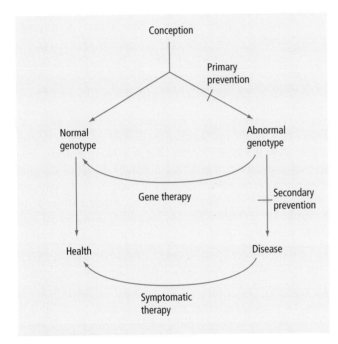

Fig. 21.2 Relationship between prevention and therapy for genetic disease.

Table 21.1 Incidence of genetic disease.

Type	Incidence	
	Number of subtypes	In 1000 live births
Chromosomal	>600	6
Single gene		
Autosomal dominant	4458	20 ⎫
Autosomal recessive	1730	2 ⎬ 24
X-linked recessive	412	2 ⎭
Multifactorial		
Major congenital malformations	>50	6*
Chronic adult	>50	10†
Mitochondrial	59	Rare
Somatic cell genetic	>100	250‡
	Total	386

* The estimated multifactorial contribution of 20% (excludes chromosomal and monogenic contributions).

† The estimated multifactorial contribution of 50% (excludes the monogenic contribution).

‡ Somatic cell genetic disorders arise after birth and occur in at least 25% of adults.

disorder such as cancer.

Hence it has been estimated that genetic and part-genetic diseases affect 1 in 20 individuals by 25 years of age and perhaps 30–40% in a lifetime.

TYPES OF GENETIC DISEASE

As indicated in Table 21.1, genetic diseases may be subdivided into chromosomal, single gene, multifactorial, mitochondrial and somatic cell genetic disorders. Numerically the multifactorial and somatic cell genetic disorders are the most important, as they account for about 20% of all congenital malformations, about one-half of all chronic conditions of adult life, and most if not all cancer (1 in 4 adults).

TREATMENT OF GENETIC DISEASE

There is a popular misconception that genetic disease is always untreatable. In practice, some symptomatic therapy is available for most genetic diseases, and in some therapy can effectively restore normal health in spite of the continued presence of the abnormal genotype.

Chromosomal disorders

For some sex chromosomal disorders sex hormone replacement will permit normal development of secondary sex characteristics, but this cannot restore fertility. Autosomal imbalance usually results in mental handicap and multiple congenital malformations for which only symptomatic therapy is possible.

Single gene disorders

Table 21.2 indicates some of the commoner single gene disorders for which effective therapy is available.

Furthermore, advances in genetic engineering have allowed the production of relatively inexpensive pure

Table 21.2 Examples of single gene disorders with effective therapies.

Disease	Therapy
Congenital adrenal hyperplasia	Hormone replacement
Phenylketonuria	Dietary restriction of phenylalanine
Galactosaemia	Dietary restriction of galactose
Haemophilia	Factor replacement
SCID	Marrow transplant
Cystinuria	High fluid intake, D-penicillamine
Polyposis coli	Colectomy
Agammaglobulinaemia	Immunoglobulin replacement
Beta-thalassaemia	Marrow transplant
Methylmalonic aciduria	Vitamin B_{12}—enzyme cofactor
Adult polycystic disease	Renal transplant
Wilson disease	D-penicillamine
Familial hypercholesterolaemia	Diet, medications
Hereditary spherocytosis	Splenectomy
Haemochromatosis	Repeated venesection

protein products (e.g. insulin, factor VIII, human growth hormone). Research is also being conducted with the goal of gene supplementation—i.e. adding a functional gene to somatic cells from a patient homozygous for a mutant gene. Successful gene supplementation therapy was first performed for severe combined immunodeficiency due to adenosine deaminase deficiency and is currently being explored in a variety of serious single gene disorders which lack effective therapy.

Multifactorial disorders

Table 21.3 indicates some of the commoner multifactorial disorders for which effective therapy is available.

Mitochondrial disorders

Only symptomatic treatment is possible for lesions of the mitochondrial chromosome at the present time.

Table 21.3 Multifactorial disorders with effective therapies.

Disease	Therapy
Cleft lip and palate	Surgery
Pyloric stenosis	Surgery
Congenital heart disease	Surgery, medication
Hydrocephalus	Surgery, medication
Diabetes mellitus	Medication
Hypertension	Medication
Epilepsy	Medication

Somatic cell genetic disorders

Most if not all cancers are now believed to be somatic cell genetic disorders. Curative therapy is available for many with palliation and symptomatic therapy in the remainder.

SECONDARY PREVENTION OF GENETIC DISEASE

Secondary prevention includes all aspects of prenatal screening with selective termination of affected pregnancies.

Chromosomal disorders

Formerly, screening was restricted to older mothers (35 years and older) and to other high-risk groups (Chapter 20). If all mothers of 35 years and over had amniocentesis then this would reduce the incidence of chromosomal disease by 30%. Although only about 6–7% of pregnant mothers are above this age, their increased incidence of aneuploidy accounts for the excess. If a maternal age of 40 years was taken as a cut-off then the reduction in chromosomal disease would be only 10%.

Table 21.4 Reproductive decisions after genetic counselling.

	Opt to have more children (%)	Refrain from further children (%)
High risk (> 1 in 10)		
Prenatal diagnosis available	87	13
Prenatal diagnosis not available	47	53
Low risk (< 1 in 10)	75	25

Table 21.5 Summary of primary prevention.

Chromosomal	Reduce non-disjunction and chromosomal breakage, genetic counselling
Single gene	Reduce mutation rate, genetic counselling
Multifactorial	Environmental prophylaxis for 'at-risk' individuals, genetic counselling

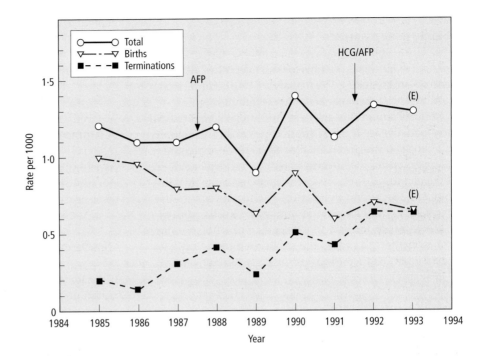

Fig. 21.3 Impact of prenatal screening on the frequency of Down syndrome in the west of Scotland on the basis of maternal age and serum alpha-fetoprotein (AFP), and maternal age, AFP and human chorionic gonadotrophin (HCG/AFP).

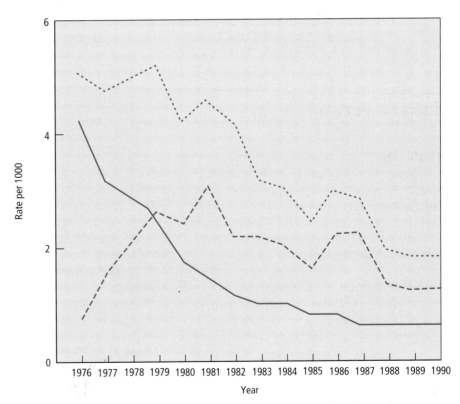

Fig. 21.4 Impact of prenatal screening on the frequency of open neural tube defects in the west of Scotland. (· · ·) total; (——) births, (- - -) terminations.

The introduction of biochemical screening to identify pregnancies at high risk of chromosomal disorders in combination with maternal age risks has markedly improved the efficacy of this prenatal programme. Combining MSAFP with maternal age increases the potential detection rate from 30% to 37% for a slight fall in the number of amniocenteses required (6.7–6.6%) and the subsequent addition of a second analyte (HCG, Chapter 20) raises the detection rate for trisomy 21 to 60–70% for a reduced amniocentesis rate of 5% (Fig. 21.3).

Single gene disorders

Prenatal diagnosis is possible for just over 6% of all single-gene disorders (using DNA analysis, biochemical analysis, ultrasound scanning and other techniques).

The problem in this group of conditions is that overall most patients are the first affected persons in that family and hence offering prenatal diagnosis in subsequent high risk pregnancies will do little to reduce the birth incidence of the condition. Carrier screening circumvents this difficulty and this approach has already had a dramatic effect in several areas. For example, amongst Greek Cypriots 1 in 6 is a carrier for beta-thalassaemia yet with screening and prenatal diagnosis the birth frequency of beta-thalassaemia has been reduced virtually to zero.

Multifactorial disorders

Secondary prevention is now possible for several congenital malformations by the combined use of maternal alpha-fetoprotein assay and detailed ultrasound scanning. With such a screening programme in the west of Scotland the birth frequency of neural tube defects has been reduced by over 74% (Fig. 21.4).

PRIMARY PREVENTION OF GENETIC DISEASE

Most couples who seek genetic counselling make an appropriate decision from the information provided (Table 21.4). Thus genetic counselling itself is a factor in primary prevention for all types of genetic disease. While its impact is real enough for the family concerned, it will have but little influence on overall gene frequencies, as most families are not known to be at special risk until a genetic disease has occurred. Although systematic counselling for an autosomal dominant trait with a low mutation rate, such as Huntington disease, may be an exception to this, other approaches need to be developed (Table 21.5).

Chromosomal disorders

As chromosomal aberrations arise by non-disjunction or chromosomal breakage, an increased understanding of these processes is the prerequisite for primary prevention.

Single gene disorders

Ultimately all single gene disorders are the result of mutation, so again research needs to be directed towards defining the causes of human mutation.

Multifactorial disorders

The multifactorial disorders offer perhaps the greatest scope for primary prevention. The goal here is to identify the environmental and genetic components. Then those with the 'at-risk' genotype can avert the disease by avoidance of the environmental factor.

Thus, for example, periconceptional folic acid supplementation can prevent neural tube defects. Two groups of women were compared, one with and one without folic acid supplementation during the periconceptional period. These women had all had a previous child with a neural tube defect, and thus a 1 in 25 recurrence risk was expected. The unsupplemented group had the expected rate of recurrence whereas the supplemented group had only a 1 in 100 recurrence rate (i.e. a 74% reduction).

Answers to Figure Questions

Fig. 3.7	(a) Suspect 1; (b) F2 is the father.
Fig. 3.12	A3, C3 and D3 are carriers; B3 is homozygous normal.
Fig. 6.2	Top left—non-informative; top right—maternal origin, first or second meiotic division; middle left—not informative but not paternal first meiotic division; middle right—non-informative; bottom left—non-informative; bottom right—maternal origin, first or second meiotic division.
Fig. 7.12	The daughter has inherited the 16.5 kb allele from her affected father and is thus not a carrier whereas the son has inherited the 14 kb allele and so is a carrier.
Fig. 8.9	The youngest daughter is predicted to be a carrier whereas the eldest is not.
Fig. 9.7	Locus A is the closest to the gene for colour blindness as it shows no recombinants in the five informative meioses (B shows one recombination and C shows three recombinations).
Fig. 9.9	Abelson oncogene locus.
Fig. 13.5(c)	From left to right, first child has a paternal X (i.e. maternal error), second family is non-informative and third child has a maternal X (i.e. paternal error).
Fig. 15.7	The second and fourth eldest sibs are carriers and a homozygous affected pregnancy is predicted.
Fig. 19.3	The male pregnancy is predicted to be unaffected and the daughter is predicted to be a carrier.
Fig. 19.5	In each parent the 700 bp allele is linked to the cystic fibrosis mutation and thus the sibs are predicted to be heterozygous, homozygous normal and heterozygous (from oldest to youngest). A homozygous normal pregnancy is predicted.

Further Reading

BASIC PRINCIPLES

Alberts B., Bray D., Lewis J., Raff M., Roberts K. & Watson J.D. (1994) *Molecular Biology of the Cell* (3rd edn). Garland Publishing, New York.

Bradley J., Johnson D. & Rubenstein, D. (1995) *Lecture Notes on Molecular Medicine*. Blackwell Science, Oxford.

Brock D.J.H. (1993) *Molecular Genetics for the Clinician*. Cambridge University Press, Cambridge.

Davies K.E. & Read A.P. (1992) *Molecular Basis of Inherited Disease* (2nd edn). IRL Press, Oxford.

Emery A.E.H. & Malcolm S. (1995) *An Introduction to Recombinant DNA in Medicine* (2nd edn). John Wiley and Sons, Chichester.

Lewin B. (1994) *Genes. V.* Oxford University Press, New York.

McKusick V.A. (1994) *Mendelian Inheritance in Man. A Catalog of Human Genes and Genetic Disorders* (11th edn). Johns Hopkins University Press, Baltimore (web address http://WWW3.ncbi.nlm.nih.gov/Omim/).

Rimoin D.L., Connor J.M. & Pyeritz R.E. (1996) *The Principles and Practice of Medical Genetics* (3rd edn). Churchill Livingstone, New York.

Trent R.J. (1993) *Molecular Medicine. An Introductory Text for Students*. Churchill Livingstone, Edinburgh.

Wilcox D.E. & Connor J.M. (1997) *An Illustrated Colour Text of Medical Genetics*. Churchill Livingstone, Edinburgh (in press).

CLINICAL APPLICATIONS

Baraitser M. & Winter R.M. (1992) *The London Neurology Database: A Database of Genetically Determined Neurological Conditions for Clinicians* (2nd edn). Oxford University Press.

Borgaonkar D.S. (1991) *Chromosomal Variation in Man: A Catalog of Chromosomal Variants and Anomalies* (6th edn). Alan Liss, New York.

Brock D.J.H., Rodeck C.H. & Ferguson-Smith M.A. (1992) *Prenatal Diagnosis and Screening*. Churchill Livingstone, Edinburgh.

Hall J.G., Froster-Iskenius U.G. & Allanson J.E. (1989) *Handbook of Normal Physical Measurements*. Oxford Medical Publications, Oxford.

Hodgson S.V. & Maher E.R. (1993) *A Practical Guide to Human Cancer Genetics*. Cambridge University Press, Cambridge.

Harper P.S. (1993) *Practical Genetic Counselling* (2nd edn). Butterworth-Heinemann, Oxford.

McKusick V.A. (1994) *Mendelian Inheritance in Man. A Catalog of Human Genes and Genetic Disorders* (11th edn). Johns Hopkins University Press, Baltimore (web address http://www3.ncbi.nlm.nih.gov/Omim/).

Rimoin D.L., Connor J.M. & Pyeritz R.E. (1996) *The Principles and Practice of Medical Genetics* (3rd edn). Churchill-Livingstone, New York.

Scriver C.R., Beaudet A.L., Sly W.S. & Valle D. (1995) *The Metabolic and Molecular Bases of Inherited Disease* (7th edn). McGraw-Hill, New York.

Whittle M.J. & Connor J.M. (1995) *Prenatal Diagnosis in Obstetric Practice* (2nd edn). Blackwell Science, Oxford.

Winter R.M. & Baraitser M. (1992) *The London Dysmorphology Database: a Computerised Database for the Diagnosis of Rare Dysmorphic Syndromes* (2nd edn). Oxford University Press.

APPENDICES

APPENDIX 1

Odds and Probabilities

The probability of an event is the *proportion* of times the event occurs in a long series of experiments. Conventionally, this is expressed as a fraction or decimal in the range 0 (event never happens) to 1 (event always happens). For example, if a coin is tossed the probability of heads is $1/2$, and similarly the probability of tails is $1/2$. In this example the outcome is either heads or tails (not both) and so these are *mutually exclusive events*. For mutually exclusive events the probability of either one outcome *or* the other outcome is the *sum* of their individual probabilities, and as there must be an outcome the sum of the probabilities of all possible outcomes is 1. Thus for the example with one throw of a dice the probability of a 5 or a 6 is $1/3$ ($1/6 + 1/6$).

In contrast, *independent events* are such that the outcome of one event has no influence whatsoever on the outcome of the other event. So, for example, if two coins are tossed and the first comes down heads the prediction about the outcome of the second coin is unchanged. For two independent events the probability of a specified outcome of the first *and* a specified outcome of the second is the *product* of their individual probabilities. Thus the probability that a toss of two coins will produce two heads is $1/4$ ($1/2 \times 1/2$).

Thus, for a couple who are both carriers for an autosomal recessive trait such as cystic fibrosis, the chance of a recessive homozygous child represents one of the four possible outcomes (see Fig. 7.8). Their chance of normal children is $3/4$ representing the sum of two mutually exclusive events: a 1 in 4 chance of a homozygous normal plus 2 in 4 chances of carriers.

In contrast, for a non-consanguineous Caucasian couple with no relevant family history the chance of a child with cystic fibrosis is 1 in 2500, which represents the combination by multiplication of three independent events: the father's carrier risk ($1/25$) × the mother's carrier risk ($1/25$) × the chance of a homozygous affected child if both are carriers ($1/4$).

APPENDIX 2

Applications of Bayes' Theorem

Bayes' theorem is used in genetic counselling to combine other information with pedigree data in the assessment of an individual's chance of being a carrier.

For example, Fig. A2.1 shows the pedigree of a family with Duchenne muscular dystrophy. In this family I2 is an obligate carrier as she has two affected sons. Thus her daughter II3 has a 1 in 2 chance of also being a carrier. If she is a carrier then one-half of her sons would be affected. She has four normal sons and thus she is either a carrier who has been lucky or, more likely, she is not a carrier. Bayes' theorem combines this conditional information (the normal sons) with the prior risk of 1 in 2 to produce a final risk (Table A2.1).

Thus the final risk that II3 is a carrier is 1 in 17, a substantial reduction from the prior risk of 1 in 2.

A normal level of creatine kinase (CK) will also reduce the risk of II3 being a carrier. For example, if her median CK was 50 i.u. l^{-1}, then from Fig. 8.3 the risk of being a carrier is 1 in 3 (from the relative heights of the two curves at this point). The conditional information (the CK level) is again combined with the pedigree risk using Bayes' theorem (Table A2.2). Her final risk of being a carrier is thus 1 in 49.

For Duchenne muscular dystrophy the risk may be modified still further with information from linked RFLPs. If the recombination fraction between the marker and the disease locus is 5%, and if the consultand (II3 in Fig. A2.1) received the non-disease-linked maternal marker her risk for being a carrier is reduced still further to 1 in 913 (Table A2.3). The close linkage of the marker to the disease locus is used to alter the prior risk ratio from $^1/_2 : ^1/_2$ to $^1/_{20} : ^{19}/_{20}$.

If information was available from two markers, and if both were on the same side of the disease locus, the closest would be most helpful. If they were on either side (flanking markers), and if no recombination was apparent with either, the error rate would at most equal the product of the individual recombination fractions (in practice, as one chiasma tends to prevent further adjacent chiasmata the chance of a double recombination between the flanking markers is probably much less than this figure).

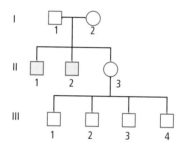

Fig. A2.1 Pedigree of a family with Duchenne muscular dystrophy.

Table A2.1 Bayes' calculation–1.

	II3 carrier	II3 not a carrier
Prior risk (Fig. A2.1)	1/2	1/2
Conditional information (four normal sons)	$(1/2)^4$	1^4
Joint odds (product of first two entries)	1/32	1/2 = 16/32
Final risk (each joint divided by the sum of the joints)	1/17	16/17

Using the same denominator in the joint entry simplifies the last calculation as it becomes each numerator over the sum of the numerators.

Table A2.2 Bayes' calculation–2.

	II3 carrier	II3 not a carrier
Prior risk	1/2	1/2
Conditional information (four normal sons and normal CK)	$(1/2)^4 \times 1/3$	$1^4 \times 1$
Joint odds	1/96	48/96
Final risk	1/49	48/49

Table A2.3 Bayes' calculation–3.

	II3 a carrier	II3 not a carrier
Prior risk	1/20	19/20
Conditional information (four normal sons, normal CK)	$(1/2)^4 \times 1/3$	$1^4 \times 1$
Joint odds	1/960	19/20 = 912/960
Final risk	1/913	912/913

APPENDIX 3

Calculation of the Coefficients of Relationship and Inbreeding

The coefficient of relationship (r) is the proportion of all genes in *two* individuals which are identical by descent. Calculation of this may be helpful in providing a recurrence risk for an autosomal recessive trait for members of an inbred family.

The coefficient is calculated from the formula:

$$r = \left(1/2\right)^n$$

where n is the number of steps apart on the pedigree for the two individuals via the common ancestor. If there is more than one common ancestor then their contributions are added to give a final r value.

For example in Fig. A3.1 first cousins have an r value of:

$$r = \left(1/2\right)^4 + \left(1/2\right)^4 \text{ or } 1/8$$

Thus, on average, 1 in 8 of the genes of first cousins are identical by descent.

The coefficient of inbreeding (F) is the proportion of loci at which *one* individual is homozygous by descent. Thus, if first cousins married, their child's proportion of loci which would be homozygous by descent would be on average one-half of the proportion of parental genes identical by descent or $r/2$. Thus:

$$F = r/2$$

In Fig. A3.2 a man by his first wife has a child with an autosomal recessive disorder. He then marries his first cousin. What is the risk of recurrence?

He is an obligate heterozygote. Since r for first cousins is 1 in 8, the chance that his wife has the same recessive allele from a common ancestor is 1 in 8. For two heterozygotes the risk of recurrence is 1 in 4. Thus the final risk is the product of these probabilities:

1 (his carrier risk) $\times$ 1/8 (her carrier risk) $\times$ 1/4 = 1/32

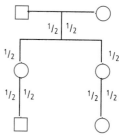

Fig. A3.1 Pedigree example of calculation of coefficient of relationship.

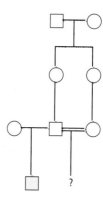

Fig. A3.2 Consanguineous pedigree with a single gene disorder.

Population Genetics of Single Gene Disorders

MAINTENANCE OF GENE FREQUENCIES

In a population the relative frequencies of different alleles tend to be kept constant from one generation to the next. This can be demonstrated mathematically and helps to explain why dominant traits do not automatically increase at the expense of recessive traits.

Consider one locus with two alleles A and a. If the frequency of the allele A is p and the frequency of the allele a is q then, since each individual must have one or other allele, the sum of these allele frequencies must be 1, or 100%. Therefore:

$$p + q = 1$$

Table A4.1 shows the frequencies of each genotype at this locus.

In the production of the next generation each of the three types of paternal genotype may mate with each of the three types of maternal genotype (Table A4.2). Table A4.3 indicates the genotypes of the offspring for each mating type, and as can be seen the relative frequency of each is unchanged and the population is said to be in genetic equilibrium. Although the actual numbers of individuals with each genotype may have increased, the relative proportions of each genotype (and allele) have remained constant (AA at p^2, Aa at $2pq$ and aa at q^2). This principle is called the Hardy–Weinberg law.

The most important application of this law is the calculation of carrier frequencies for autosomal recessive traits.

For any autosomal recessive trait, if q is the frequency of the mutant allele and p the frequency of the normal allele, then the frequency of the recessive homozygote is equal to the square of the mutant allele frequency (q^2). Thus, for cystic fibrosis:

Recessive homozygote frequency, $q^2 = 1/2500$

$$q = \sqrt{1/2500} = 1/50$$
$$p = 1 - q = 49/50$$

and so the heterozygote (carrier) frequency, $2pq \simeq 1/25$

Table A4.1 Allele and genotype frequencies at a locus with only two alleles, A and a.

	Paternal gametes	
Maternal gametes	A (p)	a (q)
A (p)	AA (p^2)	Aa (pq)
a (q)	Aa (pq)	aa (q^2)

Table A4.2 Frequencies of different parental genotypes at reproduction.

	Paternal genotypes		
Maternal genotypes	AA (p^2)	Aa ($2pq$)	aa (q^2)
AA (p^2)	AA × AA (p^4)	AA × Aa ($2p^3q$)	AA × aa (p^2q^2)
Aa ($2pq$)	Aa × AA ($2p^3q$)	Aa × Aa ($4p^2q^2$)	Aa × aa ($2pq^3$)
aa (q^2)	aa × AA (p^2q^2)	aa × Aa ($2pq^3$)	aa × aa (q^4)

Table A4.3 Frequencies of different types of offspring after reproduction.

Mating type	Frequency (from Table A4.2)	Offspring		
		AA	Aa	aa
AA × AA	p^4	p^4		
AA × Aa	$4p^3q$	$2p^3q$	$2p^3q$	
AA × aa	$2p^2q^2$		$2p^2q^2$	
Aa × Aa	$4p^2q^2$	p^2q^2	$2p^2q^2$	p^2q^2
Aa × aa	$4pq^3$		$2pq^3$	$2pq^3$
aa × aa	q^4			q^4

AA offspring $= p^4 + 2p^3q + p^2q^2$
$$= p^2(p^2 + 2pq + q^2) = p^2(p + q)^2 = p^2(1)^2 = p^2$$
Aa offspring $= 2p^3q + 4p^2q^2 + 2pq^3$
$$= 2pq(p^2 + 2pq + q^2) = 2pq$$
aa offspring $= p^2q^2 + 2pq^3 + q^4$
$$= q^2(p^2 + 2pq + q^2) = q^2$$

Glossary

Acrocentric a chromosome with the centromere near one end

Alleles alternative forms of a gene at the same locus

Allograft a graft between genetically dissimilar persons

Alternative splicing the formation of diverse messenger RNAs through differential splicing of an RNA precursor

Amniocentesis aspiration of amniotic fluid

Aneuploid any chromosome number which is not an exact multiple of the haploid number

Anticipation the apparent tendency for some diseases to begin at an earlier age and to increase in severity with each succeeding generation

Antisense RNA non-functional RNA which is complementary to an individual mRNA strand

Ascertainment identification of families with an inherited condition

Association a non-random combination of two or more structural defects which are not due to a single localized defect of embryogenesis

Assortative mating the preferential selection of a spouse with a particular genotype

Assortment random distribution of non-homologous chromosomes to daughter cells in meiosis

Autosome any chromosome other than the sex chromosomes

Bivalent a pair of homologous chromosomes as seen following synapsis prior to the first meiotic division

Burden consultant's perception of the cost (emotional, physical and financial) of a genetic disorder

Carrier a recessive heterozygote

Centimorgan length of DNA which on average has 1 cross-over per 100 gametes

Centromere the heterochromatic region within a chromosome by which the chromatids are held together

Chiasma the crossing of chromatid strands of homologous chromosomes during meiosis as a result of meiotic recombination

Chimaera an individual whose cells are derived from more than one zygote

Chorionic villus sampling a technique for prenatal diagnosis which biopsies chorionic villi

Chromatid replicated DNA prior to separation at mitosis

Chromatin the complex of DNA and associated proteins that represents the normal state of genes in the nucleus

Chromosomal aberration any abnormality of chromosome number or structure visible under the microscope

Cis location of two genes on the same chromosome

Clone a cell line derived by mitosis from a single diploid cell or gene sequences that are propagated through recombinant techniques from an identical parent gene

Codominant both alleles of a pair are expressed in the heterozygote

Codon three consecutive bases in DNA or RNA which specify an amino acid

Coefficient of inbreeding (F) the proportion of loci at which an individual is homozygous by descent

Coefficient of relationship (r) the proportion of all genes in two individuals which are identical by descent

Colinearity the parallel relationship between the base sequence of the DNA of a gene and the amino acid sequence of the corresponding peptide

Complementarity two single-stranded nucleic acid molecules are complementary when they form a succession of perfectly matched A : T and G : C base pairs in antiparallel orientation

Complementary DNA a single-stranded DNA fragment that is synthesized from the mRNA strand by reverse transcriptase

Compound an individual with two different mutant alleles at a locus

Concordant both members of a twin pair show the trait

Congenital present at birth

Consanguineous mating between individuals who share at least one common ancestor

Consensus sequence an idealized nucleotide sequence in which each position represents the base most often found when many sequences with similar function in several different genes are compared

Conserved sequence DNA sequences that are present in multiple, related members of a gene family and can be conserved between tissues or among species

Constitutive gene genes whose expression is controlled only by basal promoter activity (usually no developmental or hormonal regulation and are expressed at a constant level in most cells—see housekeeping genes)

Construct the assembly of a given set of DNA fragments in an appropriate vector using recombinant techniques

Consultand any person requesting genetic counselling

Contigs overlapping contiguous cloned DNA segments

Cosmid synthetic cloning vector which can accommodate large fragments of foreign DNA

CpG island a region of DNA often found close to the 5′ end of housekeeping genes that is relatively rich in 5′-CG-3′ oligonucleotide sequences where the C is often not methylated (see also HTF island)

Cross-over exchange of genetic material between homologous chromosomes during meiosis

Deformation alteration in shape of an organ due to unusual mechanical forces

Denaturation the separation of complementary DNA and/or RNA strands by exposure to alkali or elevated temperature

Dicentric a structurally abnormal chromosome with two centromeres

Diploid the chromosome number of somatic cells

Discordant only one member of a twin pair shows the trait

Disomy, uniparental inheritance of both homologues of a chromosome from one parent, with loss of the corresponding homologue from the other parent

Disruption a morphological defect due to breakdown of a previously normal organ or tissue

Distal elements nucleic acid sequences that are located toward the 3′ end from a reference point

Domain a segment of protein that is responsible for a specialized structure or function

Dominant a trait expressed in the heterozygote

Downstream refers to sequences that are distal or 3′ of the reference point

Empiric risk recurrence risk based on experience rather than calculation

Enhancer the region or regions of a gene that bind specific gene regulatory proteins and thus help to determine the level and cell type of gene expression

Epistasis interaction among alleles at different loci

Euchromatin the majority of nuclear DNA that remains relatively unfolded during most of the cell cycle and is therefore accessible to transcriptional machinery

Exon the segments of a gene that remain after splicing of the primary RNA transcript (5′ untranslated sequences, coding sequences and 3′ untranslated sequences)

Expressed sequence tag partial sequence of an expressed gene

Expressivity variation in the severity of a genetic trait

Familial refers to any condition which is commoner in relatives of an affected individual than in the general population

Flanking markers markers on either side of a disease locus

Flanking region the DNA sequences that are upstream (5′) of the transcriptional start site and downstream (3′) of the transcription termination signal

Flow karyotype a histogram of chromosome DNA measurements generated by a fluorescence-activated cell sorter

Gene a linear collection of DNA sequences required to produce a functional RNA molecule

Gene pool all the genes present at a given locus in the population

Gene conversion a process whereby two homologous portions of paired duplex DNA molecules become identical in sequence during recombination. In contrast to normal recombination, there is a unidirectional flow rather than an exchange of genetic information

Genetic counselling the communication of information and advice about inherited disorders

Genetic engineering the artificial production of new combinations of heritable material

Genetic epidemiology study of the role of genetic factors and their interaction with environmental factors in the distribution and determination of disease

Genetic lethal a genetic disorder in which affected individuals fail to reproduce

Genetics the scientific study of variation and heredity

Genomic imprinting parent-specific expression or repression of genes or chromosomes in offspring

Genotype the genetic constitution of the organism

Haploid the chromosome number of gametes

Haplotype a group of closely linked alleles which are inherited together as a unit

Heredity the transmission of characteristics to descendants

Heritability the fraction of the phenotypic variance due to genetic effects

Heterochromatin chromosomal regions that remain tightly folded during the entire cell cycle. These regions replicate late during S phase and do not contain actively transcribed genes

Heterogeneity similar phenotype from different genotypes

Heterozygote an individual with one normal and one mutant allele at a given locus on a pair of homologous chromosomes

Holandric Y-linked inheritance

Homologous matched

Homozygote an individual with a pair of identical alleles at a given locus on homologous chromosomes

Housekeeping genes genes which are constitutively expressed in most or all cells because they provide basic functions

HTF island cluster of *Hpa*II recognition sites resulting in *Hpa*II Tiny Fragments upon DNA digestion

Hybridization the binding of nucleic acid sequences through complementary base pairing

Idiogram a diagram of the chromosome complement

Illegitimate transcription erroneous expression of a gene

Inbreeding the mating of closely related individuals

Intron a segment of a gene that is transcribed into the primary RNA transcript but which is excised during exon splicing

Isochromosome an abnormal chromosome in which there is loss of one arm and two identical copies of the other

Isodisomy, uniparental inheritance of two copies of one homologue of a chromosome from one parent, with loss of corresponding homologue from the other parent

Isograft graft between genetically identical individuals

Isolate a genetically separate population

Karyotype the classified chromosome complement of an individual or cell

Kilobase (kb) a unit of length with 1000 bases in DNA or RNA

Kindred an extended family

Library a collection of DNA fragments which have been inserted into vector molecules

Linkage linked genes have their loci within measurable distance of one another on the same chromosome

Linkage disequilibrium the association of two linked alleles more frequently than would be expected by chance

Locus the precise location of a gene on a chromosome

Lod score logarithm of the odds score for the likelihood of two loci being within a measurable distance of each other

Malformation a primary error of normal development or morphogenesis of an organ or tissue

Megabase 1×10^6 base pairs of DNA

Meiosis reduction cell division which occurs in gamete production

Microdeletion chromosomal deletion whose size is close to the limit of resolution using the light microscope

Micronuclei separate small nuclei which contain chromosomes or chromosomal fragments which are not participating in normal mitosis

Middle repetitive DNA an intermediate class of repetitive DNA with repeat lengths of approximately 100–10 000 bp that is generally distributed widely in euchromatin

Missense mutation base-pair substitution which leads to an altered amino acid specification (cf. silent and nonsense mutations)

Mitosis somatic cell division

Monosomy one of a chromosome pair is missing

Mosaic an individual derived from a single zygote with cells of two or more different genotypes

Multifactorial inheritance due to multiple genes at different loci which summate and interact with environmental factors

Mutation a change in the genetic material

Non-disjunction failure of two members of a chromosome pair to disjoin during anaphase

Nonsense mutation base-pair substitution which results in a replacement of an amino acid codon with a termination codon (UGA, UAA or UAG)

Northern blotting filter transfer of RNA separated by size in gel electrophoresis

Nucleotide a purine or pyrimidine base attached to a sugar and phosphate group

Oncogene a gene sequence capable of causing transformation

Open reading frame series of triplet codons within a DNA sequence which does not include multiple stop or nonsense codons

Palindrome a stretch of DNA in which identical base sequences run in opposite directions

Penetrance the frequency of expression of the genotype

Pharmacogenetics the study of genetically controlled variation of response to drugs

Phenocopy an environmentally induced mimic of a genetic disease

Phenotype the outward appearance of an individual

Plasmid extrachromosomal closed circular DNA molecule found in bacteria

Pleiotropy multiple effects of a single gene

Polygenic determined by multiple genes at different loci each with a small but additive effect

Polymerase chain reaction (PCR) the amplification of a target segment of DNA

Polymorphism common (involving $\geq 2\%$ of the population) discontinuous genetic variations

Polymorphism information content (PIC) the probability that the offspring of a random mating between a carrier of a rare dominant gene and a non-carrier is informative for linkage between the locus of the dominant gene and the marker locus

Polyploid an abnormal chromosomal complement which exceeds the diploid number and is an exact multiple of the haploid number

Probability the ratio of the number of occurrences of a specified event to the total number of possible events

Proband the individual who draws medical attention to the family

Probe a radiolabelled DNA or RNA fragment used to identify a complementary sequence(s) by molecular hybridization

Prokaryote a simple unicellular organism which lacks a nuclear membrane

Promoter the region of a gene that determines where RNA polymerase binds and initiates transcription

Pseudogene a non-functional replica of a functional gene

Quasidominance the direct transmission, generation to generation, of a recessive trait if the gene is frequent or if inbreeding is intense

Race a group of historically related individuals who share a gene pool

Random mating selection of a mate without regard to genotype

Recessive a trait which is expressed only in homozygotes

Recombinant an individual in a linkage study in whom the marker and disease loci have assorted at parental meiosis

Recombination the process whereby two homologous duplex DNA molecules exchange information by crossing over

Restriction enzyme an enzyme which cleaves DNA at sequence-specific sites (the recognition site)

Restriction fragment length polymorphism (RFLP) a recognition site for a restriction enzyme which may or may not be present

Reverse transcriptase an enzyme which can make complementary DNA from messenger RNA

Ridge count the sum of ridges on the 10 fingertips by counting from the centre of each pattern to each triradius. Male mean, 145 (SD, 51), female mean, 127 (SD, 53)

Satellite DNA Highly repetitive DNA (generally repeat lengths of less than 5–10 bp) that is often found in heterochromatin and can be separated from the majority of genomic DNA by density-gradient centrifugation

RNA editing modification of mRNA sequence during processing so that it is no longer complementary to the original DNA template (e.g. production of two apolipoproteins, apoB48 and apoB100, from the same gene)

Secondary structure the proposed structural domains of a protein on the basis of its amino acid sequence (primary structure)

Segregation the separation of allelic genes at meiosis

Sequence a series of abnormalities causally related to a primary malformation

Sex-limited a trait expressed only in one sex

Sex-linked inheritance of a gene carried on a sex chromosome

Sib a brother or sister

Sibship a group of brothers and/or sisters

Single-copy DNA DNA which is present in one copy per set of haploid chromosomes (represents about 70% of the total)

Silent mutation base-pair substitution which alters a codon but does not result in altered amino acid due to degeneracy of the genetic code (e.g. GGA and GGU both code for glycine)

Sister chromatid exchange exchange of DNA by sister chromatids

Site-directed mutagenesis the production of specific mutations in a DNA fragment

Southern blotting filter transfer of DNA fragments separated by size in gel electrophoresis

Species a set of individuals who can interbreed and have fertile progeny

Sporadic no known genetic basis

Syndrome a non-random combination of features

Synteny loci on the same chromosome which may or may not be linked

Teratogen any agent which causes congenital malformations

Tertiary structure refers to the three-dimensional structure of a protein

Trait any gene-determined characteristic

Trans location of two genes on opposite chromosomes of a pair

Transcription production of mRNA from the DNA template

Transcription factors a set of proteins required for RNA synthesis

Transgenic where synthetic DNA has been introduced into the genome of an animal in order to change its genotype

Translation The process whereby protein is synthesized from a mRNA sequence

Translocation the transfer of chromosomal material between chromosomes

Triploid a cell with three times the haploid number of chromosomes

Trisomy three copies of a given chromosome per cell

Upstream refers to sequences located in the opposite direction to transcription

Untranslated regions the portions of a gene which are transcribed into mRNA but not translated into protein. By definition, untranslated regions are found in exons

Vector a plasmid, phage or cosmid into which foreign DNA may be inserted for cloning

Western blotting filter transfer of proteins separated by size in gel electrophoresis

YAC yeast artificial chromosome used for cloning of large sections of DNA

Zygote the fertilized ovum

Index

Page numbers in *italics* refer to figures, those in **bold** refer to tables.

A-gliadin 160
abdominal wall defects, anterior 185, **186**
Abelson oncogene *87*, 90
ABO antigens 152
ABO blood groups 152–3, 156
ABO gene 153
ABO incompatibility 153
abortion
   spontaneous 116, 202
   therapeutic 108, 202, 212
Abortion Act (1967) 108
acentric rings 62, *63*
acetylator status 130
beta-*N*-acetylhexosaminidase A
    mutation 147
achondroplasia 71, 130, *131*
acoustic schwannoma, bilateral 174
acquired immune deficiency syndrome *see*
    AIDS
acrocentric chromosomes 39
acute intermittent porphyria 130–1
acute lymphatic leukaemia 167–8
acute myeloid leukaemia 167, 169
adenine 9, *10*
adenoma sebaceum 175
adenomatous polyposis coli gene 163
adenosine deaminase deficiency 8, 146
adenylate kinase-1 *87*, 90, 124
adrenal cortical carcinoma 191
adrenal hypoplasia *81*, 129
adrenoleucodystrophy 131
adult polycystic kidney disease 188, 189
affective disorder, bipolar 160
agammaglobulinaemia 131
AIDS 8
albinism 3
   oculocutaneous 131–2
alcohol abuse
   congenital malformations 177
   see also fetal alcohol syndrome
alcoholism 157
alkaptonuria 5
allele-specific oligonucleotide (ASO)
    probes 29, *31*
   point mutations 27

alleles 83, 84, 155
   frequency 223
   linked 86
alpha-fetoprotein 183
   amniotic fluid 205, **206**
   biochemistry 199–200
   maternal serum 8, 204–5, *206*, **208**, *213*,
    214
Alport syndrome 132–3
Alzheimer disease 6, 157–8
amelia 189, *191*
amelogenin gene 51
amniocentesis 197–200
   chromosomal disorder detection 213–14
   de novo reciprocal translocation 117
   fetal karyotyping 117
   fetal sexing 197, *198*
   genetic 8
   mosaicism 198
   pseudomosaicism 198
   risks 200–1
amniotic band 188, *190*
amniotic fluid biochemistry 199–200
Amsterdam dwarfism 192, *193*
amyloid precursor protein mutations 158
anaphase 44–5
   lag 55
Anderson–Fabry disease *see* Fabry disease
androgen insensitivity syndrome 133
androgen receptor mutations 133
anencephaly 8, 180, *183*, 205
aneuploidy 55–6
   fetal karyotyping 198
   maternal age 212
   mitotic cell division 56
Angelman syndrome 54, 126, 128
angiokeratoma corporis diffusum 135–6
angiotensin converting enzyme 158
ankylosing spondylitis 158
anti-Rh gammaglobulin 154
antibody defects 151
antisense strand 12
alpha$_1$-antitrypsin deficiency 132
aortic aneurysm, abdominal 158
Apert syndrome 71, 133
apolipoprotein E genotype 158
apple-peel syndrome 186
arthrogryposis 189
artificial insemination by donor 108

association analysis 96
ataxia telangiectasia 170, 171
atherosclerosis 158
atopic diathesis 158
atopy locus 158
attention deficit hyperactivity disorder 158
Auer bodies 167
autism 159
autoimmune disorders 155
autosomal dominant diseases 70, **71**
autosomal dominant trait
   genetic counselling 108–9
   sex limitation 76
autosomal inheritance 69
   codominant 74
   dominant 69–71, 75
   recessive 71–3, *74*, 73
   single gene 69
autosomal recessive diseases 73, **74**
autosomal recessive trait 73
   codominant 74
   consanguinity 114
   DNA analysis 109, *110*
   ethnic association 73, **74**
   genetic counselling 109
   parents both carriers 72, *73*
   vertical transmission 73
autosomal traits, sex limitation 76, **77**
autosomes 34, 36

B-lymphocytes 150
Barr body 50, 53
   fetal sexing 197, *198*
basal cell carcionma 173–4
base pair 10
Bayes' theorem 108, 109, 220, **221**
Becker muscular dystrophy 78–9, 143–4
Beckwith–Wiedemann syndrome 191–2
beta-globin cluster 90
beta-globin gene *15*, 86
biopsy, ultrasound guidance 200–1
bladder cancer 166–7
blood
   cross-matching 156
   fetal sampling 202
   groups 152–3
blood pressure, high 160
blood transfusion, Rhesus sensitization 153,

154, 156
Bloom syndrome 170, 171
body stalk anomaly 185
bone marrow hyperplasia 154
brain stem haemangioma 176
brain tumours 169
branchio-oto-renal syndrome 187
BRCA1 mutation 170, 172
BRCA2 mutation 170, 172
breakpoint cluster region 165
breast cancer 169–70
    inherited types 172
bromodeoxyuridine 16–17
Brushfield spots 118
Bruton agammaglobulinaemia 131
Burkitt's lymphoma 165

C1 inhibitor gene mutations 140
C-banding 34, *36*
c-onc 164
café au lait patches 174
cancer 6, 162
    genetic counselling 169–71
    genetic studies 167–8
    heterozygosity loss 162, **163**, *164*
    inherited forms 209
    karyotypic abnormalities 169
    presymptomatic carriers 6
    single gene causes 171–6
    somatic cell genetic disorders 97
carcinogen metabolism 166
carrier detection 7
carrier frequency 109, 226
carrier screening 208–9
    single gene disorders 214
Carter effect 95
cataract, congenital 114
CD8+ T-cells 154
cell cycle 43
cellular immunity defects 151
central nervous system congenital
        malformations 179–84
centric fragments 65
centromere 36, 37
centromeric heterochromatin 39, 41, 43
cerebellar haemangioblastoma 176
cerebral gigantism 194
cervical carcinoma 170
Charcot–Marie–Tooth disease 140
Chargaff's rule 9
CHARGE association 192
chemical mutagens 57
chiasma formation, somatic cell 45
chiasmata 47, *49*
chimaera 67
cholinesterase 1 mutations 147
chorionic somatomammotrophin gene 6
chorionic villus sampling 8, 201–2
    fetal karyotyping 117
    maternal age 202
    mosaics 202
Christmas disease 139
chromosomal aberrations 55
    centric fragments 65
    centric fusion translocations 65
    deletions 62
    duplications 62, 64
    inversions 64–5
    numerical 55–7

ring chromosomes 62, *63*
structural 57–8, *59–60*, 61–2, *63*, 64–5
chromosomal abnormalities
    arthrogryposis 189
    fetal screening 206, *207*
    irradiation exposure 115
    likelihood ratio 206
    malignancies associated 165, *166*
    multiples of the median (MOM) 206
    rate at conception 210
chromosomal analysis 33–4, *35*, 36–7, *38*, *39*,
        40, *41*
    fetal 200
    genetic counselling 106
    recurrent miscarriages 110
chromosomal disorders 4–5, 108, 116
    45,X 116, 121–2, *123*
    46,XX 121
    47,XXX 121
    47,XXY 120–1
    47,XYY 120
    Angelman syndrome 54, 126, 128
    balanced carrier 125
    biochemical screening 213–14
    birth frequency 116, *117*
    deletions 124–6, *127–8*, 129
    duplications 124–5, *127–8*
    hydatiform changes 123, 124, **125**
    Klinefelter syndrome 110, 120–1
    marker chromosome 125–6
    microdeletions 129
    non-disjunction 123
    paracentric inversions 117–18
    pericentric inversions 117–18, *119*, 120–4
    Prader–Willi syndrome 54, 68, 126, **128**
    pregnancies at risk 213
    primary prevention 213
    secondary prevention 212–14
    treatment 211
    triploidy 56, *57*, *125*
    see also translocation; trisomy 13; trisomy
        18; trisomy 21
chromosome 4 **126**
chromosome 9
    imbalance 124, *127*
    isochromosome of short arm 65, *67*
    pericentric inversion *64*
    pericentric inversions 118
chromosome 10 58, *59*, *60*
chromosome 11
    atopy locus 158
    reciprocal translocation 58, *59*, *61*
chromosome 12
    isochromosome of short arm 65
    paracentric inversion *64*
chromosome 13
    centric fusion 58
    retinoblastoma gene 162, *163*, *164*
chromosome 14 58, *61*
chromosome 15 128
chromosome 16
    alpha-globin synthesis down-
        regulation 132
    PKD1 mutations 188
chromosome 17 90
chromosome 21 58, *61*
chromosome 22 58, *61*
chromosomes 4, 33
    3:1 segregation 58
    acrocentric 39

banding 5, 46, *49*
breakage 57
centromere 36, 37
combinations 47
condensation 46
flow cytometry 34, *39*
flow karyotyping 37, *39*, *41*
heteromorphisms 37, *39*, *40*, 41–2
homologous pairing 65
long arm 36
metaphase 33
mitochondrial 43
mosaicism 198, *199*
nonhuman primates 42–3
origin of complex structural
        rearrangements 65–6
paints 6
rearrangement and human
        oncogenes 165, **166**
ring 62, *63*
sex 34, 36, 76
short arm 36, 46
    pairing region 47
spontaneous breakage 17, 57
staining 34
sticky ends 57
structure 33, *34*
telomere 36
see also inversions; isochromosomes; X
        chromosome; Y chromosome
chronic myeloid leukaemia 165, 168, 169
cleft lip and palate 95, 185–6
clinical applications of genetics 6–8
clotting factor IX gene 25
club foot 178
codon 12, *13*
coefficient of inbreeding 222
coefficient of relationship 222
coeliac disease 160
COL4A5 132
colchicine 33
collagen mutation 132
collagen Type VII gene 135
colon cancer
    hereditary non-polyposis 170, 172
    multistage progression 163, *165*
    p53 gene mutations 163
    Peutz–Jeghers syndrome 175
colonic aganglionosis 186
colorectal cancer 170
colour blindness 6, 134
colour vision
    genes 17, 19
    red-green 90, 134
common diseases, multifactorial
        inheritance 157
complement C4 161
complement system 151, 154
concordance
    determination 92
    leprosy 151–2
    leukaemia 170
    twin studies 91–2, **93**
congenital adrenal hyperplasia 134
    ambiguous genitalia 110, **112**
    CYP21B gene 154
    Haemophilus influenzae type B 151
    selective advantage 99
Congenital Disabilities (Civil Liability) Act
        (1976) 108

congenital dislocation of the hip 178
congenital heart disease 118, 122, 184
congenital malformations 95
  aetiology 178
  autosome duplication/deficiency 178
  central nervous system 179–84
  gastrointestinal tract 184–6
  heart 118, 122, 184
  incidence 177
  kidney 186–8
  limbs 188–9
  major 178–84, *185*, 186–9
  minor 178, **179**
  multiple 110, 189, 191–6
  teratogens 194–6
  thyroid 189
  urinary tract 186–8
congenital spherocytosis 134
consanguinity 108
  genetic counselling 114
consultand 103
  follow-up 108–9
contiguous gene disorder 19, 129
copper metabolism 139
cordocentesis 202
cosmid probes 66
Coxsackie B4/B5 virus 159
CpG dinucleotides 21
CpG island 14
  housekeeping gene association 53, 90
craniosynostosis 133
creatine kinase, Duchenne muscular
    dystrophy 77, 78
CREB binding protein 193
Crohn's disease 160
cross-reacting material positive/negative
    mutations 23
crossing-over 47, 48, *50*, 82, 85
  unequal 17, 41
cystic fibrosis 134–5
  ASO probes *31*
  carrier screening 209
  mutational heterogeneity 209
  mutations **22**, 23
  prenatal diagnosis 8, 209
  probability 219
  transmembrane conductance regulator
      gene (*CFTR*) 134
cystinuria 135
cytomegalovirus 159
  congenital malformations 194
  microcephaly 180
cytosine 9, *10*
  deamination 21

de Lange syndrome 192, *193*
deafness, congenital 113–14
debrosoquine/sparteine
    polymorphism 135
deletions 17, 19
dementia, progressive 189
deoxyribonucleic acid *see* DNA
2' deoxyribose *10*
depurination/deamination repair 21
dermatoglyphic abnormalities **106**
diabetes mellitus
  insulin-dependent 6, 159
    congenital malformations 178, 178
    MHC allele association 157

limb defects 189
  non-insulin-dependent 159
diakinesis 46, 47
diaphyseal aclasis 173
dicentric rings 62, *63*
dictyotene 49
DiGeorge syndrome 193
digit fusion 188
dihydrofolate reductase 167
dihydroxyacetone phosphate
    acyltransferase 149
diploid number 46
diplotene 46–7
discontinuous traits 3
disease loci 82, *83*
disomy, uniparental 68
dispermy 56
disruption 177
dizygotic twins 91–2, **93**
DNA 4, 9
  base pairs 12
  deletions 17
  double helix 9, *11*
  fetal diagnosis 200
  fingerprint 26, *28*, 115
  flanking 14
  mismatch repair process 21
  mutations 17, 19–21, 22, 23
  polymorphisms 24
    identification 26–7, *29*
  probes 24
  repair mechanisms 21
  replication 14, 16, 43
    semiconservative 16, *18*
  sequencing 29–30, *32*
    point mutations 27
  synthesis pattern 43
DNA analysis 24
  autosomal recessive traits 109, *110*
  chorionic villus sampling 200
  direct mutant gene analysis 27, 29, *30–1*
  dominant traits 108–9
  familial hypercholesterolaemia 70
  genetic counselling 106
  indirect mutant gene tracking 24–7
  prenatal diagnosis 72
DNA-repair genes 162
DNA-repair mechanisms, genes
    involved 165–6
dominant characteristics 3
double minutes 167, *168*
Down syndrome 118, *119*
  aetiology 118
  clinical features 118, *119*
  human chorionic gonadotrophin
      (hCG) 206, *207*, 213
  maternal alpha-fetoprotein 206, *207*, 213
  prenatal screening *213*
  see also trisomy 21
Duarte-galactosaemia genetic
    compound 138
Duchenne muscular dystrophy 77–8, 143–4
  adrenal hypoplasia and glycerol kinase
      deficiency association 129
  atypical Lyonization 78
  Bayes' theorem 220
  carrier detection 77–8
  carrier female Lyonization 77–8
  DNA analysis *80*
  PCR amplification *30*

pedigree *78*, *80*
  prenatal diagnosis 8, *201*
  X–autosome translocation 78, *79*
  X-linked form 78
duodenal atresia 186
duplications 62, 64
dyslexia 161
dysmorphic features 103
  measurements **106**
dysmorphic syndromes 104–5, 189, 191–6
dystrophin
  cDNA probe **200**
  mutations 143

eclampsia 161
ectrodactyly 189, *190*
Edwards syndrome 122–3, *124*
Ehlers–Danlos syndrome 135
embryogenesis 50
encephalocele 180, 181, *183*, 188
enhancers 14
environmental factors 170
epidermolysis bullosa 135
epilepsy 159–60
  congenital malformations 178, 178
  lissencephaly 179
euchromatin 33
evolution, gene frequency change 98
exomphalos 184, *185*
exons 13
expressed tissue-specific gene replication 43

Fabry disease 135–6
facial haemangioma 194
FACS DNA sequence mapping 87, 90
factor V resistance 140
factor VIII 139
factor IX 139
familial adenomatous polyposis 171
familial atypical malignant melanoma 172
familial combined hyperlipidaemia 158
familial hypercholesterolaemia 69–70, 141,
    158
  low density lipoprotein receptor gene 74
familial spastic paraplegia 136
family correlation studies 93
family linkage studies 82–6
  cross-overs 82, 85
  disease loci 82, *83*
  gene order 86
  independent assortment 82, 83
  loci 82, **83**
  lod scores 85
  marker loci 82, *83*
  recombinants 82, 84
  recombination fraction 82–6
Fanconi syndrome 171, 172, 189
  acute leukaemia risk 170
feet, split 189
fertilization 49, 50
fetal alcohol syndrome 113, 180, 195
fetal blood sampling 202
fetal cells in maternal circulation 203
fetal chromosomal abnormality
    screening 206, *207*
fetal enzyme assay 199
fetal haemoglobin (HbF) 146
fetal karyotyping 118, 198–9

fetal liver biopsy 202
fetal skin biopsy 202
fetal visualization 8
fibrillin 1 mutations 142
fibroangiomata, facial 175
fibroblast growth factor receptor 2 gene 133
fibroblast growth factor receptor 3 130
fingerprint pattern 104, *106*
flow cytometry, dual laser 37
flow karyotype, bivariate 37, *40*
flow karyotyping 37, *39, 41*
flow sorted chromosome dot-blot
    analyses *87, 90*
fluorescence *in situ* hybridization (FISH) 6
folic acid 182
    supplementation 214
founder effect 100
fragile sites 42, 43
fragile X syndrome 23, 79, 111, 113
    facies 136, *137*
    Friedreich's ataxia 137
    inheritance 136–7
    macro-orchidism *137*
    premutation 136, 137
    prenatal diagnosis 8, 136–7
frame shift mutations 19
Friedreich's ataxia 137

G-banding 34, *35*, 37
galactosaemia 137–8
galactose-1-phosphate uridyltransferase
    (GALT) *87*, 124
    absence 137
    galactosaemia carrier detection 138
alpha-galactosidase mutations 136
gametogenesis 46
Gardner syndrome 171
gastroschisis 184, *185*
Gaucher disease 138
Gaussian distribution 93, *94*, 95
gene
    cloning
        functional *88–90*, 90
        positional 90
        strategies *90*
    conversion 19, *20*
    diversification 64
    dosage 86–7
        flow sorted chromosome dot-blot
            analyses *87, 90*
        in situ hybridization 86–7
        interspecific somatic cell
            hybridization 90
    expression 14
    frequency
        change 98
        maintenance 223
        selection 98
    mapping 90
    non-expressed tissue-specific 43
    pairs 4
    protein products *14*
    regulation 14
    size 12
    structural 10, 90
    therapy 8
    tracking 24–6
    X-linked transmission 76
    see also mutant gene; mutation

genetic assessment 7
genetic compound 73
genetic condition treatment 99–100
genetic counselling 7
    autosomal dominant traits 108–9
    Bayes' theorem 220
    cancer 169–71
    chromosomal disorders 108
    clinical examination 103–5
    communication of advice 103–8
    congenital cataract 114
    congenital deafness 113–14
    consanguinity 108, 114
    diagnosis confirmation 106–7
    diagnostic precision 108
    extended family 107, 109
    follow-up 107–8
    infertility 110
    insulin-dependent diabetes mellitus 159
    irradiation exposure 114–15
    legal aspects 108
    mental handicap 111, 113
    multifactorial disorders 110
    mutagen exposure 114–15
    paternity testing 115
    perinatal death with multiple
        malformations 110
    presymptomatic screening of adults 209
    recurrent miscarriages 110
    reproductive decisions **212**
    reproductive options 107–8
    sexual differentiation disorders 110, **112**
    short stature 115
    sickle cell disease 209
    stillbirth 110
    sudden infant death syndrome 111
    beta-thalassaemia 209
    timing 107
    X-linked recessive trait 109, *110, 111*
genetic disease
    impact 210–11
    incidence **211**
    multifactorial 212
    prevention 210, *211*
    primary prevention 214
    secondary prevention 212–14
    treatment 211–12
    types 211
genetic disorder prevalence 98
genetic engineering 211–12
genetic heterogeneity 73
genetic polymorphisms 74
genitalia, ambiguous 110, **112**
genome structure/organization *88–90*, 90
genomic DNA libraries, chromosome-
    specific 90
genomic imprinting 54
genomics 82
    family linkage studies 82–6
    gene dosage 86–7, 90
    gene mapping 82
    nucleic acid sequencing 82
germ cells, female fetus 49
Gilles de la Tourette syndrome 138
glaucoma 160
alpha-globin gene 132
beta-globin gene cluster mutations 133
glucose-6-phosphate dehydrogenase
    deficiency 99, 138
    malaria resistance 151

beta-glucosidase mutations 138
gluten enteropathy 160
glycerol kinase deficiency 129
Goldenhar syndrome 192
gonadal mosaic 67
gonadoblastoma 122
Gorlin–Goltz syndrome 173
grand mal 159
guanine 9, *10*
Guthrie bacterial inhibition assay 208

haemochromatosis 138
haemoglobin Bart's 132
haemoglobin F 147
haemoglobin H disease 132
haemoglobin S *22*, 146
    genes 71
haemolysis, glucose-6-phosphate
    dehydrogenase deficiency 138
haemolytic disease of the newborn 153–4
haemophilia 3
haemophilia A *31*, 139
haemophilia B 25, 139
Haemophilus influenzae type B 99, 151
hand–heart syndrome 189
hands, split 189
haploid number 46
haplotype 86
happy puppet syndrome *see* Angelman
    syndrome
Hardy–Weinberg equilibrium 98
Hardy–Weinberg law 223
harlequin chromosomes 17, *18*
heavy chain gene cluster 150–1
height distribution 93, *94*
hemihypertrophy 191, *192*
hepatitis, autoimmune 158–9
hepatoblastoma 191
hepatocellular carcinoma
    Fanconi syndrome 172
    p53 gene mutations 163
hepatolenticular degeneration 139
hereditary angio-oedema 140
hereditary C1-inhibitor deficiency 140
hereditary haemorrhagic telangiectasia 140
hereditary motor and sensory neuropathy
    type I 140
hereditary non-polyposis colon cancer 170,
    172
hereditary optic neuropathy, Leber 141–2
hereditary thrombophilia 140
heredity, misconceptions 107
heterochromatin 33
    centromeric *39, 41, 43*
heterogeneous RNA *see* hnRNA
heteromorphisms 37, *39*, *40*, 41–2
heteroplasmy 97
Hirschsprung disease 186
HLA B27 158
hnRNA 13
Hodgkin's disease 170
Holandric inheritance *see* Y-linked
    inheritance
holoprosencephaly 179, *180*
Holt–Oram syndrome 189
homogeneously stained chromosomal
    regions (HSRs) 167
homologous chromosome pairing 65
homoplasmy 97

housekeeping genes 14
  CpG island association 53, 90
  replication 43
HRAS gene 164, 165
human chorionic gonadotrophin (hCG) 206,
      207, **208**
  Down syndrome *213*
human gene map assignments *88–90*
human gene size 13
human genome project 6
Hunter syndrome 142, 143
Huntington disease 23, 71, 108, 140–1, 214
Hurler syndrome 142, *143*
hydatidiform mole 54
hydrocephalus 179, 180, *181*
7-hydrocholesterol reductase deficiency 194
hydrops fetalis 154
21-hydroxylase deficiency 134
21-hydroxylase deficient adrenogenital
      syndrome, salt-losing 199
4-hydroxylation, hepatic cytochrome
      P450 135
17α-hydroxyprogesterone 200
hypercholesterolaemia 141
hyperlipidaemia 141, 158
hyperparathyroidism 173
hypertelorism 104
hypertension, pregnancy-induced 161
hyperthermia of anaesthesia 141
hypertrophic cardiomyopathy 141
hypomelanosis of Ito 192
hypospadias 187
hypothyroidism, congenital 208
hypoxanthine-guanine phosphoribosyl
      transferase 142

ichthyosis vulgaris 141
IgA deficiency, selective 151
immune response components 150, *150*
immune system, genetics 150–1
immunization, genetic determination of
      response 152
immunodeficiency, inherited 151–2
immunoglobulins 150, *151*
in situ hybridization 86–7
inborn errors of metabolism 6, 8, 199
inbreeding coefficient 222
incontinentia pigmenti 79, 141
independent assortment, disturbance 82, 83
infant mortality rate 210
infantile polycystic disease 187–8
infection, genetic
      susceptibility/resistance 151–2
infertility 110
inflammatory bowel disease 160
inheritance 4
  quasidominant 73
  Y-linked 76
  see also non-Mendelian inheritance; X-
      linked inheritance
insulin, post-translational modification *17*
insulin growth factor 2 (*IGF2*) gene 54
interphase cytogenetics 199
interspersed repeats 10, *11*
intestinal atresia 186
intestinal polyposis 170
introns 13
inversions
  homologous chromosome pairing 65

paracentric 64, 65, 118–19
pericentric 64, 65, *66*, 118–19, 120–4
iris hamartoma 174
isochromosomes 65
  dicentric 65, *67*
isodisomy, uniparental 68

joint contractures, congenital multiple 189

karyotype
  gorilla *43*
  normal human 34, *35*, 36–7, *38*
  Paris nomenclature 36
  symbols 36–7
karyotyping *see* chromosomal analysis
Kayser–Fleischer rings 139
keratin gene mutations 135
kernicterus 154
kidneys, polycystic 188
Klinefelter syndrome 110, 120–1
Klippel–Feil syndrome 187, 192–3

Laemli loops 33
Leber optic neuropathy 5, *96*, 97, 141–2
length mutations 17, 19–20
  PCR 27, *29*
  Southern analysis 27
length polymorphisms 26
leprosy 151–2
leptotene 46, *48*
Lesch–Nyhan syndrome 8, 142
leukaemia 165, 167–8, 169, 170
  ataxia telangiectasia 171
  Bloom syndrome 171
  chromosomal translocation 6
  Fanconi syndrome 172
Li–Fraumeni syndrome 163, 170, 172
liability curve 95
light chain gene clusters 151
likelihood ratio for chromosomal
      abnormalities 206
linkage analysis
  multifactorial trait analysis 96
  multipoint 85
linkage disequilibrium 86, 155
lipoprotein (a) 158
lissencephaly 179
liver biopsy, fetal 202
lod scores 85
long interspersed repeats 12
low density lipoprotein receptor gene 74,
      141
lymphoedema, neonatal in Turner
      syndrome 121, *122*
lymphoma 170, 171
Lynch syndrome 172
Lyonization 50, *52*, 53
  carrier females 76, 77–9

macrocephaly 179, 192
macrosatellite repeats 11–12
major histocompatibility complex 154–5
  insulin-dependent diabetes mellitus
      association 157, 159
malaria, sickle cell disease advantage 98–9,
      151

malignant hyperpyrexia 141
malignant melanoma 171, 172
manic depression 160
mannose binding protein mutations 145
Marfan syndrome 71, 142
marker chromosome 125–6
marker loci 82, *83*
maternal age 212–14
maternal alpha-fetoprotein 204–5, *206*, **208**
  congenital malformation secondary
      prevention 214
  Down syndrome *213*
maternal circulation, fetal cells 203
maternal illness, fetal malformation 178
maternal–fetal platelet incompatibility 154
maturity-onset diabetes of youth 159
Meckel syndrome 184, 188
medical negligence 108
medium chain acyl-CoA dehydrogenase
      deficiency 142
megakaryocyte polyploidy 57
meiosis 46–8
meiotic division
  first 46–7, *56*
      resting phase 50
  second 47–8, 49, *51*
Mendel, Gregor 3–4
mental handicap
  chromosomal abnormalites 210
  fragile X syndrome 137
  genetic counselling 111, 113
  lissencephaly 179
  trisomy 21 118
messenger RNA *see* mRNA
metaphase 44, 47
methaemoglobinaemia 6
microcephaly 179–80, *182*
microsatellite 10, *11*
  instability 170
  repeats 26, 166, *167*
Miller–Dieker syndrome 179
minisatellite repeats 11, 26
miscarriage
  amniocentesis 200
  chromosomal abnormality rate 210
  recurrent 110
missense mutations 20, 23
mitochondrial chromosomes 43
mitochondrial disorders 5, *96*, 97, 212
mitochondrial DNA mutation rate 97
mitochondrial inheritance *96*
mitosis 43–5, **47**
mixed lymphocyte culture test 156
mongolism *see* trisomy 21
monosomy 55, 122
monozygotic twins 91–2, **93**
Morquio disease 142, *143*
mosaic 67
mosaicism 198, *199*
  see also pseudomosaicism
motorneurone disease 160
mRNA 12–13, *16*
mucopolysaccharidosis 142–3, **199**, 200
Mullerian duct inhibitor 53
multifactorial disorders 6, 91
  genetic counselling 110
  prevention 214
  treatment 212
multifactorial traits
  analysis 96

consanguinity 114
continuous 91, **92**, 93–4, **93**
discontinuous 91, 92, **93**, **94**, 95–6
genetic counselling 110
twins 92, *93*
multiple allelism 73
multiple endocrine neoplasia 143, 173
multiple exostoses 173
multiple sclerosis 160
multiple self-healing squamous epithelioma
syndrome 171, 173
multiples of the median (MOM) 206
muscular dystrophy
counselling 79
fascioscapulohumeral 143
genetic heterogeneity 79
X-linked 143–4
see also Becker muscular dystrophy;
Duchenne muscular dystrophy
mutagen exposure 114–15
mutant gene
direct analysis 27, 29, *30–1*
indirect tracking 24–7
unstable 71
mutation
missense 20, 23
nomenclature **22**, 23
paternal age 71
rate for single gene disorders 100
silent 20
transmission 96–7
within regulatory sequence 14
mutational analysis of candidate genes 96
MYC gene 165
myositis ossificans, progressiva 71
myotonic dystrophy 20, 23, 71, 144

NADH-dependent methaemoglobin
reductase 6
naevoid basal cell carcinoma syndrome 171,
173–4
narcolepsy 160
neck skin, redundant 121, *122*
neonatal screening 8, 207–9
nephroblastoma 176
nephrolithiasis 144
neural arch defects 184
neural groove 179
neural tube defect 179, 180–4
arthrogryposis 189
folic acid supplementation 214
frequency 181
inheritance 182
maternal AFP screening 204–5, **206**
prenatal diagnosis 183
prenatal screening *213*
risk 182–3
secondary 184, 214
neurilemmoma 174
neuroblastoma 174
neurofibroma, acoustic 174
neurofibromatosis 71, 113, 174, 189
neurofibromin 174
neuropore, closure 179, 180
neutrophil drumstick 53
non-disjunction 51, 123
meiotic 55
mitotic 55, *56*
non-expressed tissue-specific gene

replication 43
non-Mendelian inheritance 91
family correlation studies 93
mitochondrial disorders *96*, 97
multifactorial disorders 91
multifactorial trait
analysis 96
continuous 91, **92**, 93–4
discontinuous 91, 92, **93**, **94**, 95–6
somatic cell genetic disorders 96–7
twin concordance studies 91–2, **93**
non-penetrance 71
non-self antigen 155
Noonan syndrome 187, 193
nucleic acid 4
function 12–14, *15*, *16*
sequencing 82
structure 9, 11, 12
nucleolus organizer region
tandem duplication 41, *42*
see also silver NOR stain
nucleotide substitutions, single 21

oculo-auriculo-vertebral spectrum 192
oculocutaneous albinism 131–2
oesophageal atresia 186
oesophagus carcinoma 170
oligohydramnios 186, 187, 188, 189
oligonucleotide probes 90
olivopontocerebellar ataxia 147
oncogenes 162, 163–5
amplification 167
oocytes, primary 48–9
oogenesis 48–9, 51
opsonic defect 144–5, 151
optic glioma 174
optic neuropahty 5
Osler–Weber–Rendu disease 140
osteogenesis imperfecta 145
osteosarcoma 170
otosclerosis 145
ovarian cancer 170, 172
ovarian granulosa cell tumour 175

p53 gene mutations 163
pachygyria 179
pachytene 46, *49*, *51*
paint probe 66
palmar crease 104
Down syndrome 118, *119*
pancreatic cancer 170
paracentric inversions 117–18
parental characteristics, blending 3
Parkinson's disease 160–1
Patau syndrome 123, *124*
paternity testing 115
pea, Mendel's studies 3–4, *5*
pedigree
construction 103, *104*
pattern analysis 82
penetrance, dominant traits 71
pericentric inversions 117–24
perinatal asphyxia 113
perinatal death with multiple
malformations 110
peripheral myelin protein 22 gene 140
peroneal muscular atrophy 140
petit mal 160

Peutz–Jeghers syndrome 174–5
phaeochromocytoma 173
neurofibromatosis type 1 174
von Hippel–Lindau disease 176
phagocytic system defects 151
phenylalanine hydroxylase mutations 145
phenylketonuria 111, 145
congenital malformations 178, *178*
microcephaly 180
neonatal screening 8, 207, 208
Philadelphia chromosome 6, 165, 167, 168,
169
phocomelia 189, *191*
phosphate linkage 5′–3′ *9*
physical examination 103–5
phytohaemagglutinin 33
pia-arachnoid haemangioma 194
point mutations 19, 20–1, 23
demonstration 27, 32
nonsense 23
repair mechanisms 21
single gene disorders 23
tumour types 164
polycystic kidney disease, adult onset 26
polycystin 188
polydactyly 188, *190*
polymerase chain reaction 26–7, *29*
polymicrogyria 179
polymorphisms 11
polyploidy 55, 56–7
polyposis coli 171
population association studies 157
population screening 204
carrier detection 208–9, **212**
neonatal 207–9
prenatal 204–5, *207*
presymptomatic of adults 209
porphobilinogen deaminase mutations 131
porphyric crises 131
positional cloning 90
post-translational modification of
proteins 13, *17*
Potter sequence 186, *187*, 189, *191*
Prader–Willi syndrome 54, 68, 126, **128**
pre-eclampsia 161
pregnancy
at-risk 7, 197, **198**, 213–14
termination *see* abortion, therapeutic
premature vascular disease 6
prenatal diagnosis 7–8, 197, **198**
amniocentesis 197–200
chorionic villus sampling 200, 202
cordocentesis 202
fetal cells in maternal circulation 203
fetal karyotyping 198–9
fetal liver biopsy 202
fetal skin biopsy 202
genetic counselling 107–8
selective termination of pregnancy 108
ultrasonography 202
prenatal screening 204–5, *207*, *213*
secondary prevention of disease 212
presenile dementia 118
presenilin mutations 158
presymptomatic screening of adults 209
prevention of disease 210, *211*
primary 214
secondary 212–14
probability 219
proband 103

prometaphase banding 34, *35*
promoters 14
prophase 44
    suspended 49
prostatic cancer 170–1
protein biosynthesis, faults 22, *23*
protein synthesis direction 12
prune belly appearance 187
pseudoautosomal segment 46, *47*
pseudogenes, non-functional 90
pseudomosaicism 198
    single cell 199
pseudoxanthoma elasticum 146
psoriasis 161
pubertal failure 110, **112**
purine nucleoside phosphorylase 146
purines 9, *10*
pyloric stenosis, congenital 95–6, 186
pyrimidines 9, *10*, 21

Q-banding 39

R-banding 34
radial aplasia 189, *190*
ras oncogene 164
recessive characteristics 3
recessive homozygote frequency 223
recessive traits
    autosomal 100
    X-linked 79, *80*, 100
        genetic counselling 109, *110, 111*
recombination *20*
    fraction 82–6
recurrence risk 110
relationship coefficient 222
renal agenesis, bilateral 186–7
renal carcinoma 176
renal cell carcinoma 171
renal chloride channel mutations 144
renal dysplasia 187
renal hypoplasia 187
repetitive probes 66
replication, initiation *18*
replication error positive (RER⁺) 166
restriction enzymes 24, *25*
restriction fragment length polymorphisms
        (RFLPs) 25, *27*
retinal haemangioma 176
retinitis pigmentosa 146
retinoblastoma 71, 162, *163*, 175
    inheritance 175
    mutations 162, *163*, *164*
    osteosarcoma risk 170
Rett syndrome 79, 146
reverse painting 66
rhabdomyosarcoma 191
rhesus blood group system 153
rhesus incompatibility 153–4
rheumatoid arthritis 161
ribonucleic acid *see* RNA
ribose 9, *10*
ribosomal RNA *see* rRNA
rickets
    familial hypophosphataemic 148
    vitamin D resistant 79, *80*, 148
ring chromosomes 62, *63*
RNA 9
RNA polymerase promoters 14

rRNA 12
rubella 180, 194
Rubinstein–Taybi syndrome 193
Russell–Silver syndrome 194
ryanodine receptor 141

Sanfilippo syndrome 142, 143
satellite association 44
satellite DNA 10
satellite polymorphisms 39, 41, *42*
schizophrenia 161
segmental aneusomy 129
segregation 3
selection 98, *99*
sense strand 12
Sertoli cells 53
severe combined immunodeficiency 146,
        151
sex chromosomes 34, 36, 76
sex determination 53–4
sex differentiation 53–4
sex linkage 76
sex ratio 95, **96**
sex vesicle 46
sex-linked inheritance 76
    X-linked codominant *80*, 81
    X-linked dominant 79, *80*
    X-linked recessive 77–9
sexual differentiation disorders 110, **112**
short interspersed repeats 12
short stature 114, 121
sib pair analysis 96, 157
sickle cell disease 6, 22, *23*, 146–7
    autosomal recessive trait 71, *72*
    carrier screening 209
    consanguineous parents 73, *75*
    ethnic association 73, **74**
    family pedigree 71, *72*
    gene frequency 98–9
    inheritance 72
    malaria resistance 151
    mutation 86
    parents both carriers 71, *73*
    PCR amplification 27, *30*, 32
    prenatal diagnosis 72
    selective advantage 98–9
silent mutations 20
silver NOR stain 34, *36*
simian crease 104, 118
single gene disorders 5–6, *98*, *99*, 100, 130
    acetylator status 130
    altered mutation rate 100
    carrier screening 208, 214
    founder effect 100
    molecular pathology 22, *23*
    population genetics 223, **224**
    prediction of birth frequency **100**
    prenatal diagnosis 8
    primary prevention 214
    secondary prevention 214
    treatment 211–12
    see also congenital adrenal hyperplasia;
            fragile X syndrome; sickle cell
            disease; vitamin D resistant rickets
Sipple syndrome 173
sister chromatid exchange 44
    chemical mutagens 57
    ring chromosome 62
site polymorphism 24

DNA point variations 25–6
skin biopsy, fetal 202
skin cancer 171
skin colour 94
slipped mispairing 17, 19
small bowel cancer 175
Smith–Lemli–Opitz syndrome 179, 194
solute carrier family 3 member 1
        (*SLC3A1*) 135
somatic cell
    genetic disorders 6, 96–7, 212
    interspecific hybridization 87
somatic recombination in mitosis 44, 45
Sotos syndrome 194
    macrocephaly 189
Southern analysis 26–7, *29*
spastic paraplegia, familial 136
specific reading disability 161
sperm
    ovum penetration 50
    production 48
spermatids 48
spermatocyte 48
spermatogenesis 48, *51*
spermatogonium 48
spina bifida 180–1, *183*
    maternal alpha-fetoprotein screening 205
    occulta 184
spinal haemangioma 176
spindle fibres, attachment 36
spinocerebellar ataxia type I 147
spinal muscular atrophy type I 147
splicing mutations 23
Sprengel shoulder 192
squamous cell carcinoma 172
SRY gene 53
steroid sulphatase
    deficiency 147
    gene 51
stillbirth 110, 116
stomach carcinoma 170
structural genes 10
    clustering 90
Sturge–Weber syndrome 194
succinylcholine sensitivity 147
sudden infant death syndrome 111
superoxide dismutase 1 mutations 160
suxamethonium 147
synaptonemal complex 47, *50*
syndactyly 188, *190*
systemic lupus erythematosus 161

T-cell
    antigen presentation 155
    lymphomas 165
    receptor 151
T-lymphocytes 150, 151
talipes equinovarus 178
tandem duplication 41, *42*
tandem repeats 10, *11*, 19
    variable number 26
*Taq*I enzyme 24
    recognition sites 25
TAR syndrome 189
TATA box 14
Tay–Sachs disease 147
    carrier screening 209
    macrocephaly 189
    tuberculosis resistance 151

telomere 36
telophase 44
template strand 12
tendon xanthomata 69, 70
teratogens 194–6
testicular cancer 171
testicular feminization syndrome 133
testis-determining factor (TDF) 53
    inheritance 76
    region 53
    transfer to X chromosome 121
testosterone 53
tetraploidy 57
alpha-thalassaemia 8, 132, 151
alpha-thalassaemia/mental handicap
        syndrome 132
beta-thalassaemia 99, 133
    birth frequency 214
    carrier screening 208–9, 214
    malaria resistance 151
thalidomide 194
threshold effects 6
thrombocytopenia, neonatal
        alloimmune 154
thrombophilia, hereditary 140
thymidine kinase 6
    deficiency 87
thymine 9, 10
thyroid
    cancer 171
    dysgenesis 189
    medullary carcinoma 173
toxoplasmosis
    congenital malformations 194
    microcephaly 180
    treatment 195
tracheo-oesophageal fistula 186
traits 69
    codominant 69
    multifactorial analysis 96
    see also X-linked recessive traits
transcription 12–13, 16
    factors 14
    regulation 14, 17
transfer RNA see tRNA
translation 13, 16
translocation
    balanced 58, 116–17
    centric fusion 58, 61, 62, 63, 116
    imbalance 58
    insertional 58, 61–2, 63
    reciprocal 58, 59–61, 116, 117
    unbalanced offspring 117
    X-autosome 53, 78, 79
transplantation 155
Treacher Collins syndrome 148, 186

treatment of genetic disease 8, 211–12
trinucleotide repeat amplification 19–20, 23
triplets 12
triploidy 56, 57, **125**
trisomy 55, 57
trisomy 8 169
trisomy 13 123, 124
    alpha-fetoprotein levels **208**
    cleft lip/palate 186
    holoprosencephaly 179
    human chorionic gonadotrophin
        levels **208**
trisomy 16 116
trisomy 18 122–3, 124, 184
    alpha-fetoprotein levels **208**
    human chorionic gonadotrophin
        levels **208**
    radial aplasia 189
trisomy 21 5, 57, 118, 119
    acute leukaemia risk 170
    aetiology 118
    detection rate 214
    first-trimester bleeding 201
    genetic counselling 111
    karyotype 119
    maternal alpha-fetoprotein 206, 207, **208**
    mosaics 67
    recurrence risk 118
tRNA 12
tuberous sclerosis 111, 175–6
tumour suppressor genes 162–3, 164, 165
Turner syndrome 51, 65, 78, 121–2, 123
    renal hypoplasia/dysplasia 187
twin concordance studies 91–2, **93**
twinning 91
tyrosinase mutations 131

ulcerative colitis 160
ultrasonography
    high resolution 8
    prenatal 202, 206
uropathy, obstructive 187

v-onc 164
van der Woude syndrome 186
variegate porphyria 100
VATER association 191, 194
VDJ combinations 150
vitamin D resistant rickets 79, 80, 148
VJC combinations 151
von Hippel–Lindau disease 171, 176
von Recklinghausen disease 174
von Willebrand disease 148–9
von Willebrand factor 148, 149

Waardenburg syndrome 149, 194
WAGR syndrome 176
Wallace mutation 142
Werdnig–Hoffmann disease 147
Werner syndrome 173
Williams syndrome 194
Wilms' tumour 176, 191
Wilson disease 139
Wolf syndrome 126

X chromatin see Barr body
X chromosome 4–5
    active maternal/paternal 53
    female 76
    inactivation 43, 50, 51, 52, 53
    late-replicating 34
    long arm 65
    Lyonization 76
    male 76
    normal pairing 53–4
    pairing region 76
    short arm pseudoautosomal region 76
    synapsis 46
X–autosome translocation 53, 78, 79
X-linked gene transmission 76
X-linked inheritance
    codominant 80, 81
    dominant 79, 80, 81
    recessive 77–9
X-linked recessive traits 79, 80, 100
    genetic counselling 109, 110, 111
X–Y homologous loci 51
X–Y pairing region 47, 51
xeroderma pigmentosum 171, 176
Xg blood group inheritance 79
XX males 54
XY females 54

Y chromosome
    normal pairing 53–4
    pairing region 76
    short arm pseudoautosomal region 76
    synapsis 46
Y-chromatin 39, 40
Y-linked inheritance 76
YAC probes 66
Yq size 39, 40

Zellweger syndrome 149
ZFX gene 51
Zollinger–Ellison syndrome 173
zygosity 91, 92
zygotene 46, 48